ISSUES IN READING, WRITING AND SPEAKING

NEUROPSYCHOLOGY AND COGNITION

VOLUME 3

The purpose of the Neuropsychology and Cognition series is to bring out volumes that promote understanding in topics relating brain and behavior. It is intended for use by both clinicians and research scientists in the fields of neuropsychology, cognitive psychology, psycholinguistics, speech and hearing, as well as education. Examples of topics to be covered in the series would relate to memory, language acquisition and breakdown, reading, attention, developing and aging brain. By addressing the theoretical, empirical, and applied aspects of brain-behavior relationships, this series will try to present the information in the fields of neuropsychology and cognition in a coherent manner.

The titles published in this series are listed at the end of this volume.

ALFONSO CARAMAZZA

Cognitive Science Center,
The Johns Hopkins University, U.S.A.

ISSUES IN READING, WRITING AND SPEAKING

A Neuropsychological Perspective

KLUWER ACADEMIC PUBLISHERS

DORDRECHT / BOSTON / LONDON

Library of Congress Cataloging-in-Publication Data

Issues in reading, writing, and speaking : a neuropsychological
   perspective / [compiled] by Alfonso Caramazza.
        p.   cm. -- (Neuropsychology and cognition ; 3)
   Includes bibliographical references (p.
   ISBN 0-7923-0996-0 (hard : alk. paper)
   1. Language disorders. 2. Neurolinguistics.   I. Caramazza,
Alfonso. II. Series.
RC423.I85 1990
616.85'5--dc20   90-5379

ISBN 0-7923-0996-0

Published by Kluwer Academic Publishers,
P.O. Box 17, 3300 AA Dordrecht, The Netherlands.

Kluwer Academic Publishers incorporates
the publishing programmes of
D. Reidel, Martinus Nijhoff, Dr W. Junk and MTP Press.

Sold and distributed in the U.S.A. and Canada
by Kluwer Academic Publishers,
101 Philip Drive, Norwell, MA 02061, U.S.A.

In all other countries, sold and distributed
by Kluwer Academic Publishers Group,
P.O. Box 322, 3300 AH Dordrecht, The Netherlands.

Printed on acid-free paper

Printed in the Netherlands

CONTENTS

FULL REFERENCES FOR PAPERS INCLUDED IN THE VOLUME

Chapter 1
Caramazza, A. (1988). Some aspects of language processing revealed through the analysis of acquired aphasia: The lexical system. Annual Review of Neuroscience, 11, 395-421

Chapter 2
Caramazza, A., Miceli, G., Silveri, M. C. & Laudanna, A. (1985). Reading mechanisms and the organization of the lexicon: Evidence from acquired dyslexia. Cognitive Neuropsychology, 2, 81-114.

Chapter 3
Caramazza, A., Miceli, G., & Villa, G. (1986). The role of the (output) phonological buffer in reading, writing, and repetition. Cognitive Neuropsychology, 3(1), 37-76.

Chapter 4
Badecker, W. & Caramazza, A. (1987). The analysis of morphological errors in a case of acquired dyslexia. Brain and Language, 32, 278-305.

Chapter 5
Rapp, B. & Caramazza, A. (1989). General to Specific Access to Word Meaning: A Claim re-examined. Cognitive Neuropsychology, 6(2), 251-272.

Chapter 6
Goodman, R. A. & Caramazza, A. (1986). Aspects of the spelling process: Evidence from a case of acquired dysgraphia. Language & Cognitive Processes, 1(4), 263-296.

Chapter 7
Goodman, R. A. & Caramazza, A. (1986). Dissociation of spelling errors in written and oral spelling: The role of allographic conversion in writing. Cognitive Neuropsychology, 3,(2), 179-206.

Chapter 8
Caramazza, A., Miceli, G., Villa, G. & Romani, C. (1987). The role of Graphemic Buffer in Spelling: Evidence from a case of acquired dysgraphia. Cognition, 26, 59-85.

LIST OF CONTRIBUTORS

William Badecker, Cognitive Science Center, The Johns Hopkins University, Baltimore, Maryland, 21218.

Alfonso Caramazza, Cognitive Science Center, The Johns Hopkins University, Baltimore, Maryland, 21218.

Roberta A. Goodman-Schulman, Department of Speech Pathology, Loyola College, 4501 N. Charles Street, Baltimore, Maryland, 21210-2699.

Argye E. Hillis, HealthSouth Rehabilitation Center, 9512 Harford Road, Baltimore, Maryland, 21234.

Alessandro Laudanna, Istituto di Psicologia del CNR, Viale Marx, 15, 00137, Roma, Italy.

Gabriele Miceli, Neurologia, Università Cattolica del Sacro Cuore, Policlinico "A. Gemelli", Largo A. Gemelli, 8, 00168, Roma, Italy.

Brenda Rapp, Cognitive Science Center, The Johns Hopkins University, Baltimore, Maryland, 21218.

Cristina Romani, Department of Psychology, The Johns Hopkins University, Baltimore, Maryland, 21218.

M. Caterina Silveri, Neurologia, Università Cattolica del Sacro Cuore, Policlinico "A. Gemelli", Largo A. Gemelli, 8, 00168, Roma, Italy.

Giampiero Villa, Neurologia, Università Cattolica del Sacro Cuore, Policlinico "A. Gemelli", Largo A. Gemelli, 8, 00168, Roma, Italy.

A. General Introduction

"... l'état pathologique ne diffère point radicalement de l'état physiologique, à l'égard duquel il ne suarait constituer, sous un aspect quelconque, qu'un simple prolongement plus ou moins étendu des limites de variation, soit supérieures, soit inférieures, propres à chaque phénomène de l'organisme normal, sans pouvoir jamais produire de phénomènes vraiment nouveaux, qui n'auraient point, à un certain degré, leurs analogues purement physiologiques. Par une suite nécessaire de ce principe, la notion exacte et rationnelle de l'état physiologique doit donc fournir, sans doute, l'indispensable point de départ de toute saine théorie pathologique; mais il en résulte, d'une manière non moins évidente, que, réciproquement, l'examen scientifique des phénomènes pathologiques est éminemment propre à perfectionner les études uniquement relatives à l'état normal. Un tel mode d'expérimentation, quoique indirect, est, en général, mieux adapté qu'aucun autre à la vraie nature des phénomènes biologiques."
(Comte, 1838; pg 696).

The principle that an understanding of physiology can be based on the analysis of pathological states, and that, vice versa, an understanding of pathology cannot proceed without a clear formulation of the structure on normal physiological states formed the basis for the development of experimental medicine in France in the first half of the 19th century, and for the development of neuropsychology in the second half of the 19th century. The first clear formulations of the functional organization of the brain by Broca, Wernicke, and Jackson were based on the application of these principles. They can still be usefully applied today to investigate the structure of the mind/brain (and its pathologies): The analysis of the disorders of perception, cognition, and language that result from brain damage continues to provide one of the most useful windows into the organization and structure of perceptual, cognitive, and linguistic processes. The papers collected in this volume are in this tradition.

In this collection of papers written with my collaborators over the past several years, we addressed questions about the structure of lexical processing through the analysis of various forms of acquired disorders of language. In each case we asked the question: What must the structure of the normal language processing system be like so that when damaged in a particular way it leads to the observed form of lexical processing impairment in a patient? The answer to this question for any one patient consists of two parts. One part specifies the structure of the cognitive/linguistic system that is assumed to underlie normal language processing. The other part specifies a hypothesis about the type of

1

transformation--functional lesion--that the normal processing system has undergone as a consequence of brain damage. Thus, the explication of any form of cognitive pathology necessarily constitutes a claim about the nature of normal cognitive processing: In the extent to which it is possible to account for an observed pattern of cognitive dysfunction by hypothesizing a particular form of transformation to one but not another theory of normal cognitive processing, we can take that performance as support for the theory of normal cognitive function which when "lesioned" produces the observed form of pathology. In this way, cognitive pathology provides an important data base for evaluating and developing theories of normal cognitive processing.

In order to be able to use impaired performance in brain-damaged subjects to constrain claims about normal cognitive mechanisms we must assume that such performance bears a *transparent* relation to normal cognitive processes (Caramazza, 1986). The assumption of a transparent relation between impaired performance and theory of normal cognitive processing is, in fundamental respects, the same as the one that motivates the use of experimental observations of any sort to evaluate theories of cognitive processing. In the latter case, too, it is assumed that the manipulations introduced in an experiment by the investigator lead to results that bear a transparent relation to the functioning of a canonical cognitive system which underlies all performance. The only difference between the two cases is that in the laboratory situation the experimental manipulation is introduced by the experimenter, whereas in the case of pathology the manipulation is introduced by nature. Thus, we can think of the performance of a brain-damaged patient as the result of an "experiment of nature," but an experiment nonetheless. However, unlike laboratory experiments where experimental conditions are under the control of the experimenter, in experiments of nature the manipulations introduced by nature--the functional lesions--are *unknown* and must be inferred from the performance of the patient. As a consequence, inferences about normal cognition from the performance of brain-damaged subject are necessarily mediated by hypotheses about the nature of the unknown functional lesion introduced by nature. This difference between experiments of nature and laboratory experiments has important methodological consequences which if not properly appreciated can render the study of brain-damaged subjects a useless enterprise.

The most important consequence is that the significant event for analysis in experiments of nature is the "single brain-damaged subject." The reason for this conclusion is straightforward. The interpretation of results in experiments are necessarily mediated by assumptions about the effects of the experimental conditions under which observations are made. Two sets of observations made under different experimental conditions cannot be treated as equivalent. Thus, the significant event for analysis is "the individual experiment"--a set of observations made under specifiable experimental conditions. This constraint on the interpretation of results applies both to laboratory experiments and to experiments of nature. Since the experimental conditions introduced by nature in its experiments --brain-damaged subjects--are unknown, we are not licensed to treat such experiments as equivalent and, therefore, must begin with the presumption that each brain-damaged subject constitutes a different experiment. The implication is that valid inferences about the structure of cognitive processes from the performance of brain-damaged subjects are only possible for single-patient studies (see Caramazza, 1986, for detailed discussion). The papers in this volume strictly adhere to this methodological imperative.

Another overarching feature of the papers in this volume is the explicit commitment to a "computational" approach to the study of cognitive/ linguistic mechanisms--an approach that attempts to specify both the overall functional architecture of a cognitive system and the representations that are computed at each stage of a cognitive process. The core assumption in this theoretical framework is that we can think of a cognitive process (e.g., comprehending a sentence, spelling a word, and so forth) as a series of transformations of mental representations. In this framework, the assumption is generally made that cognitive mechanisms may be distinguished in terms of whether their functional burden is to compute a representation from some input or whether their function is merely that of temporarily holding a representation for further processing. An example of the former type of processing component is the phonology to orthography conversion mechanism which, in the course of spelling unfamiliar words, is hypothesized to compute a graphemic representation --a set of abstract letter identities--from a phonological representation (Beauvois & Dérouesné, 1981; Goodman & Caramazza, 1986). The other type of processing components are working memory systems. A working memory system is hypothesized at those junctures in the cognitive architecture where the unit of representation of the output of one component is incommensurate with the unit of representation of a subsequent component (Caramazza, Miceli, & Villa, 1986). Thus, for example, since the output of the orthographic output lexicon consists of morpheme- or word-sized graphemic representations (usually several graphemes) whereas the input to the allographic conversion mechanism consists of single graphemes, we must hypothesize the existence of a working memory system (the graphemic buffer) which temporarily holds the graphemic string computed by the orthographic output lexicon while the allographic conversion mechanism sequentially processes the graphemes that comprise the lexical string (Caramazza, Miceli, Villa, & Romani, 1987; Ellis, 1982; Wing & Baddeley, 1980).

A further theoretical distinction among processing components is based on the type of representation computed by a hypothesized mechanism in the system. Thus, for example, the cognitive mechanism referred to as "orthographic output lexicon"--the stored knowledge of the graphemic structure of words--is distinguished from other mechanisms principally on the basis of the type of representation it takes as input (semantic) and the type of representation it computes for output (graphemic). These considerations serve to motivate the functional architecture of a cognitive system--the set of cognitive processes that are engaged in the execution of a task. An example of such a functional architecture is the one schematically represented in Figure 1 for the spelling process.

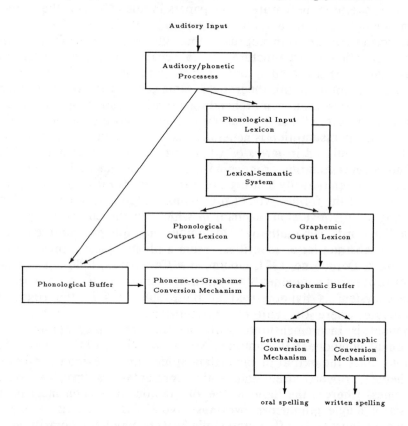

Figure 1. Schematic diagram of the spelling process.

Inferring the structure of normal cognition from pathology: The case of spelling

The model of spelling summarized in Figure 1 is not only the result of considerations such as those above, but, and more importantly, the result of the effort to explicate the patterns of spelling impairments found in brain-damaged subjects. The differential disruption of spelling for different types of stimuli or tasks (e.g., impaired performance in spelling familiar words in the face of spared ability to spell nonwords, or impaired performance in written but not oral spelling) has been interpreted as support for the hypothesized functional architecture of the spelling process. For example, the dissociation in overall accuracy in spelling familiar and unfamiliar words (the latter operationally represented by nonwords)--impaired performance in spelling nonwords in the face of normal performance with words in some brain-damaged subjects, and the reverse pattern of performance in other brain-damaged subjects--has been used to argue for a distinction between lexical and nonlexical procedures in spelling. Various dysgraphic patterns have been recorded which would seem to be explicable by assuming damage to one or another of the following components of the spelling process: the allographic conversion mechanism (Goodman & Caramazza, 1986b; Kinsbourne & Rosenfield, 1974), the graphemic output lexicon (Baxter & Warrington, 1987; Beauvois & Dérouesné, 1981; Goodman & Caramazza, 1986a; Patterson, 1987; Sanders & Caramazza, 1990), the phoneme-grapheme conversion mechanism (Bub & Kertesz, 1982; Roeltgen, Sevush, & Heilman, 1983; Shallice, 1981), the phonological output buffer (Bub, Black, Howell, & Kertesz, 1987; Caramazza, Miceli, & Villa, 1986), and the graphemic output buffer (Caramazza, Miceli, Villa, & Romani, 1987; Hillis & Caramazza, 1989; Miceli, Silveri & Caramazza, 1985; Posteraro, Zinelli, & Mazzucchi, 1988). It would seem, then, that there is considerable support for the principal components of the proposed functional architecture of the spelling process (see Ellis, 1988; Margolin, 1984, for discussion of more peripheral mechanisms in spelling).

Cognitive models of the type schematically represented in Figure 1 have, not without some justification, been derided by those who find the effort to articulate the functional architecture of a cognitive system--the "boxology" of information processing models--too general and unspecific to serve the desired explanatory function (e.g., Seidenberg, 1988). Furthermore, there are those who believe that cognitive neuropsychology can do no more than address general issues about the functional architecture of cognitive systems--that neuropsychological evidence (as well as certain types of experimental results with normal subjects) "relates to the overall organization of subsystems rather than to the details of their operation" (Shallice, 1988, p. 24). Taking these two claims together, it would seem that cognitive neuropsychology not only has failed to contribute significantly to our current understanding of normal cognition (Seidenberg), but it could not be otherwise given the intrinsic limitations of the evidence used in this area of investigation (Shallice). However, I believe that this indictment and the pessimism about the prospects of cognitive neuropsychology's contribution to the development of detailed theories of normal cognitive functioning is unjustified. Consider in this context the case of the spelling process.

Although it is true that research on different forms of dysgraphia has mostly, but not entirely (e.g., see Caramazza & Miceli, in press), been concerned with charting the overall configuration of the component processes that comprise the spelling system, this objective is far from unimportant or trivial. The point here is that specifying an empirically defensible functional architecture of the spelling process is an integral part of the development of a nontrivial theory of the process. This is necessarily true if one adopts the view that even the simplest spelling performance involves the concerted activity of a number of independent processing mechanisms. For example, something as "simple" as the spelling-to-dictation of single words involves sensory and perceptual processing mechanisms, attentional mechanisms, various sorts of lexical knowledge (phonological, semantic, and orthographic), working memory components, and motor mechanisms. Furthermore, a theory of the functional architecture of a cognitive process implicitly constrains theories of the processing structure of the components that comprise the system.

To illustrate this claim consider the contrast between models that assume that familiar and unfamiliar words are spelled through distinct lexical and nonlexical processing components, respectively, and those models that assume that familiar and unfamiliar words are processed through a single processing component. The processing structure of those components that produce orthographic representations for spelling in the two types of functional architectures are obviously different. For the class of functional architectures that distinguish between lexical and nonlexical processing, spelling familiar words involves the activation of semantic representations which serve as the input to a process that specifies particular lexical-orthographic representations, whereas spelling unfamiliar words involves converting phonological strings into graphemic representations through a set of sub-morphemic, phonology-to-orthography mapping rules. For the class of functional architectures that hypothesize a common mechanism for spelling familiar and unfamiliar words, the computations performed by this component involve converting phonological strings into orthographic representations through a lexically-based, non-semantic procedure (e.g., Campbell, 1983). It is quite obvious that decisions about the functional architecture of the spelling process have highly specific consequences for the computational structure of its component parts.

To this point I have argued that important evidence for the functional architecture of the spelling system schematically represented in Figure 1 has been provided by the analysis of the acquired dysgraphias: There are various dysgraphic patterns which are all explicable by hypothesizing some (local or restricted) transformation or other of the proposed functional architecture.[1] However, the reasoning that has motivated the use of dysgraphic performance to constrain hypotheses about the structure of the normal spelling process is indifferent to the level of theoretical detail that may be supported by such observations. That is, there is no reason for supposing that the motivation for using the analysis of acquired dysgraphia to chart the functional architecture of the spelling process should not apply equally to the case of the analysis of dysgraphic patterns to inform detailed hypotheses about the representations computed in the course of spelling, or to inform detailed hypotheses about the processing structure

---

[1]One criticism that has been raised against the effort to explicate various patterns of impaired performance by reference to functional lesions to one or more components of a cognitive system is that this type of analysis too easily lends itself to the unprincipled proliferation of processing components. There is the temptation, it is argued, to explain problematic new patterns of impaired performance by hypothesizing a "new box" in the cognitive system. This criticism is not altogether unjustified for a sizeable proportion of current neuropsychological research (see Rapp & Caramazza, in press, for discussion). However, this limitation of current practice is not beyond repair. Although it may be easy to "explain" the performance of a single patient (or single experiment) by postulating still another distinction in a complex functional architecture, it is much more difficult to account for the diverse patterns of impairment in different patients by postulating still further distinctions in a cognitive system. This expectation is motivated by the fact that we are held to having to explain not only the results of the patient whose performance motivated the new distinction, but also the results of all patients whose performance is relevant to a particular cognitive system. Consequently, although the postulation of an arbitrary new distinction may account for the performance of a particular patient it will ultimately conflict with the performance of patients whose performance is relevant to the cognitive processes where the arbitrary distinction was drawn.

of individual components of the system. And, if inferences about the functional architecture of the spelling process from the analysis of dysgraphic performance are, in principle, legitimate, they should be no less so when they concern the structure of representations computed in the course of spelling, or the processing structure of specific components of the system. Consider in this context the case of a dysgraphic subject whose performance suggests a functional lesion at the level of the graphemic buffer.

The function of the graphemic buffer is to hold temporarily the orthographic representations computed by the lexical or non-lexical components for subsequent, more peripheral spelling processes (e.g., allographic conversion). Damage at this level of the system has far-reaching but highly specific consequences for spelling performance: 1) spelling should be impaired in all tasks and for all types of stimuli; 2) spelling performance should be quantitatively the same across modalities of input (e.g., writing-to-dictation vs written naming) or output (e.g., oral vs written spelling), and across types of stimuli matched for length (e.g., words of different grammatical class or familiar vs unfamiliar words); 3) the same types of errors should be produced across all spelling tasks and for all types of stimuli; and, 4) since the type of representation involved at the level of the hypothesized deficit is orthographic in nature, errors should be explicable by appeal to strictly orthographic (and not lexical, semantic, or phonological) principles. These expectations about the consequences of damage to the graphemic buffer follow directly from the type of functional architecture that has been assumed for the spelling process. The reason for expecting that spelling should be impaired in all tasks and in equivalent extents is because in the proposed functional architecture the graphemic buffer is implicated in all spelling tasks (see Figure 1). (By contrast, damage to any other (single) component of the spelling system should result in a dissociation in performance between spelling tasks or types of stimuli; for example, damage to the allographic conversion mechanism should result in impaired writing performance in the context of spared ability to spell orally; damage to the orthographic output lexicon should result in impaired spelling of familiar words (primarily those that are orthographically irregular) in the context of spared ability to spell nonwords; and so forth.) Similarly, the reason for expecting that lexical, semantic, or phonological factors should not affect spelling performance in subjects with selective damage to the graphemic buffer is that the representations processed at the level of this component consist of orthographic representations. Since, by hypothesis, the information stored in the graphemic buffer consists of orthographic representations, damage to this component of the system should result in the loss of orthographic information and, consequently, should lead to errors characterized by orthographic deviations from the target response --errors should be explicable by appeal to strictly orthographic principles. A dysgraphic subject whose spelling performance satisfies conditions (1-4) may be assumed to have a selective deficit at the level of the graphemic buffer--that is, the existence of such a pattern of performance (in the context of other patterns of spelling impairment) may be taken as support for a functional architecture of the spelling process that includes the hypothesized graphemic buffer as one of its components (see Caramazza et al., 1987, for detailed discussion).

Loosely speaking, there are two aspects of a dysgraphic subject's performance that are relevant to determining the locus of damage to the spelling process: Performance levels across tasks or stimulus types (items (1-3), above) and the types of errors produced in various tasks (item (4), above).[2] Thus, while the analysis of the dissociation or association of spelling impairments may serve to identify in broad terms the locus of damage in the functional architecture of the spelling process, it is the detailed analysis of error types that provides the crucial evidence regarding the nature of the representations that are computed at some stage of the spelling process--it is the fact that the spelling errors produced by a subject with putative damage to the graphemic buffer are presumably explicable by appeal to orthographic principles that warrants the conclusion that damage is at a level that involves processing of orthographic representations.[3] And, since the nature and distribution of

---

[2]The distinction drawn here between two aspects of a patient's performance is an artificial one that does not have theoretical motivation. It is mentioned only for expository purposes: The distinction between performance levels across tasks or stimuli and types of errors serves to illustrate the importance of error analysis in drawing inferences about the structure of mental representations from the analysis of impaired performance. There is no principled basis for an a priori distinction between types of performance for informing and constraining cognitive theory. What counts as relevant evidence cannot be decided independently of the theories we are willing to entertain.

[3]To illustrate this claim consider the case where a patient's spelling performance satisfied conditions (1-3) above--that is, the patient had quantitatively and qualitatively similar spelling difficulties in all spelling tasks and for all types of stimuli. Suppose further, however, that the patient's errors all involved substitutions of letters (or spelling units) with

errors are, by hypothesis, constrained by the structure of the representations processed at the level where the system is damaged, the detailed analysis of errors in subjects with putative damage to the graphemic buffer can serve to inform hypotheses about the structure of the orthographic representations that are processed at that level of the spelling system. In other words, the analysis of acquired cognitive disorders may be used not only to constrain theoretical claims about the functional architecture of a complex system such as spelling, but also to constrain detailed claims about the structure of cognitive representations (see Caramazza & Miceli, 1989; in press).

Overview of the volume

The papers collected in this volume are organized into four sections. The paper in Section 1 serves as a general introduction to cognitive neuropsychology. It is a review chapter that first appeared in the *Annual Review of Neuropsychology* (1988). Although the principal focus of the paper is to review results on disorders of lexical processing, I also briefly discuss the scope of cognitive neuropsychology as well as matters of methodology. Sections 2, 3, and 4 collect papers on disorders of reading, writing, and speaking, respectively. Each of the latter three Sections is preceded by an introduction which briefly summarizes current views on these topics, including the work of my colleagues and myself.

Although I appear as the sole author of the volume, the work reprinted here is the result of collaboration with a group of colleagues. Most of the papers were written together with Gabriele Miceli from the Clinica Neurologica, Università Cattolica, Roma, with whom I have been collaborating since 1983. Without Gabriele's immense clinical knowledge and deep insight into the nature of clinical phenomena none of these papers would have been written. The remaining papers were written with Bill Badecker, Roberta Goodman-Schulman, Argye Hillis, and Brenda Rapp from the Cognitive Neuropsychology Laboratory, The Johns Hopkins University. In this case, too, I am indebted to my collaborators for sharing with me their experimental and clinical knowledge. I am

---

phonologically related letters or letter clusters such as favor --> *vavor*, date --> *dape*, match --> *madge*, and so forth. Since in this hypothetical case the impairment seems to involve phonological and not orthographic representations we cannot conclude that damage is at the level of the graphemic buffer. Clearly, the nature of errors plays a crucial role in constraining hypotheses about the structure of cognitive systems.

indeed fortunate to have colleagues such as Gabriele, Bill, Bobbi, Argye, and Brenda--I have learned much from them, both about neuropsychology and about friendship. I am also grateful to the other collaborators on these papers, Alessandro Laudanna, Cristina Romani, Caterina Silveri, and Giampiero Villa, for their contribution to the papers reprinted in this volume. To all my co-authors in the papers collected in this volume I am indebted for allowing me to reprint our joint work under my name. I would like to thank Helen Reilly and Kathy Yantis for typing and organizing the materials for this volume.

References

Baxter, D. M. & Warrington, E. K. (1987). Transcoding sound to spelling: Single or multiple sound unit correspondence? Cortex, 23, 11-28.

Beauvois, M. F. & Dérouesné, J. (1981). Lexical or orthographic agraphia. Brain, 104, 21-49.

Bub, D., Black S., Howell, J. & Kertesz, A. (1987). Speech outlet processes and reading. In M. Coltheart, G. Sartori, & R. Job (Eds). The cognitive neuropsychology of language. London: Lawrence Erlbaum Associates Ltd.

Bub, D. & Kertesz, A. (1982). Evidence for lexicographic processing in a patient with preserved written over oral single word naming. Brain, 105, 697-717.

Campbell, R. (1983). Writing nonwords to dictation. Brain and Language, 19, 153-178.

Caramazza, A. (1986). On drawing inferences about the structure of normal cognitive systems from the analysis of patterns of impaired performance: The case for single-patient studies. Brain and Cognition, 5, 41-66.

Caramazza, A., Miceli, G. & Villa, G. (1986). The role of the (output) phonological buffer in reading, writing, and repetition. Cognitive Neuropsychology, 3, 37-76.

Caramazza, A. & Miceli, G. (in press). The structure of graphemic representations. Cognition.

Caramazza, A., Miceli, G., Villa, G. & Romani, C. (1987). The role of the Graphemic Buffer in Spelling: Evidence of a case from acquired dysgraphia. Cognition, 26, 59-85.

Caramazza, A., Miceli, G. (1989). Orthographic structure, the graphemic buffer and the spelling process. In C. von Euler, I. Lundberg, & G. Lennerstrand (Eds.). Brain and Reading. MacMillan/Wenner-Gren International Symposium Series.

Ellis, A. W. (1982). Spelling and writing (and reading and speaking). In A. W. Ellis (Ed.), Normality and pathology in cognitive functions. London: Academic Press.

Ellis, A. W. (1988). Normal writing processes and peripheral acquired dysgraphias. Language and Cognitive Processes, 3, 99-127.

Goodman, R. A. & Caramazza, A. (1986a). Phonologically plausible errors: Implications for a model of the phoneme-grapheme conversion mechanism in the spelling process. In G. Augst (Ed.), Proceedings of the International Colloquium on Graphemics & Orthography, pp. 300-325. Berlin/NY: Walter de Gruyter.

Goodman, R. A. & Caramazza, A. (1986b). Dissociation of spelling errors in written and oral spelling: The role of allographic conversion in writing. Cognitive Neuropsychology, 3, 179-206.

Hillis, A. & Caramazza, A. (1989). The graphemic buffer and attentional mechanisms. Brain and Language, 36, 208-235.

Kinsbourne, M. & Rosenfield, D. B. (1974). Agraphia selective for written spelling. Brain and language, 1, 215-225.

Margolin, D. I. (1984). The neuropsychology of writing and spelling: Semantic, phonological, motor and perceptual processes. Quarterly Journal of Experimental Psychology, 36A, 459-489.

Miceli, G., Silveri, M. C. & Caramazza, A. (1985). Cognitive analysis of a case of pure dysgraphia. Brain and Language, 25, 187-212.

Patterson, K. E. (1987). Acquired disorders of spelling. In: G. Denes, C. Semenza, P. Bisiacchi & E. Andreewsky (Eds.). Perspectives in Cognitive Neuropsychology. London: Lawrence Erlbaum Associates.

Posteraro, L., Zinelli, P. & Mazzucchi, A. (1988). Selective impairment of the graphemic buffer in acquired dysgraphia: A case study. Brain and Language, 35, 274-286.

Rapp, B. & Caramazza, A. (in press). Cognitive neuropsychology: From impaired performance to normal cognitive structure. In R. Liser & H. Weingartner (Eds.), Cognitive Neuroscience, Oxford University Press.

Roeltgen D. P. , Sevush S. & Heilman, K. M. (1983). Phonological agraphia, writing by the lexical-semantic route, in Neurology, 33, 755-765.

Sanders, R. & Caramazza, A. (1990). Operation of the phoneme-to-grapheme conversion mechanism in a brain-injured patient. Reading and Writing, 2, 61-82.

Seidenberg, M. S. (1988). Cognitive neuropsychology and language: The state of the art. Cognitive Neuropsychology, 5, 403-426.

Shallice T. (1981). Phonological agraphia and the lexical route in writing, in Brain, 104, 413-429.

Shallice, T. (1988). <u>From Neuropsychology to Mental Structure</u>. Cambridge: Cambridge University Press.

Wing, A. M. & Baddeley, A. D. (1980). Spelling errors in handwriting: A corpus and distributional analysis, in U. Firth (a cura di), <u>Cognitive processes in spelling</u>, London: Academic Press.

CHAPTER ONE

SOME ASPECTS OF LANGUAGE PROCESSING REVEALED THROUGH THE ANALYSIS OF ACQUIRED APHASIA:
The Lexical System

INTRODUCTION

Acquired aphasia is the loss of some aspect of language processing consequent to brain damage. The specific form of aphasia observed in a patient is determined by the locus of cerebral insult. However, given the complexity of the language processing system, involving as it does complex linguistic mechanisms--phonological, lexical, syntactic, semantic, and pragmatic--as well as associated cognitive systems (e.g., working memory), a vast number of different forms of aphasia may be observed. Each form of aphasia observed is presumed to result from the particular type of damage to a component or combination of components of the language processing system. It is unrealistic, therefore, in the limited space available here, to attempt a review of the full range of possible language deficits in aphasia. A more manageable task is to focus the review on just one subsystem of the language faculty. This review will focus on the lexical system.

Under normal circumstances at this point I could have moved directly to a presentation of the main theoretical and empirical developments in the area of lexical processing and the analysis of diverse forms of aphasia involving lexical deficits. However, developments over the past decade have led to a reconsideration of the theoretical and methodological underpinnings of the then dominant approach in neuropsychological research with the result that the approach has been challenged and the interpretability of most of its empirical findings questioned. The full implications of this challenge are only now becoming apparent and it is necessary, therefore, to briefly consider the nature of this critique so as to motivate the selection of material reviewed here (as well as the exclusion of certain materials).

The organization of this chapter is as follows. First I present a brief critique of the classical approach in neuropsychological research and a discussion of the theoretical and methodological assumptions of a new approach identified as Cognitive Neuropsychology. I then review the major empirical and theoretical developments in the area of lexical processing and lexical deficits in aphasia. A brief discussion of the implications of these results for a functional neuroanatomy of language concludes the review.

METHODOLOGICAL AND THEORETICAL ASSUMPTIONS FOR A COGNITIVE NEUROPSYCHOLOGY OF LANGUAGE

The modern study of acquired language disorders is based on a set of theoretical and methodological principles which distinguish it from, and even put it in opposition to, the classical study of aphasia. This latter approach is primarily concerned with establishing clinico-pathological correlates for different forms of aphasia. By contrast, the modern study of acquired aphasia has as its objective that of specifying the computational structure of normal language processing. Within this framework, those relationships between the cognitive/linguistic mechanisms comprising the language faculty and brain structures that may emerge from the analysis of aphasia, while very important, do not constitute the principal objective of research. That is, although research on aphasia will undoubtedly serve to provide an important source of constraints on a functional neuroanatomy for language processing it need not, and in much recent work it appears not to, be explicitly committed to such a goal. This does not mean that Cognitive Neuropsychology is unconcerned with the problem of relating cognitive mechanisms to the brain. To the contrary, the relationship of cognition to the brain is one of its objectives, but such a goal cannot take precedence over that of specifying the nature of the cognitive mechanisms that must be neurally implemented. To state the problem differently, the objective of cognitive neuropsychology is to articulate and attempt to answer the correct type of empirical questions about brain/cognition relationships--questions that can only be formulated through an explicit theory of cognitive functioning. Thus, a "neuroscientific" theory of cognitive abilities will not be formulated by directly relating behavior to neural events but through the mediation of cognitive operations. Cognitive neuropsychology rejects as prejudicial the eliminative materialism of some neuroscientists (and philosophers - cf. Churchland, 1986) and operates instead with the assumption that a neuroscientific theory of cognition will be a theory about cognitive mechanisms and not directly about behavior--cognitive descriptions of mental events will not be replaced by neural descriptions but may be reduced to this latter level of description should such a day arrive.

Classical neuropsychological research operated within a medical-model framework mostly uninformed by cognitive or linguistic theory, and certainly unconcerned with the objective of developing a computationally explicit account of language processing. The syndromes that were correlated to anatomical sites for clinico-pathological analyses were based on impoverished notions of language processing using clinically-derived, common sense classification schemes for language impairments (e.g., Benson, 1985; Damasio, 1981; Kertesz, 1985). The symptoms that comprised the syndromes were grossly nonanalytic behavioral categories such as poor repetition, poor auditory language comprehension, poor naming ability, and so forth--behavioral conglomerates that are subserved by highly complex sets of cognitive and linguistic mechanisms. There are several reasons for rejecting this approach as a framework within which to explore the structure of the cognitive/linguistic mechanisms that subserve language processing and their relationship to the brain. However, before briefly presenting the details of this critical analysis I should like to consider one major accomplishment that has been achieved through research carried out within this framework.

Despite the serious limitations of this approach, what little is known about the functional neuroanatomy for language has come to us principally through clinico-pathological correlations for the aphasias. Although it has been known at least since the time of Hippocrates (ca 400 B.C.) that insult to the brain may result in disturbances of the language faculty, it was not until the detailed analysis of Broca, Wernicke, Charcot, Lichtheim, Dejerine and others in the second half of the 19th century that a firm foundation was laid for relating language processes to the brain. Indeed by the end of that century French and German neurologists had described all the major aphasia syndromes at a level of detail that seemed to allow little opportunity for improvement. These investigators, under the influence of Gall's phrenological hypothesis, which proposed that distinct areas of the cerebral cortex subserve different cognitive faculties, set out to chart the functional burden of distinct parts of the cortex; that is, to localize the language faculty and its principal subcomponents in particular areas of the brain. Their labors and those of other students of aphasia since that time have not gone unrewarded. Neuropsychologists have amassed a systematic body of observations relating locus of brain damage to patterns of language dysfunction. These observations have established not only that language processing is subserved by neural structures in the left hemisphere (in most people) but that there is a highly articulated functional organization within this hemisphere, with different parts assumed to subserve different components of language processing. These results are well known and have been reviewed many times (e.g., Caplan, in press; Caramazza & Berndt, 1982; Damasio & Geschwind, 1984).

The general picture to emerge from this research program may be summarized thus: The linguistic components of language processing--syntactic, morphological, lexical-semantic, and phonological--are subserved by neural structures in the perisylvian region of the left hemisphere (see Figure 1); other regions of the brain, notably the right hemisphere, play a less important, supportive role in language processing. Thus, there is now considerable evidence that an intact right hemisphere may be needed for subtle interpretation of language such as the appreciation of irony, metaphor, and humor as well as the emotional content of a linguistic act, but not for strictly linguistic processing (e.g., Brownell et al., 1984; Gardner et al., 1983.

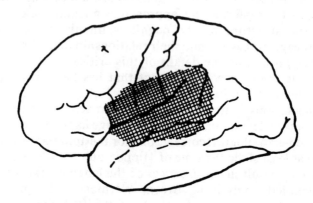

Figure 1. Schematic representation of the lateral surface of the left hemisphere with shading of the perisylvian region.

This general view of the neural representation of language processes has received considerable support from neuropsychological research with other methodologies and techniques. Research with split-brain patients-- patients whose two cerebral hemispheres have been disconnected for medical reasons--where the capacities of the two hemispheres may be investigated in relative isolation, has confirmed that linguistic capacities are represented exclusively in the left hemisphere. A similar conclusion has been reached through electrical stimulation research of the exposed cerebral cortex during neurosurgical procedures. This latter research has shown that electrical stimulation of the cortex results in temporary linguistic impairments only when the stimulation is applied to the perisylvian region of the left hemisphere. And, finally, studies of regional cerebral blood flow using emission tomography during language activities in normal subjects have also led to a similar conclusion. These studies, which measure the metabolic (blood flow) activity in different regions of the brain during the performance of language tasks, have shown that it is the perisylvian region of the left hemisphere that is most directly implicated in language processing (cf. Caplan, in press).

Without in the least intending to minimize the importance of that which has been learned about the neuropsychology of language through the methods currently at our disposal it should be emphasized, nevertheless, that we have only succeeded in providing a gross, nonanalytic mapping of the language faculty onto the brain--at best a gross functional neuroanatomy. Is this the most that may be achieved through the analysis of language disorders consequent to brain damage? This question receives different answers depending on whether we place the focus on the neural or the cognitive part of the brain/cognition equation. Let us consider first the brain part of the equation.

The answer here is not an entirely encouraging one. The effort to relate functional disorders of language to locus of brain damage, no matter how fine-grained an analysis, can only result in a "modern phrenology." This is not to say that such an achievement would be insignificant. Quite the contrary: A fine-grained mapping of component parts of the language processing system onto neural structures would place important constraints on theories of the neurophysiological bases for language. But the type of observation at our disposal cannot lead to a neurophysiology of language. Furthermore, the fact that natural language is a uniquely human ability severely restricts the range of experimental opportunities for exploring the neurophysiological mechanisms for language processing--for example, we cannot use those experimental procedures currently within the armamentarium of the neurophysiologist for the analysis of neural activity in non-human animals. Does this mean that we must abandon the hope for a neurophysiology of language? Although current opportunities are limited, there is the hope that technological developments will eventually make it possible to directly investigate neural activity in humans with ethically acceptable means. In the meantime, we are not completely disarmed. We could rely on a bootstrap strategy that exploits whatever brain/cognition principles might emerge from the analysis of diverse cognitive processes in various non-human species to develop a computational neurophysiology of language processing; that is, a theoretical neurophysiology which relies on principles of neuronal functioning to develop neuronal-net models of specific linguistic processes--an approach that has received considerable attention in recent years (Arbib, Caplan, & Marshall, 1982; Hinton & Anderson, 1981; Rumelhart & McClelland, 1986). I will return to this general issue in the concluding section of this review.

By contrast to the less-than-optimistic conclusion about the possibility of an experimental neurophysiology of language, the outlook for progress in developing a detailed functional theory of language processing through the analysis of different forms of acquired aphasia is very encouraging. The pragmatic motivation for using language deficits to inform and constrain theories of normal language processing comes from the observation that brain damage does not result in undifferentiated loss of language ability but in the selective loss of some ability in the face of otherwise normal performance. Thus, for example, brain damage may selectively impair language processes while sparing other perceptual and cognitive abilities. However, if brain damage were to result in dissociations of functions that are no finer than global cognitive systems (e.g., language, calculation, etc.), the resulting patterns of impaired performance would be of little value in determining the processing structure of these systems. Fortunately for our enterprise, brain damage may result in highly specific patterns of dysfunction, presumably reflecting the componential structure of cognitive systems. We can use these highly articulated patterns of impaired performance to evaluate and develop models of normal language processing. However, such an enterprise cannot be carried out within the framework of classical neuropsychology. To fully appreciate this claim we must consider, albeit very briefly here, the assumptions that motivate the possibility of drawing meaningful inferences about normal language processing from patterns of language disorders (see Caramazza, 1986, for detailed discussion).

As already noted, the object of cognitive neuropsychology is to develop a theory of cognitive functioning through the analysis of patterns of cognitive dysfunction consequent to brain damage. The theoretical assumption that motivates the use of impaired performance as the basis for inferring the structure of normal processes is that the transformations of the normal system under conditions of damage are not indefinite or random but, instead, obey precise constraints determined by the intrinsic structure of the normal system: A pattern of impaired performance reflects a discoverable (and specifiable) transformation of the normal cognitive system (what I have called elsewhere the assumption of "transparency"; Caramazza, 1984; 1986). In this framework, a pattern of impaired performance is taken as support for a theory of the processing structure of a cognitive system (over some alternative theory) if it is possible to specify a transformation--a functional lesion--in the proposed theory (but not in some alternative theory) of the cognitive system such that the transformed system may account for the observed pattern of performance. This procedure allows a precise criterion for the empirical evaluation of a cognitive theory through the analysis of the performance of cognitively impaired brain-damaged patients.

It may be noted that the role played by "functional lesions" in the proposed framework for research is analogous to that played by "experimental conditions" in a typical experimental paradigm; that is, in a regular experiment the relationship between data and theory is mediated by specific experimental conditions and in research with brain-damaged patients it is mediated by functional lesions (as well as experimental conditions). However, the two situations are disanalogous in one crucial respect: Whereas experimental conditions are under the control of the experimenter (and, therefore known a priori), functional lesions are not known a priori but must themselves be inferred from the performance of patients. Thus, although we may consider a brain-damaged patient as constituting an "experiment of nature," where the functional lesion represents some of the experimental conditions of the experiment, these latter conditions are not known a priori, as would be the case in a regular experiment, and therefore raise particular problems whose solution has important methodological consequences. Specifically, given that functional lesions may only be specified a posteriori--that is, once all the relevant performance for inferring a functional lesion in a cognitive system is available--there can be no theoretical merit in a classificatory scheme of patients' performance which is based on any arbitrary subset of a patient's performance. Two important consequences follow from these observations: 1) patient classification cannot play any significant role in cognitive neuropsychological research and 2) patient-group studies do not allow valid inferences about the structure of normal cognitive processes.

On the issue of patient-classification-based research not only are there methodological arguments against its validity but, in addition, there are theoretical and practical considerations which undermine its usefulness (see Badecker & Caramazza, 1985; Caramazza, 1984; Caramazza & Martin, 1983; Marshall, 1982; 1986). The great majority of classification-based research has used theoretically-uninformed behavioral categories for patient classification. Patients are classified as being of a particular type on the basis of criteria such as the following: whether or not a patient has poor repetition performance, or poor language comprehension performance, and so forth. However, since performance of such complex tasks as repetition or comprehension involves many cognitive mechanisms, impaired performance on these tasks may be due to damage to any one or combination of the cognitive mechanisms implicated in the performance of the task as a whole. Thus, poor performance in such tasks does not guarantee a theoretically useful homogeneity of the patients classified by these criteria. Furthermore, there is little value in reviewing classification -based research on aphasia for strictly pragmatic reasons. This research has led to little if any insight into the structure of normal language processes despite over a century of work.

The second major consequence of recent analyses of the logic of research in cognitive neuropsychology is that valid inferences about the structure of cognitive systems from patterns of cognitive dysfunctions are only possible for single-patient studies (Caramazza, 1984; 1986; Caramazza & McCloskey, in press; Shallice, 1979). The arguments for this contention are straightforward but too long to present here. Suffice it to say that the principal argument is based on the observation that functional lesions can only be postulated a posteriori--that is, on the basis of all the relevant evidence needed to fix a functional lesion in a cognitive system.

Thus far I have focused on some negative conclusions of recent methodological and theoretical developments in cognitive neuropsychology; that is, I have presented recent conclusions concerning the impossibility of using the clinically-based, classical methods of research on aphasia for learning about the structure of normal language processes and their neural correlates. A focus on these negative conclusions has been found necessary because of the need for clearly identifying the type of theoretical questions that may profitably be addressed through investigations of patients with cognitive deficits and for specifying the attendant methodology for addressing these issues. These developments may also be viewed positively, however: They offer us a theoretically coherent basis for a productive cognitive neuropsychology which increasingly interacts with other subdisciplines of the cognitive and neural sciences.

THE LEXICAL SYSTEM

Even though the focus of this review has been restricted to just a single subsystem of the language processing system, the ground to be covered is still quite extensive. The lexical system is very complex involving many linguistic and cognitive dimensions as well as being implicated in many different types of cognitive functions such as sentence comprehension and production, reading, writing, and naming. Consequently a further restriction of focus is necessary. The primary focus will be on single-word processing tasks, although an effort will be made to link the account of the lexicon that emerges from the review to the broader issue of sentence processing. Three sets of issues will be dealt with in this review: the general architecture of the lexical system; the representational content in different lexical processing components; and the processing structure within components. Although these issues are not entirely independent, it is useful to draw these distinctions for purposes of exposition.

The functional architecture of the lexical system

The dominant view of the functional architecture of the lexical system is that it consists of a distributed but interconnected set of lexical components (e.g., Allport & Funnell, 1981; Caramazza, in press; Morton, 1981; Shallice, 1981). Over the past 10 to 15 years an impressive range of theoretical arguments and empirical evidence has been amassed in support of this view. The modal model that has emerged has the following structure. A major distinction is drawn between input and output lexical components; that is, lexical components involved in the comprehension (recognition) or production of words, respectively. A second major distinction is drawn between modality-specific input or output lexical components: The orthographic input lexicon, those mechanisms involved in processing written words, is distinguished from the phonological input lexicon, those mechanisms involved in processing spoken words. These modality-specific input lexicons are distinguished from their corresponding output lexicons, those mechanisms involved in the production of written and spoken words. It is further assumed that modality-specific lexical components are interconnected through a lexical-semantic system which stores the semantic representations for words. A schematic representation (as a visual aid) of these processing components is shown in Figure 2.

The evidence in favor of this view of the architecture of the lexical system is quite compelling. On strictly theoretical grounds the distinction between modality-specific components is unimpeachable--the mechanisms involved in processing visual and acoustic signals and the orthographic and phonological lexical representations these give rise to, are computationally independent. In one case--reading--the computational problem involves

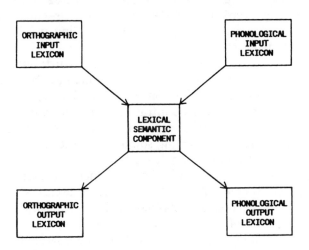

Figure 2. Schematic structure of the lexical system.

computing a lexical representation on the basis of visual information and subsequently letters or graphemes; in the other--listening--the computational problem involves computing a lexical representation on the basis of acoustic information and subsequently phonetic and phonemic information. Obviously, the computed representations must be different objects--orthographic or phonological lexical representations. A similar argument may be made for the input/output lexicon distinction.

The available empirical evidence is no less compelling. Two types of evidence have been reported: patients who present with selective damage to one or another lexical component (e.g., Basso, Taborelli, & Vignolo, 1978; Hier & Mohr, 1977; Miceli, Silveri, & Caramazza, 1985; Michel, 1979) and patients who present with different patterns of impairments to different components (e.g., Beauvois & Dérouesné; 1981; Goodman & Caramazza, 1986a). Both kinds of evidence may be taken as support for a distributed view of the lexical system. Thus, for example, Goodman & Caramazza (1986b) have reported a patient who presents with damage to the output graphemic lexicon but who has normal access to other components of the lexical system (e.g., the output phonological lexicon and the lexical-semantic component). This pattern of performance is strong evidence against any theory of the lexicon which assumes a nondistributed, unitary lexical system. Equally supportive of the distributed theory of the lexicon are those patterns of performance where different types of dysfunctions are found for different components of the lexicon. To give just one example of this type of result, Beauvois & Dérouesné (1979) have reported a patient whose impaired reading performance was radically different from his impaired spelling performance. This patient's impairment in reading involved only those cognitive mechanisms required for converting print-to-sound for novel or unfamiliar words--the patient could not read nonwords but essentially had no difficulty in reading words (see also Goodman & Caramazza, 1986a). Thus the graphemic input lexicon must be intact, as must be the phonological output lexicon. By contrast, this patients spelling impairment resulted from damage to the graphemic output lexicon sparing those mechanisms involved in converting sound-to-print and the phonological input lexicon (see also Goodman & Caramazza, 1986a). This pattern of dissociation of deficits can only be explained by assuming selective damage to different components of a distributed lexical system. There is now a vast cognitive neuropsychological literature which demonstrates differential patterns of impairments for different parts of the lexical system (see also Allport & Funnell, 1981; Shallice, 1981, for reviews).

Lexical representations

The distributed lexical system under consideration here distinguishes between modality specific lexical components. These distinctions capture the most salient (perceptual) features of lexical information--phonological and orthographic information are represented in distinct processing components. However, there are other important lexical feature that must be accounted for in a more general theory of the lexicon. These include form class or categorial information (i.e., noun, verb, etc.), morphological structure (root/stem and affixes), thematic structure (the argument structure of predicates), and semantic information (the meaning of words and morphemes). This information must be captured at some level of the lexical system. In this section I will review some of the experimental evidence in favor of these representational distinctions. I will also briefly review theoretical arguments and empirical evidence which bear on the issue of which lexical components may be assumed to capture the hypothesized lexical features.

FORM CLASS   Although words have an independent status, their primary function is to convey meaning in sentential contexts. It is only when words are used in sentences that the full range of their syntactic, semantic, morphological, and phonological properties become apparent. Thus, for example, the word jump may be used as a noun (I watched the jump with trepidation) or as a verb (I watched him jump with trepidation). The two uses of jump have distinct grammatical roles (noun vs. verb), different meanings, and accept different inflectional affixes (the noun accepts -s for plural, the verb accepts -s, -ing, and -ed to mark person and tense).   The grammatical class of a word and its subcategorization features (e.g., transitive/intransitive) also determine the type of derivational affixes it accepts (e.g., only verbs accept the -able derivational affix, as in enjoyable but not *windowable and, furthermore, this applies only for transitive verbs as in enjoyable but not *appearable). Clearly, then, the lexicon must represent not only the phonological and orthographic structure of words but also their syntactic, semantic, and morphological properties (e.g., Chomsky, 1965).

As already indicated a crucial property of lexical items is their form (grammatical) class; that is, whether a word is (functions as) a noun, a verb, an adjective, an adverb, or a function word. These lexical properties play a determining role in the organization of the lexicon. Already in the classical literature there were clear indications for the dissociability of impairment of different form classes of words. The strongest evidence was for the dissociability of function words (articles, auxiliaries, prepositions, etc.) from other form classes (nouns, verbs, and adjectives) (e.g., De Villiers, 1978; Goodglass, 1976; Stemberger, 1984; see Berndt & Caramazza, 1980; Lesser, 1978, for reviews). Patients clinically classified as agrammatic aphasics--that is, patients whose spontaneous speech is characterized by the relative omission of function words--could be argued to have a selective impairment in lexical access of function words (this position has been argued most forcefully by Bradley, Garrett, & Zurif, 1980). However, this type of deficit does not allow us to distinguish between a deficit at some level of sentence production (where a syntactic frame for sentence production is specified) and a pure lexical access deficit (Caramazza & Berndt, 1985; Miceli & Caramazza, 1987). Nonetheless, independently of whether the deficit in any one patient who makes errors with (or omissions of) function words in sentence production is ultimately found to be at the level of specifying a sentence frame or in lexical access, such patterns of language impairment are prima facie evidence for a representational distinction between function words and other word classes, and hence for a particular form of organization of the lexicon.

There does exist more direct evidence for the selective impairment of lexical access of function words. There are reports of patients whose performance in single word processing--reading, writing or repetition of single words--is either relatively poor or relatively good when compared to other form classes (e.g., Bub & Kertesz, 1982; papers in Coltheart, Patterson, & Marshall, 1980; Friederici & Schoenle, 1980; Nolan & Caramazza, 1982; 1983). Although it initially appeared that a deficit in function word processing was associated with a more general morphological processing impairment (Beauvois & Dérouesné, 1979; DeBastiani, Barry, & Carreras, 1983; Patterson, 1982), it is now clear that these two types of deficits are dissociable (Caramazza, Miceli, Silveri, & Laudanna, 1985; Funnell, 1983). Thus, we have evidence for at least one type of organizational distinction at some level of the lexicon (I will take up the issues of the level at which these distinctions may be represented below).

Evidence for other organizational distinctions within the lexicon has also been obtained. There are numerous reports of patients whose oral reading or writing performance is differentially affected for nouns, verbs, and adjectives (see papers in Coltheart et al 1980). The typical result reported is for better performance for nouns relative to verbs and adjectives. The systematicity of this result raises the possibility that a lexical dimension other than form class is responsible for this ordering of performance difficulty. Indeed, patients who present with the form class effect described, typically show greater difficulties in processing abstract than concrete (or high imageability) words. This association of deficits allows the possibility that the relevant dimension affected by brain damage in the patients in question is not form class but concreteness/abstractness. However, an effect of form class has been obtained even when concreteness/abstractness is controlled for (e.g., Baxter & Warrington, 1985; Shallice & Warrington, 1975). Furthermore, there is evidence in the literature on naming disorders for a double dissociation in naming difficulty for verbs and nouns (Baxter & Warrington, 1985; McCarthy & Warrington, 1985; Miceli, Silveri, Villa, & Caramazza, 1984). Some patients have considerably greater difficulty naming nouns than verbs, other patients present with the reverse pattern in naming difficulty for nouns and verbs. This result suggests that, at least in some patients, the underlying cause of their naming impairment is selective damage to different subsets of the lexicon--subsets defined by form-class membership. The double dissociation of processing difficulty for nouns and verbs has also been documented for a word comprehension task (Miceli, Silveri, Nocentini, & Caramazza, 1986). In this latter case the reported dissociation for form class also concerned a dissociation by modality of use. That is, some patients presented with selective impairment in comprehension of verbs without a corresponding difficulty in naming of this class of words.

The results reviewed in this section are unequivocal in one regard: they support the view that the lexicon is organized by grammatical class. They do not provide as compelling a basis, if at all, for determining where in the lexical system form class information is represented. Nonetheless, I will propose that, at this time, our best answer to this latter question is that form class information is represented in each modality-specific lexicon (i.e., in the phonological input and output lexicons, and in the orthographic input and output lexicons). Although empirical support for this position--modality specific form class effects in lexical processing (e.g., Baxter & Warrington, 1985)--is scanty, there are good theoretical reasons for adopting it. Basically, the argument is that since morphological structure is strictly dependent on form class information, this latter information must be represented at the same lexical level as that at which morphological structure is represented. And, as we will see below, morphological structure is represented in modality specific lexicons.

MORPHOLOGICAL STRUCTURE Words are not unanalyzable units-- they have phonological (and orthographic) and morphological structure. The word "nationalized" is considered to be composed of the verb stem nationalize plus the inflectional affix -ed (past tense). In turn, the verb nationalize is derived from the adjective national by the addition of the derivational affix -ize, which is itself derived from the noun nation by the addition of the adjectival derivational affix -al. Thus, we may analyze words into stems (or roots), derivational affixes (affixes that serve to specify the form class of the derived word; e.g., nation (noun) → national (adjective)) and inflectional affixes which mark the tense, number, and gender of a word (See Scalise, 1984, for review). A crucial issue for a theory of the lexicon is whether morphological structure is explicitly represented in the lexicon and how it is represented and used in language processing.

Various theoretical positions have been taken on this issue. A major contrast is between the view that words are represented in the lexicon in morphologically decomposed form (e.g., Taft, 1985) versus the view that words are represented as nondecomposed wholes (e.g., Butterworth, 1983). A second distinction, relevant only for the case of morphologically decomposed lexical representations, is whether lexical access is only possible after a word stimulus is parsed into its morphological components (stems or roots and affixes) (e.g., Taft, 1979) or whether lexical access may proceed through both whole-word and morphemic access procedures (e.g., Caramazza et al., 1985). Other issues concern the proper relationship between derivational and inflectional morphology and whether inflectional morphology is represented in the lexical or syntactic system (e.g., Anderson, 1982). In the limited space available here I will consider only the general issue of morphological decomposition as it emerges through the analysis of the word-processing performance in brain-damaged patients.

Various reports in the literature have dealt with morphological processing in brain-damaged patients. Some of this research has focused on the patterns of omissions (e.g., De Villiers, 1978; Gleason, 1978; Goodglass, 1976; Goodglass & Berko, 1960) or substitutions (e.g., Miceli, Mazzucchi, Menn, & Goodglass, 1983) of inflectional affixes in patients clinically classified as agrammatic aphasics. These reports have clearly documented a dissociation in processing inflectional affixes (impaired) versus word stems ("intact"). The reverse pattern of dissociation, impaired stem production and spared inflectional affix production, has also been reported (e.g., Caplan, Keller, & Locke, 1972). On the face of it these patterns of result would appear to be prima facie evidence for morphological decomposition in the lexicon. However, as in the case of function word omission (or substitution) in spontaneous sentence production (discussed above), these results are ambiguous with respect to the locus of deficit: A patient may fail to produce (or fail to produce correctly) an inflectional affix because of damage to the inflectional component of a morphologically decomposed representation or because of damage to a component of the syntactic frames computed in the course of sentence production. The relevant data needed to resolve this issue involves patterns of selective impairment in single word processing. Such data are available.

An important source of evidence comes to us from the oral reading errors in patients with acquired dyslexia. An often noted feature in dyslexic patients in the presence of morphological errors--that is, errors such as reading walked for walking (inflectional error) or kindness for kindly (derivational error). Errors of this type were first most clearly documented in patients clinically classified as deep dyslexic. These are patients who in addition to morphological errors also make semantic (read priest for minister) and visual (read bear for fear) errors as well as presenting with other processing impairments (i.e., a form class effect, a concreteness/abstractness effect, a frequency effect, and disproportional difficulties in reading nonwords; see Coltheart, Patterson, & Marshall (1980) for review and discussion). Although the presence of morphological errors as part of the complex clinical picture in these patients may be suggestive, it does not permit an unequivocal conclusion regarding the issue in question; namely, whether or not lexical representations are morphologically decomposed. After all, the putative morphological errors may be no more than visual or semantic errors. However, the existence of "morphological" reading errors may be used in more focused analyses to address the question of concern here.

Patterson (1980; 1982) and Job & Sartori (1984) have described in some detail patients whose reading errors were almost exclusively of the morphological type. These authors interpreted the highly selective impairment in their patients (essentially restricted to the production of morphological paralexias) as evidence for a selective deficit to the morphological component of the lexicon. This conclusion has been challenged, however. Badecker & Caramazza (1986) have argued that the mere production of "morphological" paralexic errors is not sufficient grounds for concluding that the basis for the impairment is a deficit to the morphological component of the lexicon. Equally plausibly these errors could be considered to be highly similar visual errors or highly similar semantic errors. The ambiguity of interpretation could be resolved only if it turned out that a pattern of errors is only explicable by appeal to a morphological and no other lexical (semantic) or perceptual dimension. Note that this objection does not imply that the cases described by Patterson and Job and Sartori may not, after all, truly be cases of selective deficit to a morphological processing component. All that is asserted is that the presented evidence is not sufficient to unambiguously decide the issue. Fortunately, there is at least one case report of a patient whose impaired lexical processing performance is unequivocally the result of a selective deficit to the morphological component of the phonological output lexicon.

Miceli & Caramazza (1987) have described a patient, F.S., who makes morphological errors in spontaneous sentence production and in repetition of single words. The great majority of this patient's single word repetition errors were morphologically related to the target response. Crucially, these morphologically related responses were almost all inflectional errors (97%). The massive presence of morphological errors restricted to the inflectional category is only explicable by appeal to a morphological principle--a distinction between inflectional and derivational morphology: The evidence for a true morphological processing impairment. The highly selective deficit for inflectional morphology in a single-word processing task reported for F.S. allows the conclusion that lexical entries are represented in morphologically decomposed form--stems (or roots) are represented independently of their inflectional and derivational affixes which, in turn, constitute independent components within the lexicon.

In this section I have reviewed evidence in support of the view that the lexical system represents words in morphologically decomposed form. As a final issue in this area I will argue that morphological structure is represented directly in modality-specific lexicons. However, the evidence for this conclusion is, at best, indirect.

Caramazza, Miceli, Silveri, & Laudanna (1985) have described a patient with a selective deficit in reading nonwords. The patient could read all types of words but made on the order of 40% errors in reading nonwords. However, when his reading performance for "morphologically legal" nonwords (e.g., walken, composed of the inappropriately combined morphemes, walk- and -en) was assessed, it was found that he read these nonwords much better than comparable nonwords that did not have any morphological structure (e.g., wolkon). Since we may safely assume that nonwords do not have permanent entries in the lexical system, the better performance for the "morphologically legal" nonwords must be due to the activation of morphemic representations (e.g., walk- and -en) in the orthographic input lexicon. If this argument is correct them we must conclude that morphological structure is represented in modality specific lexicons.

In conclusion, the evidence from the analysis of language impairments in brain damaged patients taken together with results in the literature on normal word processing (e.g., Stemberger, 1985; Taft, 1985) and linguistics (e.g., Scalise, 1984) strongly argues for the autonomous representation of morphological structure in the lexical system.

LEXICAL SEMANTICS   That of various features of a word its meaning is the most important is quite obvious. Despite this and despite the fact that word meaning is increasingly seen as playing a determining role in linguistic theory (e.g., Chomsky, 1981; Wasow, 1985), we do not have the detailed theory of lexical meaning that would be commensurate with the crucial role of this dimension of lexical items. The absence of theory has left empirical work in this area in disarray so that we do not have anything like a coherent research program in the analysis of disorders of lexical meaning. Consequently, in this section I will focus on an interesting empirical phenomenon concerning semantic organization of the lexicon, without attempting to provide a general model of this component of the lexicon (in contrast to what I have attempted to do for other components of the lexical system). The phenomenon I will consider here is that of category-specific deficits.

We have seen in previous sections that brain damage may result in highly specific deficits. The patient with a selective deficit of inflectional morphology or the patients with selective deficit in processing function words are cases in point. Results such as these allow us to articulate the functional architecture of the modality-specific lexicons. In recent years Warrington and her colleagues (Warrington, 1975; 1981; Warrington & McCarthy, 1983; Warrington & Shallice, 1984), following an earlier observation by Goodglass, Klein, Carey, & Jones (1966), have described a number of patients with selective deficits to specific semantic categories. These results provide evidence relevant to the organization of the semantic lexicon.

Goodglass et al. (1966) provided a quantitative analysis of a large number of patients in which they show that different patients present with different patterns of relative difficulty in auditory comprehension of semantic categories. Warrington and her colleagues in a series of detailed single-patient analyses have documented selective dissociations between concrete (impaired) and abstract words (spared) (the reverse pattern is commonly reported), inanimate (impaired) and animate words (spared), and living things and foods (impaired) and inanimate words (spared). Perhaps the most striking result in this domain is one reported by Hart, Berndt, & Caramazza (1985). The patient, M.D., presented with a very selective disturbance of the ability to name items from two related semantic categories. Despite normal naming performance with the items from many different semantic categories, the patient showed a striking and consistent naming deficit for the categories 'fruits' and 'vegetables.' Thus, as can be seen in Table 1, the patient performed poorly in naming fruits and vegetables in the face of spared ability to name items from other categories.

The patient's difficulties in processing the members of the categories fruits and vegetables extended to a number of other tasks. Thus, the patient presented with difficulties in sorting pictures of fruits and vegetables into the appropriate categories--i.e., sorting together fruits separately from vegetables; he had difficulties in generating the names of members of the two categories when given the category--i.e., producing apple, orange, peach, etc. in response to the category "fruits"; and he showed a selective difficulty in naming fruits and vegetables from definition as well as from tactile presentation. By contrast, he showed normal performance with these categories in a word-picture matching task and in judgments of category, size, texture, and shape when given the name of individual fruits and vegetables. Normal performance on these

A. Caramazza

latter tasks demonstrates that the patient's knowledge of these categories is intact but can only be accessed from the lexicon.

Table 1. Number of correct naming responses*

| | Semantic category | | |
	Fruit	Vegetables	Other**
Line drawings	5/11	7/11	11/11
Colored drawings	4/6	5/7	18/18
Photographs	11/18	12/18	222/229
Real objects	10/13	13/23	11/11
TOTAL	30/48 (0.63)	37/59 (0.63)	262/269 (0.97)

* From Hart et al. (1985).
** The 'other' category includes vehicles, toys, tools, animals, body parts, food products, school, bathroom, kitchen and personal items, clothing, colors, shapes and trees.

Although the absence of a well developed theory of lexical semantics makes it difficult to provide a systematic interpretation of these category (semantic)-specific deficits, they provide a provocative source of data on which far reaching speculations about the structure of lexical organization may be based. Thus, at the very least, these results strongly argue for a highly structured lexical organization based on semantic categories. The implication of these results for neural organization will be considered below.

Processing Principles

The material reviewed thus far has allowed us to address issues concerning the architecture of the lexical system and the types and organization of information represented in lexical components. I turn now to a consideration of the processing principles that govern the access of this information.

Two general classes of lexical processing models have been proposed: serial search models and passive, parallel activation models (activation, for short). Of these two classes, the activation models have clearly emerged dominant over the past decade. The basic assumption of activation models is that a stimulus (or input at some level of the lexical system) activates in parallel all stored representations. The degree of activation of any representation is proportional to the overall similarity between the input and the stored representation. Thus, for example, the stimulus word car will activate the representations 'cat', 'tar', 'cart', 'cord', etc., to different degrees. In this example, 'car', will be activated most strongly and 'cat' will be activated more than 'cord' and so forth. When the level of activation of a representation reaches a set, threshold value, the representation becomes available for further processing to other components of the processing system. Models of this type are known as serial stage models. If we relax the assumption that only the representation that reaches a threshold value can serve to activate subsequent stages of processing and we allow all representations that reach a minimal level of activation to activate representations in other components of the system, we have what are called cascade models of processing (McClelland, 1979). Here I will assume, for the sake of simplicity, a serial stage model (although it is quite likely that the cascading principle is a more realistic characterization of the processing sequence).

A distributed model of the lexical system, as that discussed in this review, which operates on the principle of passive, parallel activation, provides a natural framework for considering various features of impaired language performance. Two such features are the ubiquitous frequency effect (words of higher usage frequency are in many cases relatively spared in comparison to words of lower frequency) and certain types of error responses produced by patients in single-word processing tasks.

It is a well established phenomenon in the psychological literature that reaction time to recognize a word or to decide that a string of letters forms a word (lexical decision) is inversely proportional to the frequency of usage of a word (and, similarly for error rates) (see Gordon, 1983, for review). Activation models account for this effect by assuming that the activation threshold of a representation is lowered with repeated presentations of the stimulus or input (Morton, 1970). Thus, high frequency words have lower thresholds than low frequency words and, therefore, can be activated more easily, resulting in lower RTs and lower error rates, than low frequency words. This differential effect of word frequency is also found in aphasic patients' performance (see Gordon & Caramazza, 1982). To give just one example, many dyslexic patients make more errors in reading low frequency words than in reading high frequency words. What is important for our present concern, however, is that the presence of a frequency effect may be associated with certain types of error responses allowing us to identify the locus of deficit responsible for a patient's impaired performance. That is, we may take the presence of a word frequency effect as an indication of a deficit to the lexical system and the type of error (e.g., visual or semantic) as an indication of a deficit at a specific level within the lexical system.

I have already indicated that two types of errors produced by dyslexic patients are visual and semantic paralexias. Various accounts have been offered as the basis for these errors types (e.g., Caramazza, in press; Marshall & Newcombe, 1973; Morton & Patterson, 1980; Nolan & Caramazza, 1982; Shallice & Warrington, 1980). I will argue that, at least in some cases, these errors arise from independent deficits to the graphemic input lexicon, and the phonological output lexicon for visual and semantic paralexic errors, respectively.

Recall that visual paralexic errors are errors such as reading bead for head and semantic paralexic errors are errors such as reading airplane for ship. In an indepth investigation of a single patient, F.M., Gordon, Goodman-Schulman, and Caramazza (1987) asked the patient to read several thousand words in order to obtain a reliable data base of errors for detailed analysis. The patient's responses were scored either as correct or as an error of one of the following types: visual, semantic, inflectional, derivational, or other--where this last category consists of ambiguous errors, visual-to-semantic errors or word responses that could not be classified in any of the previously listed error categories. Here I first wish to focus on the evidential role of visual and semantic errors to constrain a model of the lexical system.

A priori it is unlikely that these two types of errors have a common basis: A semantic error can only occur if the correct lexical entry has been activated; that is, in order to produce "minister" for "bishop," the lexical entry for "bishop" had to be activated. There is no such constraint for visual errors. This latter type of error most likely arises from damage to the input graphemic lexicon where an inappropriate lexical representation is activated. To explore this issue consider the following argument. A word that is read correctly is one that successfully activates a lexical entry in the input graphemic lexicon and the output phonological lexicon. By contrast a word that gives rise to a visual error is one that fails to activate its lexical entry in the input graphemic lexicon and instead activates a visually similar entry in this lexicon. Similarly, a word that gives rise to a semantic error is one that successfully activates a correct lexical entry in the input graphemic lexicon, but fails to activate its lexical entry in the output phonological lexicon, and instead activates a semantically related entry. Note that this argument makes two obvious, but important assumptions: 1) The access procedure for the input graphemic lexicon is orthographically based; 2) The access procedure for the output phonological lexicon is semantically based.

This proposed architecture of the lexical system and, more specifically, the assumptions we have made about the address procedures for the input graphemic lexicon and the output phonological lexicon, (i.e., parallel activation) allow us to make a precise prediction about F.M.'s performance on re-reading words read correctly, incorrectly produced responses, words to which he made visual errors and words to which he made semantic errors on the first reading. The prediction is that he should read very well words he read correctly the first time as well as the incorrectly produced responses but should read poorly words to which he previously made errors. Furthermore, the new errors for words that gave rise to visual errors should predominantly be visual whereas those for words which gave rise to semantic errors should predominantly be semantic. These predictions were borne out.

To further substantiate the claim that visual and semantic errors arise due to difficulties in addressing lexical representations in the input graphemic lexicon and the output phonological lexicon, respectively, we assessed F.M.'s ability to comprehend words which were on a previous occasion read correctly or had resulted in visual or semantic errors. The model of the lexical system proposed here leads to the prediction that F.M. should understand both the words he previously read correctly and those to which he made semantic errors, but he should fail to comprehend the words to which he had made visual errors. This prediction too was borne out.

The implication of these results for claims concerning the processing structure of the hypothesized lexical components is clear cut. It would appear that a visual error is made when a particular lexical entry in the graphemic input lexicon cannot reach threshold and instead a visually similar representation reaches threshold. Similarly, a semantic error occurs when a representation in the phonological output lexicon cannot reach threshold and instead a semantically related response reaches threshold. This interpretation of the basis for F.M.'s visual and semantic errors is only possible if we assume that lexical representations are activated in parallel and in proportion to the similarity between the input and the stored representation.

CONCLUSION

In this all too brief and highly condensed review I have dealt with three aspects of the structure of the lexical system: the general architecture of the system, the types of representational content in each hypothesized component, and the processing principles that allow access of the information stored in the lexicon. The evidence reviewed not only provides empirical support for the model but, in addition, the model serves as a guide for the interpretation and analysis of cognitive/linguistic disorders. Our discussion has focussed, however, entirely on functional (cognitive) aspects of the process. We may wish to ask, therefore, whether or not the types of observations available to us from the analysis of cognitive deficits will be relevant to the formulation of a truly *neuro*psychological theory of cognitive functioning. That is, is a *neuro*psychology of language possible? In a previous section of this review I sounded a pessimistic note with respect to this question. Here, by way of conclusion, I would like to take up this issue in a little more detail.

As I have indicated the classical study of aphasia has failed to lead to any significant insights into the structure of language processing mechanisms and their neural instantiation, other than the gross clinical-pathological mapping already available at the end of the last century. This work clearly established the importance of the perisylvian region of the left hemisphere for language processing but could not go beyond this general phrenological statement. Theoretical and methodological developments over the past decade have introduced the possibility for significant progress for one part of the brain/cognition equation. We have see that we now have a clearly articulated justification for drawing inferences about normal cognitive processing from the analysis of patterns of cognitive dysfunction, as well as a powerful theoretical and methodological basis for the analysis of cognitive dysfunctions. This development, by itself, is not sufficient to lead to any significant insights into the nature of the neural mechanisms that subserve language processing. It may be sufficient, however, to provide a set of principled constraints on the possible form of a neuropsychological theory of language processing.

Recent work (some of it reviewed here) in cognitive neuropsychology has provided an impressive set of results on the nature of language dysfunctions. It has been possible to demonstrate that language dysfunction may be highly selective affecting a single component (e.g., Miceli & Caramazza, 1987) or even a single representational dimension within a component (e.g., Warrington, 1981). Such observations provide a natural set of constraints for a theory of language processing as amply demonstrated above. However, since the observations that enter into this theory-construction process consist of brain/behavior pairs, we may use them to constrain the formulation of a neuropsychological theory of language. Thus far little use has been made of this opportunity. But we may already state an important constraint that has emerged from this research: Given the highly selective and systematic dissociations of function observed in brain-damaged patients, we may conclude that there is a high degree of specialization of cognitive function in the brain--that is, the observations reported support a strong localizationist view of brain organization. This conclusion needs some elaboration.

We have seen that brain pathology may selectively damage one or another component of a distributed lexical system. These results support a modular theory of lexical components (Allport & Funnell, 1981; Shallice, 1981). They also suggest, however, that distinct neural structures subserve the hypothesized lexical components. Indeed, the evidence on hand shows a fine-grained localization of function well beyond the level of gross lexical component all the way down to single representational dimensions. This does not necessarily mean (although such may be the case) that distinct neuroanatomical loci are associated with different components of the lexicon. All that is asserted is that a distinct neural process is associated with different cognitive mechanisms and that these neural processes may be selectively damaged. What is clear, however, is that the neuropsychological data do not support an indefinitely plastic, nonlocalizationist model of neural functioning. This is a nontrivial conclusion about neural processing that has emerged from cognitive neuropsychological research.

Cognitive neuropsychological analyses may also be used to provide a fine-grained mapping of cognitive mechanisms to neural structures or processes. That is, we may be able to go beyond the level of merely specifying general constraints for a neural theory of language processing. But this is not possible without a profound transformation of the social organization of scientific investigation in this area.

We have seen that valid inferences about the structure of normal cognition are only possible for single-patient studies. The highly detailed investigation of single patients allows us to infer a functional lesion to a model of a cognitive system and thereby provide support for that model. And, while the analysis of single patients is well-suited for drawing conclusions about cognitive structure, this methodology is not sufficient for drawing conclusions about brain/cognition relationships. For this latter purpose we need to accumulate enough cases with "identical" functional lesions in order to correlate the identified cognitive mechanisms with the neural structures that support the identified functions. This entails the accumulation of large numbers of cases. However, since the most useful, clear information is likely to come from patients with highly selective deficits and since such cases are relatively rare, it is extremely unlikely that any single investigator or laboratory will have enough cases to carry out the correlational analyses needed for this purpose. This limitation of the cognitive neuropsychological method in relating cognitive mechanisms to neural structures is not an in-principle limitation of the method but only a practical one which may be overcome if adequate measures are taken. Specifically, as I have argued elsewhere (Caramazza & Martin, 1983), cognitive neuropsychologists will have to create research consortia, as have done high energy physicists and astronomers in their respective domains. This step will permit the accumulation of cases with the desired characteristics for the needed correlational analysis. (It must be emphasized here, if there is any need, that this proposal in no way implies an indirect justification for the group-study methodology. The frequency analysis proposed here is based on single-patient analyses and does not require the averaging of patients' performance, a methodologically invalid procedure.)

In this concluding section I have identified a procedure for relating language processing mechanisms to brain structures within the methodology of cognitive neuropsychology. We should note, however, that even in the best of all possible worlds this methodology can only lead to a fine-grained, modern phrenology--it will not provide information directly relevant to a neurophysiology of language. This latter goal may be unattainable even with technological developments. The most promising avenue open to us at this time is the development of a computational neuropsychology; that is, the development of neural network models of language processing (e.g., Arbib, Caplan, & Marshall, 1982). It is not difficult to imagine how the interaction of increasingly-detailed, neurally-constrained models of language processing that emerge from cognitive neuropsychological research with neural network models of language processes may lead to a theoretical neurophysiology of language.

ACKNOWLEDGEMENTS

The research reported here was supported in part by NIH grants NS23836 and NS22201, as well as The Seaver Institute and The Lounsbery Foundation. I would like to thank Marie-Camille Havard, Kathy Yantis and Olivier Koenig for their help in the preparation of this manuscript.

REFERENCES

Allport, A. & Funnell, E. (1981). Components of the mental lexicon. Philosophical Transactions of the Royal Society of London, 295, 397-410.

Anderson, S. (1982). Where's morphology? Linguistic Inquiry, 13, 571-612.

Arbib, M. A., Caplan, D. & Marshall, J. F., Eds. (1982). Neural models of language processes. New York, NY: Academic Press.

Badecker, W. & Caramazza, A. (1985). On considerations of method and theory governing the use of clinical categories in Neurolinguistics and Cognitive Neuropsychology: The case against Agrammatism. Cognition, 20, 97-115.

Badecker, W. & Caramazza, A. (1986). The analysis of morphological errors in a case of acquired dyslexia. Reports of the Cognitive

Neuropsychology Laboratory.   The Johns Hopkins University, Baltimore, MD.

Basso, A., Taborelli, A. & Vignolo, L. A. (1978). Dissociated disorders of speaking and writing in aphasia. Journal of Neurology, Neurosurgery, and Psychiatry, 41, 6, 556.

Baxter, D. M. & Warrington, E. K. (1985). Category-specific phonological dysgraphia. Neuropsychologia, 23, 653-666.

Beauvois, M.-F. & Dérouesné, J. (1979). Phonological alexia: Three dissociations. Journal of Neurology, Neurosurgery and Psychiatry, 42, 1111-1124.

Beauvois, M.-F. & Dérouesné, J. (1981). Lexical or orthographic agraphia. Brain, 104, 21-49.

Benson, D. F. (1985). Aphasia. In K. M. Heilman & E. Valenstein (Eds.), Clinical Neuropsychology. New York, NY: Oxford University Press.

Berndt, R. S. & Caramazza, A. (1980). A redefinition of the syndrome of Broca's aphasia: Implications for a neuropsychological model of language. Applied Psycholinguistics, 1, 225-278.

Bradley, D., Garrett, M. & Zurif, E. (1980). Syntactic deficits in Broca's aphasia. In D. Caplan (Ed.), Biological Studies of Mental Processes. Cambridge, MA: MIT Press.

Brownell, H. H., Potter, H. H., Michelow, D. & Gardner, H. (1984). Sensitivity to lexical denotation and connotation in brain-damaged patients: A double dissociation? Brain and Language, 22, 253-265.

Bub, D. N. & Kertesz, A. (1982). Deep agraphia. Brain and Language, 17, 147-166.

Butterworth, B. (1983). Lexical representation. In B. Butterworth (Ed.), Language Production, Vol. 2. New York, NY: Academic Press.

Caplan, D. (in press). Neurolinguistics and linguistic aphasiology: An Introduction. Cambridge: Cambridge University Press.

Caplan, D., Keller, L. & Locke, S. (1972). Inflection of neologisms in aphasia. Brain, 95, 169-172.

Caramazza, A. (in press). The structure of the lexical system: Evidence from acquired language disorders.   In R. H. Brookshire (Ed.), Proceedings of the Clinical Aphasiology Conference.

Caramazza, A. (1984). The logic of neuropsychological research and the problem of patient classification in aphasia. Brain and Language, 21, 9-20.

Caramazza, A. (1986). On drawing inferences about the structure of normal cognitive systems from the analysis of patterns of impaired performance: The case for single-patient studies. Brain and Cognition, 5, 41-66.

Caramazza, A. & Berndt, R. S. (1982). A psycholinguistic assessment of adult aphasia. In S. Rosenberg (Ed.), Handbook of applied psycholinguistics, 477-535. Cambridge: Cambridge University Press.

Caramazza, A. & Berndt, R. S. (1985). A multicomponent deficit view of agrammatic Broca's aphasia. In M.-L. Kean (Ed.), Agrammatism. Orlando, FL: Academic Press.

Caramazza, A. & Martin, R. (1983). Theoretical and methodological issues in the study of aphasia. In J.B. Hellige (Ed.), Cerebral hemisphere asymmetry: Method, theory and application, 18-45. New York, NY: Praeger Scientific Publishers.

Caramazza, A. & McCloskey, M. (in press). The case for single-patient studies. Cognitive Neuropsychology.

Caramazza, A., Miceli, G., Silveri M., & Laudanna, A. (1985). Reading mechanisms and the organization of the lexicon: Evidence from acquired dyslexia. Cognitive Neuropsychology, 2, 81-114.

Chomsky, N. (1965). Aspects of the theory of syntax. Cambridge, MA: MIT Press.

Chomsky, N. (1981). Lectures on government and binding. Dordrecht, Netherlands: Foris Publications.

Churchland, P. (1986). Neurophilosophy: Toward a unified science of the mind/brain. Cambridge, MA: The MIT Press.

Coltheart, M., Patterson, K. & Marshall, J. (Eds.) (1980). Deep Dyslexia. London: Routledge & Kegan Paul.

Damasio, A. (1981). The nature of aphasia: Signs and syndromes. In N. T. Sarno (Ed.), Acquired Aphasia. New York, NY: Academic Press.

Damasio, A. R. & Geschwind, N. (1984). The neural basis of language. Annual Review of Neuroscience, 7, 127-147.

DeBastiani, P., Barry, C. & Carreras, M. (1983). Mechanisms for reading nonwords: Evidence from a case of phonological dyslexia in an Italian reader. Paper presented at the First European Workshop on Cognitive Neuropsychology, Bressanone, Italy.

De Villiers, J. G. (1978). Fourteen grammatical morphemes in acquisition and aphasia. In A. Caramazza & E. B. Zurif (Eds.), Language acquisition and language breakdown: Parallels and divergences, pp 121-144. Baltimore, MD: The Johns Hopkins University Press.

Friederici, A. D. & Schoenle, P. W. (1980). Computational dissociation of two vocabulary types: Evidence from aphasia. Neuropsychologia, 18, 11-20.

Funnell, E. (1983). Phonological processes in reading: New evidence from acquired dyslexia. British Journal of Psychology, 74, 159-180.

Gardner, H., Brownell, H. H., Wapner, W. & Michelow, D. (1983). Missing the point: The role of the right hemisphere in the processing of complex linguistic materials. In E. Pereceman (Ed.), <u>Cognitive Processes in the right hemisphere</u>. New York, NY: Academic Press.

Gleason, J. B. (1978). The acquisition and dissolution of the English Inflectional System. In A. Caramazza & E. B. Zurif (Eds.), <u>Language acquisition and language breakdown: Parallels and divergences</u>, pp 109-120. Baltimore, MD: The Johns Hopkins University Press.

Goodglass, H. (1976). Agrammatism. In H. Whitaker & H. A. Whitaker (Eds.), <u>Studies in neurolinguistics</u>, Vol. 1. New York, NY: Academic Press.

Goodglass, H. & Berko, J. (1960). Agrammatism and inflectional morphology in English. <u>Journal of Speech and Hearing Research</u>, <u>3</u>, 257-267.

Goodglass, H., Klein, B., Carey, P. & Jones, K. J. (1966). Specific semantic word categories in aphasia. <u>Cortex</u>, <u>2</u>, 74-89.

Goodman, R. A. & Caramazza, A. (in press). Aspects of the spelling process: Evidence from a case of acquired dysgraphia. <u>Language and Cognitive Processes</u>.

Goodman, R. A. & Caramazza, A. (1986). Dissociation of spelling errors in written and oral spelling: The role of allographic conversion in writing. <u>Cognitive Neuropsychology</u>, <u>3</u>, 179-206.

Gordon, B. (1983). Lexical access and lexical decision: Mechanisms of frequency sensitivity. <u>Journal of Verbal Learning and Verbal Behavior</u>, <u>22</u>, 146-160.

Gordon, B. & Caramazza, A. (1982). Lexical decision for open- and closed-class items: Failure to replicate differential frequency sensitivity. <u>Brain and Language</u>, <u>15</u>, 143-160.

Gordon, B., Goodman-Schulman, R. A. & Caramazza, A. (1987). Separating the stages of reading errors. Submitted to <u>Brain</u>.

Hart, J., Berndt, R. S. & Caramazza, A. (1985). Category-specific naming deficit following cerebral infarction. <u>Nature</u>, <u>316</u>, 439-440.

Hier, D. B. & Mohr, J. P. (1977). Incongruous oral and written naming: Evidence for a subdivision of the syndrome of Wernicke's aphasia. <u>Brain and Language</u>, <u>4</u>, 115-126.

Hinton, G. E. & Anderson, J. A.(Eds.), (1981). <u>Parallel models of associative memory</u>. Hillsdale, NJ: Erlbaum.

Job, R. & Sartori, G. (1984). Morphological decomposition: Evidence from crossed phonological dyslexia. <u>The Quarterly Journal of Experimental Psychology</u>, <u>36</u>, 435-458.

Kertesz, A. (1985). Aphasia. In P. J. Vinken, J. W. Bruyn, & H. L. Klawans (Eds.), <u>Handbook of Clinical Neurology</u>. New York, NY: Elsevier Science Publishing Company.

Lesser, R. (1978). <u>Linguistic investigations of aphasia</u>. New York, NY: Elsevier North-Holland.

Marshall, J. (1982). What is a symptom-complex. In M. A. Arbib, D. Caplan, & J. F. Marshall (Eds.), Neural models of language processes. New York, NY: Academic Press.

Marshall, J. C. (1986). The description and interpretation of aphasic language disorder. Neuropsychologia, 24, 5-24.

Marshall, J. C. & Newcombe, F. (1973). Patterns of paralexia: A psycholinguistic approach. Journal of Psycholinguistic Research, 2, 175-199.

McCarthy, R. & Warrington, E. K. (1985). Category-specificity in a agrammatic patient: The relative impairment of verb retrieval and comprehension. Neuropsychologia, 23, 709-727.

McClelland, J. L. (1979). On the time-relations of mental processes: An examination of systems of processes in cascade. Psychological Review, 86, 287-330.

Miceli, G. & Caramazza, A. (1987). Dissociation of inflectional and derivational morphology. Reports of the Cognitive Neuropsychology Laboratory. The Johns Hopkins University, Baltimore, MD.

Miceli, G., Mazzucchi, A., Menn, L. & Goodglass, H. (1983). Contrasting cases of Italian agrammatic aphasia without comprehension disorder. Brain and Language, 19, 65-97.

Miceli, G., Silveri, M. C., Nocentini, U. & Caramazza, A. (1986). Patterns of dissociation in comprehension and production of nouns and verbs. Aphasiology. In press.

Miceli, G., Silveri, M. C., Villa, G. & Caramazza, A. (1984). On the basis for the agrammatic's difficulty in producing main verbs. Cortex, 20, 207-220.

Miceli, G., Silveri, M. C. & Caramazza, A. (1985). Cognitive analysis of a case of pure dysgraphia. Brain and Language, 25, 187-212.

Michel, F. (1979). Préservation du langage écrit malgré un deficit majeur du langage oral. Lyon Médical, 241, 141-149.

Morton, J. (1970). A functional model of memory. In D. A. Normal (Ed.), Models of human memory. New York, NY: Academic Press.

Morton, J. (1981). The status of information processing models of language. Philosophical Transactions of the Royal Society of London, 295, 387-396.

Morton, J. & Patterson, K. E. (1980). A new attempt at an interpretation, or, an attempt at a new interpretation. In M. Coltheart, K. E. Patterson, & J. C. Marshall (Eds.), Deep Dyslexia. London: Routledge & Kegan Paul.

Nolan, K. A. & Caramazza, A. (1982). Modality-independent impairments in word processing in a deep dyslexic patient. Brain and Language, 16, 237-264.

Nolan, K. A. & Caramazza, A. (1983). An analysis of writing in a case of deep dyslexia. Brain and Language, 20, 305-328.

Patterson, K. (1980). Derivational Errors. In M. Coltheart, K. Patterson, & J. Marshall (Eds.), Deep Dyslexia. London: Routledge & Kegan Paul.

Patterson, K. (1982). The relation between reading and phonological coding: Further neuropsychological observation. In A. W. Ellis (Ed.), Normality and Pathology in Cognitive Functions. London: Academic Press.

Rumelhart, D. E. & McClelland, J. L. (1986). Parallel distributed processing: Explorations in the microstructure of cognition, Vol. 1: Foundations. Cambridge, MA: Bradford Books/MIT Press.

Scalise, S. (1984). Generative morphology. Dordrecht, Netherlands: Foris Publications.

Shallice, T. (1979). Case study approach in neuropsychological research. Journal of Clinical Neuropsychology, 1, 183-211.

Shallice, T. (1981). Phonological agraphia and the lexical route in writing. Brain, 104, 413-429.

Shallice, T. & Warrington, E. K. (1975). Word recognition in a phonemic dyslexic patient. Quarterly Journal of Experimental Psychology, 27, 187-199.

Shallice, T. & Warrington, E. K. (1980). Single and multiple component central dyslexic syndromes. In M. Coltheart, K. E. Patterson, & J. C. Marshall (Eds.), Deep Dyslexia. London: Routledge & Kegan Paul.

Stemberger, J. P. (1984). Structural errors in normal and agrammatic speech. Cognitive Neuropsychology, 1, 281-313.

Stemberger, J. P. (1985). An interactive activation model of language production. In A. W. Ellis (Ed.), Progress in the psychology of language, pp 143-183 (Vol. 1). London: LEA Limited.

Taft, M. (1979). Recognition of affixed words and the word frequency effect. Memory and Cognition, 7, 263-272.

Taft, M. (1985). The decoding of words in lexical access: A review of the morphographic approach. In D. Besner, T. Waller, & G. Mackinnon (Eds.), Reading research: Advances in theory and practice (Vol. 5). New York, NY: Academic Press.

Warrington, E. K. (1975). The selective impairment of semantic memory. Quarterly Journal of Experimental Psychology, 27, 635-657.

Warrington, E. K. (1981). Concrete word dyslexia. British Journal of Psychology, 72, 175-196.

Warrington, E. K. & McCarthy, R. (1983). Category-specific access dysphasia. Brain, 106, 859-878.

Warrington, E. K. & Shallice, T. (1984). Category-specific semantic impairments. Brain, 107, 829-854.

Wasow, T. (1985). Postscript. In P. Sells, <u>Lectures on contemporary syntactic theories: An introduction to government-binding theory, generalized phrase structure grammar, and lexical-functional grammar.</u> Stanford, CA: Center for the Study of Language and Information.

B. Reading

Introduction to Section on Reading

The study of acquired disorders of reading occupies a special place in modern cognitive neuropsychology. It was Marshall and Newcombe's "Patterns of paralexia" in the early 1970's (1973) that captured the imagination and interest of cognitive psychologists leading to a large number of empirical and theoretical papers on the nature of reading disorders and the structure of the cognitive mechanisms that underlie reading. In that paper, Marshall and Newcombe clearly distinguished between two patterns of reading deficits and attributed them to damage to different components of the reading process. A number of papers followed, attempting to refine and enrich these initial observations (see Coltheart, Patterson & Marshall, 1980; Patterson, Marshall, & Coltheart, 1985), as well various efforts to identify new patterns of reading impairment. Thus, in addition to the original syndromes of deep and surface dyslexia described by Marshall & Newcombe, phonological dyslexia (Beauvois & Dérouesné, 1979), letter-by-letter reading (Patterson & Kay, 1982), and attentional dyslexia (Shallice & Warrington, 1977) were identified as distinct neurological syndromes. And, in each case, specific proposals were made about possible underlying functional causes for the observed disorders.

To be sure, not all the research in this area has led to significant insights into the structure of the reading process or the nature of reading disorders. A considerable amount of effort was devoted to discussions about the underlying functional causes of various syndrome types, such as deep and surface dyslexia. These efforts could not but be unproductive. As I have extensively argued elsewhere (e.g., Caramazza, 1984; 1986), the application of the "medical model" of research to cognitive disorders, and in particular its reliance on syndromes, is of dubious value. Syndromes are theoretically arbitrary constructs which hinder more than help in understanding the structure of cognitive systems or their dissolution in conditions of brain damage.

Nonetheless, there has also been major progress made in the development of a theory of the reading process, both in specifying the overall architecture of the cognitive/linguistic components involved in reading as well as in understanding the processing structure of the individual components that comprise the reading system. Thus, there is now considerable agreement that the principal components of the reading process are those schematically represented in Figure 1. This model assumes that reading aloud may be accomplished either through the activation of lexical-phonological representations for familiar words or the

45

conversion of a graphemic string into a phonological representation by the application of sub-lexical orthography-to-phonology mapping rules (e.g., Coltheart, 1978; Patterson& Morton, 1985; Shallice & McCarthy, 1985). The model also assumes that graphemic representations in input and phonological representations in output are temporarily held in a graphemic and a phonological buffer, respectively, for subsequent processing (e.g., Caramazza, Miceli, & Villa, 1986). Finally, the model shown in Figure 2 also assumes that information from the semantic component and the orthography-to-phonology conversion procedure can summate in the activation of lexical-phonological representations for output (e.g., Saffran, 1985; Hillis & Caramazza, in press).

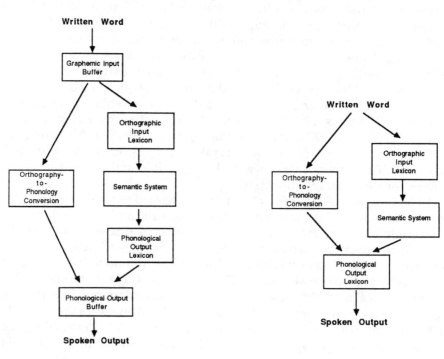

Figure 1.   Figure 2.

There has also been progress in describing the processing structure of various components of the reading system. Thus, for example, there are a number of interesting proposals about the nature of the orthography-to-phonology conversion procedure (e.g., see Coltheart; Shallice & McCarthy, 1985), and about the nature of lexical-orthographic input representations (Caramazza, Miceli, Silveri & Laudanna, 1985) and lexical-phonological output representations (Badecker & Caramazza, in press). Unfortunately, though, progress in this area has been slow, reflecting, I think, insufficient reliance on developments in linguistic theory, on the one hand, and failure to carry out sufficiently detailed analyses of patients' performance, on the other hand.

The papers in this section concern a disparate set of issues within the general area of reading. Chapter 2, written with Gabriele Miceli, Caterina Silveri, and Alessandro Laudanna, reports the analysis of two patients, AG and LB, who made reading errors virtually only for nonwords. This dissociation of performance between words and nonwords (see also Funnell, 1983) was interpreted as undermining Patterson's (1982) proposal that morphological paralexias result from a disorder of phonological processing. The latter hypothesis was based on the observation that deficits of nonword reading and morphological paralexias co-occur (Beauvois & Dérouesné, 1979; Patterson, 1982). The performance obtained for AG and LB showed that the association between nonword reading deficit and morphological paralexias was not a necessary one. A more interesting aspect of this report was the observation that LB performed better in reading those nonwords that could be parsed exhaustively into legal morphemes of the language even though their combination resulted in nonwords (e.g., walken) than in reading nonwords that could not be parsed into morphemes. The effect of morphological structure on reading performance was interpreted as support for the hypothesis that the orthographic input lexicon represents information in morphologically decomposed form--stems are represented independently of inflections. Another conclusion reached in this paper was that the deficit responsible for LB's nonword reading performance was to the orthography-to-phonology conversion mechanism. The latter conclusion may be incorrect, however. Further analyses of LB's performance revealed a deficit in spelling which could be explained as arising from damage to the graphemic buffer (Caramazza, Miceli, Villa, & Romani, 1987). More recently we have argued that a deficit at the level of graphemic representations can result in differential performance for words and nonwords in reading (Caramazza & Hillis, in press). Thus, it is entirely possible that contrary to our earlier proposal the deficit responsible for LB's reading performance is damage at the level of the graphemic buffer and not damage to the orthography-to-phonology conversion mechanism. Independently of which account of the locus of deficit in LB is the correct one, the conclusions reached about the structure of lexical representations and lexical access operations seem to be correct: we have obtained additional, independent support for these conclusions in experiments with normal subjects (see Caramazza, Laudanna, & Romani, 1988; Laudanna, Badecker, & Caramazza, 1989), and we have also reported other patterns of impairment which support the view that the phonological output lexicon (Miceli & Caramazza, 1988; Badecker & Caramazza, in press) and the orthographic output lexicon (Badecker, Hillis, & Caramazza, 1990) represent information in morphologically decomposed form.

The inferences drawn from the performance of subject LB about the morphological structure of lexical representations does not depend on specific assumptions about damage to the component of processing about which inferences are made. By contrast, the inferences drawn about the role of the phonological buffer in the architecture of the reading process from the performance of subject IGR (Chapter 3, written with Gabriele Miceli and Giampiero Villa) does depend on assumptions about the possibility of damage to a particular component of that process. IGR was impaired in reading, writing, and repetition of nonwords, but not words. Furthermore, the pattern of errors made in each of the three tasks was the same. In each case responses were phonologically related to the stimulus (e.g., brelve → prelve; ledria → letria; and cadata → gadata; in reading, writing, and repetition, respectively). This performance suggests a common, phonological basis for the obtained error pattern. Since the only component of processing common to the three tasks is the phonological buffer, the invited inference is that the locus of damage responsible for the observed impairment is to the phonological buffer (see also Bub, Black, Howell, & Kertesz, 1987). It is worth noting that unlike the case for LB where the inference was based on a dissociation of performance, the inference in this case is based on a pattern of association of impairments. The obvious implication is that both dissociations and associations of performance may be used to infer the structure of cognitive systems and their disorder.

The conclusions reached from IGR's performance are consistent with computational considerations and other experimental results. Thus, we have recently reported the performance of an Italian brain-damaged subject (CLB) who was severely impaired at the level of the phonological output lexicon, but who could read very many words and virtually all nonwords (Miceli & Caramazza, 1990). Because Italian orthography is segmentally transparent (i.e., orthography-to-phonology mapping at the level of single syllables is unambiguous) the patient could produce correctly the phonological segments associated with a given graphemic sequence by the application of sub-lexical orthography-to-phonology conversion procedures. However, in Italian, stress is assigned lexically (e.g., macchina → makkina; but tacchina → takkina), so that although the patient could correctly produce the segmental structure of a word by sub-lexical conversion procedures, he could not assign stress correctly. Indeed, almost all the reading errors produced by the patient were stress errors. Nonetheless, stress assignment was not random, but tended to respect the distribution of the stress pattern in Italian. This implies that in those cases where lexical information was not available, stress was assigned syllabically, and, therefore, we must assume that in the latter case this procedure had to operate over the full syllabic string for production--a phonological representation presumably held temporarily in a phonological buffer.

Morphological paralexias (e.g., walking → walked) are a relatively common feature of reading impairments. The question arises whether these errors might not reflect a deficit to specifically morphological processes. This issue is addressed in Chapter 4. In this paper, Badecker and I analyzed in some detail the reading performance of a brain-damaged subject, FM, whose performance could be clinically classified as deep dyslexia (Gordon, Goodman, & Caramazza, 1987): FM produced semantic, visual, and morphological paralexias in reading, and performed very poorly in reading nonwords; he also showed marked word-class and concreteness effects. The specific issue we addressed was whether morphological errors could be attributed to a specific deficit in morphological processing. Although it was easy to demonstrate that morphological structure affected performance it was not possible to rule out the possibility that these effects were the result of combined visual, form class, semantic, and concreteness effects. To be sure, we were able to show that each of the latter factors alone, as revealed through the use of specially designed word lists, could not account for the production of morphological paralexias; however, the possibility that some combination of these factors could account for the production of morphological paralexias could not be ruled out in this case. The results obtained with FM allowed us to question the conclusions drawn by Patterson (1982) and Job & Sartori (1984) that the morphological paralexias produced by their patients were in fact the result of damage to morphological processing mechanisms. The issues addressed in this paper are not without methodological interest beyond questions about the role of morphology in lexical representation. The general issue is whether the superficial characterization of an error allows direct inferences about the possible locus of damage responsible for the error type in question. That is, the issue is whether categorizing an error as morphological, visual, or semantic implies necessarily a morphological, visual-perceptual, or semantic level of deficit, respectively. We have seen that, at least for morphological paralexias, this is not the case. In a recent paper we were able to show the same for semantic paralexias--semantic errors may be produced even when the semantic system can be shown to be essentially undamaged

(Caramazza & Hillis, 1990). We suspect that the same conclusion can be extended to the production of visual errors.

The last paper in this section--Chapter 5, written with Brenda Rapp-- also addresses the question of what inferences are legitimate from a pattern of reading impairment about the structure of lexical processes. In a series of papers, Warrington, Shallice, and McCarthy (Warrington, 1975; Warrington & McCarthy, 1983; Warrington & Shallice, 1979) proposed that access to word meaning proceeds progressively from the activation of superordinate to increasingly specific information in a hierarchically organized semantic network. The clearest evidence for this hypothesis was obtained from a case of so-called "semantic access dyslexia." The principal feature of this disorder is good performance in judging the superordinate class of an item the patient is otherwise unable to identify. Although this dissociation would, on the face of it, seem to suggest the conclusion reached by Warrington and her collaborators, there are some problems with it, ranging from theoretical to methodological to empirical problems. The theoretical difficulty concerns the possibility of deriving a coherent explanation for semantic access based on sequential access of superordinate followed by more specific information. Our attempts to derive such an explanation were unsuccessful. The methodological problem concerns the legitimate inferences that are possible from a comparison of performance on tasks that require only a category judgment versus performance on tasks that require the identification of an object or word. We point out that the amount of information required for good performance on the two tasks are unequal, allowing the possibility that performance would be good in one task but not on another, without requiring that the crucial information needed for good category membership performance concern specifically superordinate information. And, finally, we show that in a patient, JE, who satisfies the stated criteria for classification as a "semantic access dyslexic", his performance in a word/picture categorization task, in which semantic and orthographic factors are controlled, did not favor predictions derived from the hypothesis of sequential access of superordinate to specific semantic information.

References

Badecker, W., Hillis, A. & Caramazza, A. (1990). Lexical morphology and its role in the writing process: Evidence from a case of acquired dysgraphia. Cognition, 34, 205-243.

Badecker, W. & Caramazza, A. (in press). Morphological composition in the lexical output system. Cognitive Neuropsychology.

Beauvois, M. F. & Dérouesné, J. (1979). Phonological alexia: Three dissociations. Journal of Neurology, Neurosurgery, and Psychiatry, 42, 1115-1124.

Bub, D., Black, S., Howell, J. & Kertesz, A. (1987). Speech output processes and reading. In M. Coltheart, G. Sartori & R. Job (Eds), The cognitive neuropsychology of language. London: Lawrence Erlbaum Associates, Ltd.

Caramazza, A. (1984). The logic of neuropsychological research and the problem of patient classification in aphasia. Brain and Language, 21, 9-20.

Caramazza, A. & Hillis, A. (in press). Levels of representation, coordinate frames, and unilateral neglect. Cognitive Neuropsychology.

Caramazza, A. & Hillis, A. (1990). Where do semantic errors come from? Cortex, 26, 95-122.

Caramazza, A., Miceli, G., Silveri, M. C. & Laudanna, A. (1985). Reading mechanisms and the organization of the lexicon: Evidence from acquired dyslexia. Cognitive Neuropsychology, 2, 81-114.

Caramazza, A. (1986). On drawing inferences about the structure of normal cognitive systems from the analysis of impaired performance: The case for single-patient studies. Brain and Cognition, 5, 41-66.

Caramazza, A., Miceli, G. & Villa, G. (1986). The role of the (output) phonological buffer in reading, writing, and repetition. Cognitive Neuropsychology, 3, 37-76.

Caramazza, A. Miceli, G., Villa, G. & Romani, C. (1987). The role of the Graphemic Buffer in Spelling: Evidence from a case of acquired dysgraphia. Cognition, 26, 59-85.

Caramazza, A., Laudanna, A. & Romani, C. (1988). Lexical access and inflectional morphology. Cognition, 28, 297-332.

Coltheart, M. (1978). Lexical access in simple reading tasks. In G. Underwood (Ed.), Strategies of Information Processing. London: Academic Press.

Coltheart, M., Patterson, K. & Marshall, J. C. (Eds.). (1980). Deep Dyslexia. London: Routledge and Kegan Paul.

Coltheart, M. (1985). Cognitive Neuropsychology and the study of reading. In M. I. Posner & O. S. M. Marin (Eds.), Attention and Performance. (Vol. 11). Hillsdale, NJ: Erlbaum.

Funnell, E. (1983). Phonological processes in reading: New evidence from acquired dyslexia. British Journal of Psychology, 74, 159-180.

Gordon, B., Goodman-Schulman, R. & Caramazza, A. (1987). Separating the stages of reading errors. Reports of the Cognitive Neuropsychology Laboratory. The Johns Hopkins University, Baltimore, MD 21218.

Hillis, A. & Caramazza, A. (in press). The Reading Process and Its Disorders. In D. Margolin (Ed.). Cognitive Neuropsychology In Clinical Practice. New York, NY: Oxford University Press.

Job, R. & Sartori, G. (1984). Morphological decomposition: Evidence from crossed phonological dyslexia. Quarterly Journal of Experimental Psychology, 36A, 435-458.

Laudanna, A., Badecker, W. & Caramazza, A. (1989). Priming homographic stems. Journal of Memory & Language, 28, 531-646.

Marshall, J. C. & Newcombe, F. (1973). Patterns of paralexia: A pyscholinguistic approach. Journal of Psycholinguistic Research, 2, 175-199.

Miceli, G. & Caramazza, A. (1988). Dissociation of inflectional and derivational morphology. Brain & Language, 35, 24-65.

Miceli, G. & Caramazza, A. (1990). The assignment of word stress: Evidence from as case of acquired dyslexia. Unpublished manuscript, The Johns Hopkins University, Baltimore, MD.

Patterson, K. E. (1982). The relation between reading and psychological coding: Further neuropsychological observations. In A. W. Ellis (Ed.), Normality and pathology in cognitive functions. London: Academic Press.

Patterson, K. E., Marshall, J. C. & Coltheart, M. (Eds.). (1985). Surface dyslexia. London: Lawrence Erlbaum Associates.

Patterson, K. E. & Kay, J. (1982). Letter-by-letter reading: Psychological descriptions of a neurological syndrome. Quarterly Journal of Experimental Psychology, 34A, 411-442.

Patterson, K. E. & Morton, J. (1985). From orthography to phonology: An attempt at an old interpretation. In K. E. Patterson, J. C. Marshall & M. Coltheart (Eds), Surface dyslexia: Neuropsychological and cognitive studies of phonological reading. London: Lawrence Erlbaum Associates Ltd.

Saffran, E. M. (1985). Lexicalisation and reading performance in surface dyslexia. In K. E. Patterson, M. Coltheart & J. C. Marshall (Eds.), Surface dyslexia. London: Lawrence Erlbaum Associates.

Shallice, T. & McCarthy, R. (1985). Phonological reading: From patterns of impairment to possible procedures. In K. E. Patterson, M. Coltheart & J. C. Marshall (Eds.), Surface dyslexia. London: Lawrence Erlbaum Associates.

Shallice, T. & Warrington, E. K. (1977). The possible role of selective attention in acquired dyslexia. Neuropsychologia, 15, 31-41.

Warrington, E. K. (1975). The selective impairment of semantic memory. Quarterly Journal of Experimental Psychology, 27, 635-657.

Warrington, E. K. & McCarthy, R. (1983). Category specific access dysphasia. Brain, 106, 859-878.

Warrington, E. K. & Shallice, T. (1979). Semantic access dyslexia. Brain, 102, 43-63.

CHAPTER TWO

READING MECHANISMS AND THE ORGANISATION
OF THE LEXICON
EVIDENCE FROM ACQUIRED DYSLEXIA

INTRODUCTION

The study of patients with acquired reading disorders has contributed significantly to the formulation and development of models of the normal reading process (e.g., Coltheart, 1981; Patterson, 1981; Saffran, in press; Shallice, 1981; Martin & Caramazza, in press). Various forms of acquired dyslexia have been described providing a rich source of constraints on the structure and organisation of the lexicon and of the cognitive mechanisms implicated in the reading process. The explanation within a single, coherent framework of such diverse symptoms as the production of semantic (e.g., reading "table" as "chair") or morphological (e.g., reading "walked" as "walking") paralexias or the ability to read some types of words (e.g., nouns or regularly spelled words) but not other types (e.g., function words or irregularly spelled words), and so forth, severely reduces our options in formulating a model of normal reading which when appropriately lesioned produces the various symptoms and symptom complexes observed.

A reading impairment that has played an important role in recent discussions of models of reading is phonological dyslexia. The major characteristic of this disorder is a severe limitation in the ability to read nonwords relative to the ability to read all types of words (Beauvois & Dérouesné, 1979; Shallice & Warrington, 1980; Patterson, 1982). The marked dissociation between word and nonword reading ability in this patient type has led some investigators to consider this form of dyslexia a single-component deficit disorder. That is, in contrast to deep dyslexia (Marshall & Newcombe, 1973), which is now widely considered to be a multi-component deficit disorder involving impairments to several processing components (Shallice & Warrington, 1980; Morton & Patterson, 1980; Nolan & Caramazza, 1982), phonological dyslexia has been considered to represent a disorder arising from a disruption to a single component of processing. A characterisation of this processing component will contribute to our understanding of phonological dyslexia as well as to our understanding of the structure of the normal reading process. To this end, an important step is to identify clearly the nature of the disorder. Specifically, it is important to determine whether the ability to read words dissociates completely from the ability to read nonwords.

While the original well-documented cases of phonological dyslexia (cases RG and AM by Beauvois & Dérouesné (1979) and Patterson (1982), respectively) did present with a marked inability to read nonwords relative to words, these cases also evidenced other reading difficulties. Both patients presented with two additional symptoms: morphological (derivational and inflectional) paralexias (e.g., *love* → "lover" and *love* → "loved," respectively) and errors in reading free-standing grammatical morphemes, often leading to so-called "functor substitutions" (e.g., *that* → "which"). It is a matter of considerable importance to determine whether these latter two symptoms necessarily co-occur with a deficit in reading nonwords. If the deficit in reading nonwords necessarily co-occurs with impairments in processing grammatical markers (both bound and free-standing), then the nature of the mechanism assumed to be disrupted must reflect this fact. In other words, the mechanism normally implicated in reading nonwords could also be implicated in the processing of grammatical markers. In contrast, if the nonword reading deficit dissociates from the grammatical marker processing deficit, we would ascribe the locus of impairment for these two deficits to different processing mechanisms (or different levels within a mechanism).

Since Beauvois & Dérouesné (1979) first presented a case (RG) of phonological dyslexia, several other cases have been described in sufficient detail to permit a consideration of whether the nonword reading deficit dissociates from the grammatical marker reading deficit. We have already mentioned case AM (Patterson, 1982) who, like RG, presented with difficulties in reading morphologically complex words and functors in addition to an inability to read nonwords. Several Italian cases of phonological dyslexia have been described. Two of these (case Leonardo: Job & Satori, 1982; and case AMM: DeBastiani, Barry, & Carreras, Note 1.) had considerable difficulties in processing grammatical markers in addition to severe problems in reading nonwords. One patient (Beatrice: Sartori, Barry, & Job, 1984) appears to have made disproportionately few morphological paralexic errors in relation to her difficulty in reading nonwords, but she did make a substantial number of function word substitution errors.

Another case that suggests the dissociability of nonword reading and grammatical marker processing difficulties is an English patient (WB) reported by Funnell (1983). WB presents with severe difficulties in reading nonwords but only a relatively mild difficulty in processing affixes and function words. Specifically, the patient's rate of function word substitutions and morphological paralexias was relatively low and comparable to other types of word reading errors (e.g., to the rate of semantic paralexias). Funnell interpreted this pattern of results as demonstration that the nonword reading deficit dissociates from the grammatical marker processing deficit. However, a more cautious conclusion may gave been appropriate since, although it was clear that the patient was unable to read nonwords (100% errors), he did make a not insignificant number of errors in word reading (15% overall), including a fair share of morphological paralexias and functor substitutions. The interpretation of a discrepancy in performance in reading words and nonwords must be made cautiously in languages like English because of the complexity of the relationship between orthography and sound. The complexity of this relationship appears to create difficulties in nonword reading even in neurologically unimpaired subjects (Martin, Caramazza, & Berndt, Note 3). and, thus, we must interpret with caution quantitative differences among individuals in word/nonword reading performance. Nonetheless, WB certainly represents the clearest demonstration to date that nonword reading may be disrupted selectively.

Several explanations have been offered for the patterns of reading difficulties in phonological dyslexics. A major difference among these explanations concerns whether a single- (e.g., Marcel, 1980) or a dual-route (e.g., Shallice, 1981) model of reading is assumed. Within the class of dual-route models the explanation of the phonological dyslexic's selective inability to read nonwords has been in terms of a disruption to a mechanism that converts graphemes or clusters of letters into phonological representations--a disruption to a non-lexical or phonological route. It is assumed that this patient type can read words because an independent mechanism normally used in retrieving a word's phonology through a lexical-orthographic address--the lexical route--is unimpaired (Beauvois & Dérouesné, 1979; Shallice & Warrington, 1980). Patterson (1982) extended this account to deal with the observed co-occurrence of morphological paralexias and function word reading errors with the nonword reading deficit. Patterson's proposal is based on a critical assumption: The phonological representation of affixes and functors cannot be retrieved directly through an orthographic address but must be assembled through the application of procedures in the non-lexical route.[1] With this assumption the disruption of the non-lexical route must result not only in the failure to read nonwords but also, *necessarily*, in the failure to read affixes and functors. In this way, Patterson was able to provide a unitary account for seemingly disparate symptoms considered to be necessarily a part of the phonological dyslexia syndrome.

Explanations based on a single-route model of reading have assumed that the nonword reading deficit reflects the disruption of a lexically-based, phonological assembly mechanism that is essential for nonword reading but which can be bypassed in word reading because the phonological representation for words can be addressed as a whole (e.g, DeBastiani, Barry, & Carreras, Note 1). DeBastiani et al.'s explanation for the co-occurrence of the nonword reading deficit with the grammatical marker processing deficit is based on the assumption that orthographic segmentation and phonological assembly for morphemically complex words and functors are disrupted. Presumably, then, the phonology of these words cannot be retrieved as a whole as is the case for other words.

The explanations that have been proposed to account for the cooccurrence of the nonword reading deficit and morphological paralexias and function word errors have made theoretically unmotivated assumptions. There is no independent motivation offered by Patterson in support of her claim that the phonology of function words and derivational and inflectional affixes cannot be addressed directly through an orthographic-lexical code; nor is there independent motivation offered by DeBastiani et al. for their claim that the phonology of function words and morphemically complex words cannot be addressed as a "whole" as is the case for other types of words.

Given the lack of a clearly motivated account for the constellation of symptoms in phonological dyslexia it seems more reasonable to assume that two distinct impairments are responsible for the co-occurrence of the symptoms that have been considered to constitute the syndrome: an impairment to a mechanism needed in reading nonwords and an impairment to a subcomponent of the lexicon needed in processing derivational morphology as well as bound and free-standing grammatical markers. There are clear theoretical and empirical consequences associated with this alternative conception of the cognitive basis for the type of phonological dyslexia discussed.

On the empirical side, this account leads to the prediction that the two symptoms should dissociate completely so that we should find patients who are impaired in reading nonwords but who have no difficulties in reading derivational and inflectional affixes and function words. Funnell's patient, WB, could be considered to be an example of such a dissociation. In this paper we describe two Italian dyslexic patients (AG and LB) who demonstrate a clear dissociation between the ability to read affixes and function words and nonwords, strongly supporting the dual-deficit hypothesis for the phonological dyslexia syndrome. On the theoretical side, the major consequence of hypothesising that the deficits in reading nonwords and in reading affixes and function words result from impairments to distinct cognitive mechanisms is the type of assumption we must make about the organization of the lexicon and the nature of the lexical access mechanisms compatible with the assumed structure of the lexicon. Specifically, since, by assumption, the ability to process affixes and function words is independent of the ability to process the root morphemes of words (and the ability to process nonwords), we must assume that there is a level within the lexical system in which the two types of information (root morphemes and affixes and function words) are represented independently. Furthermore, the assumption that the lexicon represents words in morphological decomposed form (root morphemes and affixes) requires that the lexical access mechanism be structured in a manner that is compatible with the assumed organisation of the lexicon. These issues are addressed in this paper through an analysis of the reading performance of two patients clinically classified as phonological dyslexics.

CASE 1

Case History

AG is a 43-year-old, right-handed missionary nun. As a child she was educated until the fifth grade. When she was 30, she went back to school and obtained a diploma as a kindergarten teacher. She was admitted to the Neuropsychology Service of the Catholic University in September 1981, two months after a cerebrovascular accident, sustained while she was in Africa. On admission, neurological examination failed to reveal motor weakness or sensory defect. Visual fields were full on confrontation as well as on campimetric and perimetric exam.

CT scan showed a low-density area, involving the middle and the posterior portions of the left middle temporal gyrus, and extending deeply into the white matter (Plate 1, p.61).

Neuropsychological Status Two Months Post-onset

Language Evaluation. Speech was fluent and well articulated, with occasional semantic paraphasias and anomias. Object naming was sometimes slow but accurate. A very mild colour anomia was also present. Repetition of words, nonwords, and sentences, including complex sentences (e.g., centre-embedded sentences) was error-free. Discrimination and labelling (mapping phonetic segments onto graphemic segments) of phonemes, discrimination among semantically related pictures and comprehension of semantically reversible (declarative and embedded) sentences, both in the active and the passive voice, were all within normal limits.

Neuropsychological Exam.   AG scored 27/36 on Raven's Coloured Progressive Matrices.   Memory for meaningless visual patterns and for pictured objects was normal.   Memory for unrelated lists of auditorily presented words was at the lower end of the normal range.   Digit span was five forward, three backward.   No apraxic signs, right-left disorientation, finger agnosia or disorders of the body schema were detected.   Visual-perceptual and visual-spatial abilities were spared.   Calculation was poor.   Astereognosis was absent, but a mild agraphesthesia in the right hand was discovered.   A mild agraphia was also present on writing to dictation, consisting of spelling errors on words (10/100) and nonwords (6/20).

At this stage, AG's reading showed features of both letter-by-letter reading and phonological dyslexia.   She read correctly 114/160 words (71.2%) but only 14/40 nonwords (35%).   Her reading was very slow and laborious.   The patient did not actually spell the stimuli aloud, but a clear-cut relationship between stimulus length and reading time was shown for both words and nonwords.   Thus, for example, average reading time for four-, six-,eight-letter stimuli were 2.0, 4.0 and 7.6 seconds, respectively. AG did not produce inflectional or derivational paralexias, nor functor substitutions.

Neuropsychological Status 18 Months Post-onset

AG was followed as an outpatient.   Her condition improved steadily.   Her reading abilities were tested extensively at 18 months post-onset.

At that time, no aphasic signs could be detected.   Her speech was fluent and she displayed a normal range of word choice and syntactic constructions.   AG scored 30/36 on Raven's Coloured Progressive Matrices.   Memory functions were normal.   The only remaining deficits were a mild acalculia and a mild agraphia (spelling errors on words, 6%, and nonwords, 8.5%).   AG's reading deficit is described below.   The tests used to assess her reading behaviour were constructed keeping in mind the clinical picture shown in the acute stage (i.e., letter-by-letter and phonological dyslexia.

EVALUATION OF READING ABILITIES 18 MONTH POST-ONSET

Reading Briefly Exposed Words and Nonwords

On hundred words and 100 nonwords randomly intermixed were presented tachistoscopically for 150msec followed immediately by a pattern mask. The patient was asked to read aloud the presented stimuli.

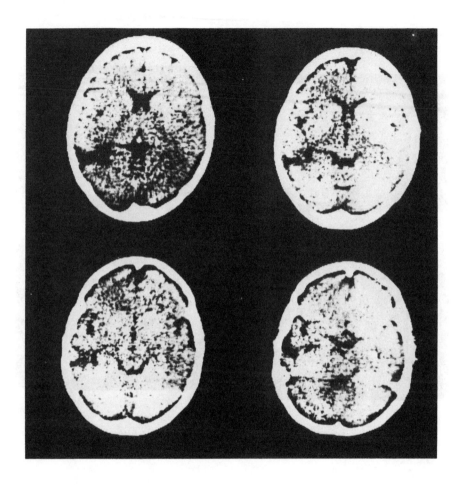

Plate 1. CT scan sections showing an area of hypodensity in the middle and posterior portions of the middle temporal gyrus, extending deeply into the white matter.

A. Caramazza

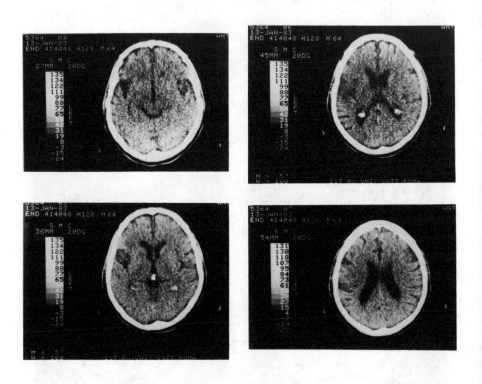

Plate 2. CT scan sections showing an area of low-density in the pre- and post-rolandic gyri, extending deeply in the white matter.

AG read correctly 90/100 words but only 30/100 nonwords. The difference between mean length of words read correctly (5.1 letters) andincorrectly (5.3) was not significant (*t*=1.06). By contrast, nonwords read correctly (4.7) and incorrectly (6.0) differed significantly (*t*=5.71; P<.001). The fact that AG was able to perform relatively well in reading words presented tachistoscopically (150msec) and the fact that no relationship was found either between word length and accuracy or between word length and reading time, argue against letter-by-letter reading being a relevant component of her dyslexia at this stage.

Reading Words and Nonwords

The patient was asked to read three different lists of words and nonwords on three separate occasions.

List 1. The first list consisted of 220 words and 30 nonwords. The stimulus features controlled in this list included: word class (nouns, verbs, adjectives, and function words), frequency, concreteness, and letter length. The nonwords varied in letter length.

AG was able to read all but one (0.4%) of the 220 words but made 10 errors (33%) in reading nonwords. Her responses were given promptly and no relationship was found between stimulus length and reading time. The single word reading error was her reading of *tavola* as "tavolo" (both correct forms of the Italian word for table). Two out of the 10 errors in reading nonwords resulted in words. All error responses were visually similar to the nonword stimulus and often retained the orthographic structure; that is, vowels were exchanged for vowels and consonants for consonants.

List 2. The second list consisted of 120 nouns and 120 nonwords randomly intermixed. Sixty nouns were of high frequency (occur more than 100 times per million in written language; Bortolini, Tagliavini, & Zampolli, 1979) and 60 of low frequency (<10 per million). Within each frequency range one-third of the stimuli were four or five letters long, one-third six or seven letters long, and the remaining third eight or nine letters long. The nonwords were matched to the words in length. These stimuli were constructed by changing one or two letters equally frequently at the beginning, middle, or end of a word.

AG read 118/120 words correctly (98.3%). Errors were produced for low frequency words. By contrast, she read correctly 85/120 nonwords (70.8%). The two errors on words and 29/35 errors on nonwords (82.9%) resulted in nonwords. Mean length of nonwords read correctly (6.5) and incorrectly (6.6) did not differ (*t*=0.56). All the error responses were visually similar to stimulus items, often preserving the orthographic structure of the stimulus.

List 3. This list consisted of 120 words and 120 nonwords randomly intermixed. Sixty words were verbs (20 high-frequency forms of verbs of high-frequency root, 20 low-frequency forms of verbs of high-frequency root, and 20 low-frequency forms of verbs of low-frequency root). Of the remaining 60 words, 27 were nouns, 21 were adjectives, 12 were functors, matched (with the exception of function words) to verb forms in frequency and length. The nonwords differed from words by one or two letters; some of the nonwords derived from verb forms preserved their suffixes.

AG gave prompt responses to all stimuli. She read correctly 115/120 words (95.8%), missing three low-frequency verbs (root) and two nouns, one in the high-and one in the low-frequency range. The errors were: *depurato* (cleaned) → "deputato" (deputy); *lasciato* (abandoned) → "laschiato" (nonword); *capello* (hair) → "cappello" (hat); lettere (letters) → "lettera" (letter); *decaduto* (decayed) → "depatuto" (nonword). It is clear that AG did not show any particular difficulty in reading multi-affixed (for mood, tense, and person) words such as verbs. The only error that could be construed as morphological was produced in response to a noun (*lettere* → "lettera"). However, considering that analogous errors were made on nonwords (e.g. *fievane* → "fievani"; *piccofe* → "piccovi"), we are inclined to consider this single error as a visual error.

Once again AG performed poorly in reading nonwords responding correctly only to 82/120 nonwords (68.3%). Only 4/38 errors on nonwords resulted in words. All errors were visually similar to the stimulus items.

AG's overall reading performance for the three word lists is summarised in Table 1.

Table 1. Summary of AG's reading of words and nonwords.

	Words			Nonwords		
	Correct	Incorrect	Total	Correct	Incorrect	Total
List 1	219	1	220	20	10	30
List 2	118	2	120	85	35	120
List 3	115	5	120	82	38	120
Total	452	8	460	187	83	270
%	98.3	1.7	100	69.3	30.7	100

She read correctly 98.3% of the words but only 69.3% of the nonwords presented. The few errors the patient made in reading words resulted equally frequently in nonwords and words (four of each). In contrast, errors in reading nonwords resulted almost always in nonwords (71 of 83 errors were nonwords, 85.5%). Finally, although ample opportunities were present for function word reading errors (52 function words were presented) and morphological paralexias (all Italian words except for function words and proper nouns are inflected), the patient's performance was strikingly free of such errors.

DISCUSSION

Two features of the performance of patient AG are of particular interest. The first is the striking dissociation between the ability to read words and nonwords. The patient was able to read essentially all words (98.3% correct), including morphologically complex verbs, but made a considerable number of errors in reading nonwords (69.3% correct) even though the orthography/phonology relationship in Italian is unambiguous. The second important feature concerns the type of errors the patient produced for nonword stimuli. Unlike previously reported cases of phonological dyslexia (e.g., DeBastiani et al., Note 1; Funnell, 1983; Patterson, 1982), our patient produced mostly nonword responses (86%) in reading nonwords. These results have important implications for models of reading and for the explication of the bases for different forms of reading impairments.

The clear dissociation between word/nonword reading abilities in our patient supports the thesis that different cognitive mechanisms are implicated in the reading of affixes and function words, on the one hand, and nonwords, on the other. Thus, cases RG (Beauvois & Dérouesné, 1979), AM (Patterson, 1982), and AMM (DeBastiani et al., Note 1.)-- patients who presented with marked deficits in reading both nonwords and affixes and function words--should be considered to have had impairments to two independent (and, hence, dissociable) cognitive mechanisms.[2] The implication of this conclusion is that there is a level of processing or mechanism that is specifically implicated in the processing of nonwords (Funnell, 1983).

The selective disruption of nonword reading finds a natural explanation within a dual-route model of reading. The nonword deficit is explained by assuming that there is a disruption to the mechanism that converts letters and letter clusters into phonological representations (e.g., Shallice, 1981). This mechanism can be disrupted to different extents leading to different forms of reading errors for nonwords. When the disruption of this mechanism is extensive relative to the disruption of the word reading mechanism, the patient will be forced to use the lexical route in reading nonwords--that is, the patient will use the orthographic structure of the stimulus to "guess" at a possible phonological form with the lexicon.[3] In this case the responses to nonword stimuli will be mostly words (or omissions) and the patient should manifest considerable uncertainty about his response (e.g., Funnell, 1983; Patterson, 1982). When the nonword reading mechanism is impaired only partially, nonwords can be read through this mechanism, leading to nonword errors which reflect the malfunctioning of the orthography to sound conversion process. Our patient AG falls into this latter category.

On this account, the co-occurrence of morphological and function word reading errors in the presence of nonword reading difficulties reflects the additional disruption to a subcomponent of the lexicon. The selective difficulty with a subset of the lexicon reveals organisational properties of the lexicon and not characteristics of the nonword reading mechanism. In particular, it suggest an organisation of the lexicon that distinguishes between root morphemes, on the one hand, and derivational and inflectional affixes and function words, on the other. It must be emphasised that there is independent evidence in the literature on lexical processing in normal subjects (e.g., Murrell & Morton, 1974; Taft & Forster, 1975; Stanners, Neirser, Hernon & Hall, 1979; Kempley & Morton, 1982) and aphasic subjects (e.g., agrammatism; see Caramazza & Berndt, 1985, for discussion) for the view that lexical entries are represented in morphologically decomposed form.

Even though the selective disruption of nonword reading is given a straightforward explanation within a dual-route model of reading, this result is not incompatible with single-route models of reading. Single-route models of reading explain the nonword reading deficit by assuming that the mechanism that assembles *lexically activated* phonological segments, corresponding to variously sized orthographic segments of nonwords, is disrupted (e.g., Marcel, 1980; DeBastiani et al., Note 1). In addition, to explain the selective (only nonwords) nature of the deficit, the assumption must be made that the phonology of a word can be addressed as a whole and that this process is unimpaired in phonological dyslexics. The selective difficulty in reading function words and affixes in some phonological dyslexics can be explained by assuming that these patients have, additionally, a disruption to a subcomponent of the lexicon (either in terms of a storage or retrieval deficit).

While it is clear that both the single-and dual-route models of reading can be elaborated to account for the patterns of performance in different forms of phonological dyslexia, it is less clear whether the two models truly constitute alternative accounts when elaborated in the manner we have here. To be sure, the dual-route model distinguishes between two distinct mechanisms in the processing of words and nonwords while the single-route model distinguishes between word and nonword processing only in the level of processing that these two types of stimuli receive within the same mechanism--the phonology of a word can be addressed as a whole while the phonology of a nonword *must* be assembled from lexically activated phonological segments. The critical point, however, is that both models distinguish between a phonological assembly process for nonwords and a whole word phonology activation process for words. The difference between the two models is reduced, then, to the mechanism by which nonwords are processed. In one case, the single-route model, nonwords are read by assembling a set of lexically based phonological segments while in the other, the dual-route model, the phonological segments assembled are not lexically derived but are computed through the application of a set of rules for conversion of letters and letter clusters to phonological segments. While this difference may be far from theoretically unimportant when fully articulated, it is at the present time of little empirical consequence in the analysis of reading disorders. Because of this we will not pursue this issue any longer here and focus instead on the potentially more productive issue of the implications for the reading process of assuming that words are represented in the lexicon in morphologically decomposed form. Specifically, we will focus on the question of how morphologically complex forms are processed in reading.

The issue of particular interest here is whether morphologically decomposed lexical forms are addressed or computed (Taft & Forster, 1975; Kempley & Morton, 1982; Manelis & Tharp, 1977); that is, whether the morphemes in a word (e.g., *walk-* and *ed*) are derived subsequent to access of the whole word address (e.g. *walked*) or whether the morphemes are computed independently in the process of lexical access of a word.

The proposition that the lexicon must represent the morphological structure of words can be motivated on both logical and empirical grounds. Speakers of a language make productive use of the morphological properties of their language; that is, they produce "novel" words by the correct application of morphological principles to known root morphemes. Furthermore, empirical results obtained with various experimental paradigms in word perception (e.g., Murrell & Morton, 1974; Stanners et al., 1979) and word production (e.g., MacKay, 1978) tasks as well as evidence from different patterns of language breakdown (e.g., Patterson, 1982; Caramazza & Berndt, 1985) has confirmed the need to assume that words are represented in the lexicon in morphologically decomposed form (but, see Butterworth, 1983, for a dissenting view). More problematical is the issue of the level at which morphological information is represented

A. Caramazza

in the lexicon and the mechanism by which lexical representations are accessed by a whole word address.

The primary source of evidence for the Morphological Parsing Model is a set of results which show that lexical decision times are affected by the morphological structure of the stimuli. For example, pseudo-root nonwords (e.g., *nings* in *innings*) are easier to reject than real root nonwords (e.g., *sults* in *insults*) and pseudo-prefixed nonwords composed of prefix+root morpheme (e.g., *dejuvenate* from *rejuvenate*) are rejected more slowly than pseudo-prefixed nonword composed of prefix+pseudo-root morpheme (e.g., *deligion* from *religion*) (Taft & Forster, 1975). Results of this type have been interpreted to favour a model of lexical access in which, first, a word input is stripped of its affix(es) (prefixes and suffixes) and, then, the remaining root morpheme is used to address a lexical entry. Since the Morphological Parsing Model assumes that lexical representations are accessed through root morphemes, an expectation derived from this model is that root morpheme nonwords (*sults*) and prefixed nonwords composed of prefix+root morpheme (*dejuvenate*) should be rejected as words more slowly than nonwords that do not constitute or contain a real root morpheme (*nings* and *deligion*)[4]-- just the result reported by Taft and Forster. The validity of these results has not gone unchallenged, in particular those concerning the decision times for root morpheme and pseudo-root morpheme nonwords.

Manelis and Tharp (1977) have noted that while Taft and Forster chose root morphemes and pseudo-root morphemes from words equated for frequency, the frequency considered was that for single words from which the root morphemes and pseudo-root morphemes were derived (e.g., *insults* and *innings*, respectively). However, there is evidence that lexical decision times are affected not only by the frequency of individual words but also by the overall frequency of morphologically related sets of words, e.g., *insults, results, consults* (Taft, 1979). When the frequency of the root morpheme and pseudo-root morpheme nonwords used by Taft and Forster (1975) are computed, including all morphologically related words, the frequency for the two sets of stimuli are no longer equal; the mean frequency for root morpheme nonwords was 84 and for pseudo-root morpheme nonwords was 14. It is possible, therefore, that the difference in reaction time between root morpheme and pseudo-root morpheme nonwords may reflect no more than a difference in frequency (Manelis & Tharp, 1977).

The logic used to motivate expectations about lexical decision times for root morpheme and pseudo-root morpheme nonwords from the Morphological Parsing Model also allows predictions concerning lexical decision times for affixed and pseudo-affixed words; and, here, the bulk of the empirical evidence is incompatible with this model of lexical access. Specifically, the model predicts that, everything else being equal, the time to decide that a pseudo-affixed word (e.g., *religion*) is a word should be longer than that for an affixed word (e.g., *rejuvenate*). This expectation is based on the assumption that there is a cost associated with the process of parsing a word into a prefix+pseudo-root and the consequent failure to find an address in the lexicon for the pseudo-root. The prediction derived from the Morphological Parsing Model for affixed and pseudo-affixed words has not been confirmed: lexical decision times do not differ for affixed and pseudo-affixed words (e.g., Manelis & Tharp, 1977; Rubin, Becker, & Freeman, 1979; Henderson, Wallis, & Knight, 1984; but, see Taft, 1979). On the whole, then, the Morphological Parsing Model of lexical access can hardly be considered to have met with overwhelming empirical support.

The Addressed Morphology Model assumes that lexical entries are accessed through whole word addresses and further that the accessed lexical representations consist of morphologically decomposed forms. Models of this type make a distinction between the address system which consists of whole word "addresses" and lexical representations which represent root morphemes independently of affixal elements.

This model accounts naturally for the lack of difference in lexical decision times for affixed and pseudo-affixed words (e.g., Henderson et al., 1984). The model is much too underspecified, however, with respect to the way in which new words, morphologically related to known words, are recognised or the way in which nonwords are rejected. Indeed, an empirical issue that must be confronted by models that postulate a whole word address system is Taft and Forster's (1975) finding that, in a lexical decision task, pseudo-prefixed nonwords composed of prefix+root morpheme are rejected more slowly than pseudo-prefixed nonwords composed of prefix+pseudo-root morpheme. This result has been extended to pseudo-suffixed nonwords (Laudanna & Caramazza, Note 2.). Elaborating the model in order to deal with these latter two issue leads to an interesting conclusion; namely, that in addition to a whole word address system we must postulate an independent morphological parsing procedure. In turn, the postulation of an independent parsing procedure logically implies the assumption that root morphemes and affixes are represented as independent addresses in the lexical address system. Thus to be able to recognise new words that are morphologically related to known words (e.g., *walking* from *walked*) the lexical processing system must be able to parse *walking* into walk+ing and, therefore, must include addresses for *walk* and *-ing* (where "-" indicates that *ing* is a bound morpheme and can only be accessed by a graphemic representation that

A. Caramazza

satisfies the condition of being bound to a root)[5] in order to access their respective representations in the lexicon.

By augmenting the Addressed Morphology Model to include an independent morphological parsing procedure the model can account for the observed effects in lexical decisions with pseudo-affixed nonwords. Specifically, the explanation given within this model for the reported effect with pseudo-affixed nonwords (Taft & Forster, 1975; Laudanna & Caramazza, Note 2.) is of the same type as that already discussed for the Morphological Parsing Model--the nonword is parsed morphologically and lexical decisions are slowed for nonwords composed of prefix+root morpheme or root morpheme+suffix because both the affix and root morpheme activate entries in the address system and can only be rejected as nonwords at the level of lexical representation, a level later in the course of lexical processing than the point at which pseudo-affixed nonwords composed of prefix+pseudo-root morpheme or pseudo-root morpheme+suffix would be rejected as nonwords.

The two major components of the proposed Addressed Morphology Model are the Lexical Address Procedure and the Orthographic Input Lexicon. The Orthographic Input Lexicon is the repository of the lexical information concerning the orthographic structure of words. This information is represented in morphologically decomposed form; in other words, root morphemes are represented independently of affixal elements. However, root morpheme representations include specifications for the permissible affixations that each root may undergo. Thus, for example, the lexical entry for walk (V=verb) would specify permissible affixations with *-ed, -s, -ing,* and *-er.*

The other major component of the Addressed Morphology Model is the Lexical Address Procedure. This component of the system consists of two independent procedures operating in parallel. One procedure operates directly on whole word inputs in a passive, logogen-like, activation fashion (e.g., Morton, 1979; Gordon, 1983). The activated whole word address specifies a morphologically decomposed, root morpheme+affix representation in the Orthographic Input Lexicon. The other part in this system is the morphological parsing procedure which operates in parallel with the whole word address procedure and functions, also, along the principle of passive activation. That is, orthographically "regular" affixed words (e.g., *walked → walk+ed,* but not *took → take+ed*) activate the morphemic elements that comprise it (*walk* and *-ed* in this example). We assume, however, that because the morphological parsing procedure is a complex process relative to the whole word address procedure, it is a relatively slow process. Consequently, the effects of the morphological parsing procedure are unlikely to be revealed in lexical access of words in normal circumstances since the lexical representation of a word would be addressed quickly and efficiently through the whole word address procedure. Hence, the lack of an effect in a comparison of lexical decision times for pseudo-suffixed words like *sister* and suffixed words like *maker* (Rubin et al., 1979).

The lexical access procedure described constitutes only one part of the input process of the reading system. The other part, as noted already, is the nonlexical system which consists of a procedure for converting submorphemic graphemic clusters into phonological segments. A complete model of reading will also have to include a lexical-semantic component and an output component. We assume that the output component has a parallel structure to the input component; that is, the Phonological Output Lexicon represents lexical entries in morphologically decomposed form which in turn can activate "preassembled" whole word phonological forms. A schematic representation, intended as a graphic summary of the proposed model, is presented in Figure 1 (p.72).

The model of lexical access and reading we have presented is anything but parsimonious in terms of the types of processes it assumes. However, the complex architecture of the proposed system may be unavoidable; certainly, the available data cannot be reconciled either with a simple Morphological Parsing Model or with the exclusively whole word form of the Addressed Morphology Model. More direct evidence in favour of the proposed model can be adduced by considering in detail the reading performance of dyslexic patients who present with a selective disruption of the nonword reading mechanism.

Consider what could happen when a patient of this type is asked to read an "Italian" nonword such as *chiediva*, which contains the root morpheme *chied-* (to ask) and the inappropriate but legal suffix *-iva* (an example in English might be *walken* from *walk*), versus a nonword such as *chiadova* (an English example: *wolkon*) which does not contain a real word root morpheme or legal affix (actually, the string can be parsed into *chiadov-* and *-a* but *chiadov-* is not a root morpheme in Italian). If morphologically decomposed forms are accessed only through whole word addresses (the exclusively whole word form of the Addressed Morphology Model) the patient should perform equally poorly on the two types of nonwords since in neither case is there a lexical address for the stimulus. Both types of nonwords must be processed through the nonword reading mechanism which is impaired in these patients and, thus, should lead to an equal number and type of reading errors in the two cases. If, instead, morphologically decomposed forms are only and always computed (the Morphological Parsing Model) the mechanism that carries out this process (if unimpaired) should be able to parse successfully the morphologically

A. Caramazza

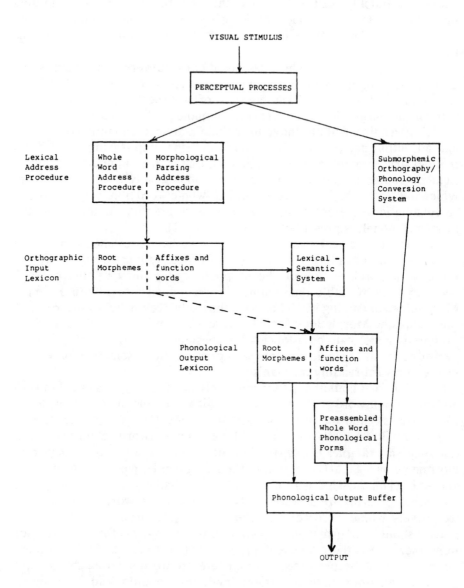

Figure 1. Schematic representation of Addressed Morphology Model of reading.

"legal" (e.g., *chiediva*) but not "illegal" (e.g., *chiadova*) letter strings.[6] In such a case we expect the patient to perform better in reading morphologically "legal" than morphologically "illegal" nonwords since the former allow access to lexically based phonological representations (e.g., *chied-* and *-iva*) that are unimpaired in these patients. However, in this case we also expect that there should be no difference in reading performance between words and morphologically "legal" nonwords since in both cases a successful parsing of the letter string is possible.

Finally, consider the expectations derived from the proposed Addressed Morphology Model. Because of the availability of a whole word address procedure in the Lexical Access System we expect this type of patient to read words better than any type of nonword including morphologically "legal" nonwords (see the Discussion section). Furthermore, since the Access System also allows entries in the Orthographic Input Lexicon to be addressed through a morphological parsing procedure, we expect that the patient should read morphologically "legal" nonwords better than morphologically "illegal" nonwords.

We address the issue of the morphological organisation of the lexicon and the reading mechanisms compatible with this form of lexical organisation through the analysis of the reading performance of another case of selective disruption of the nonword reading process.

CASE 2

Case History

LB is a 65-year-old, right-handed male. He has university degrees in engineering and in mathematics and is a top-ranking officer in the Italian Air Force. Six months prior to his retirement, he had a CVA in the left hemisphere and was admitted to the Neuropsychology Service of the Catholic University in Rome. In the acute phase, he showed very frequent anomic pauses in spontaneous speech, with occasional phonemic and semantic paraphasias. Repetition of words was almost normal; repetition of nonwords was impaired. Repetition of sentences was mildly impaired. On the receptive side, discrimination and labelling of phonemes, comprehension of isolated words presented auditorily or visually, and auditory comprehension of reversible sentences were poor. LB gave 19/36 correct responses to the shortened version of the Token Test. Memory for word lists was very poor: digit span was five forward, three backward. He scored 21/36 on Raven's Coloured Progressive Matrices. He also presented with a severe dyslexia of the phonological type, and with a severe dysgraphia, with production of neologisms. A mild buccofacial apraxia was present, but disturbances of limb praxis were not detected. Visual-spatial and visual-perceptual abilities were speared. Constructional praxis was preserved.

The present study was conducted eight months post-onset. At that times, aphasic signs had essentially disappeared. Spontaneous speech was occasionally hesitant, but free from phonemic and semantic paraphasias. Repetition of words, nonwords and sentences was normal. Receptive abilities were normal at the phonemic, semantic and syntactic levels. LB obtained normal scores on the shortened Token Test (30/36 correct) and on Raven's Progressive Matrices (31/36). Digit span was seven forward and four backward. Memory of word lists was at the lower normal level. A marked dysgraphia (although improved with respect to the acute stage) was still present, consisting of spelling errors on words (33.3%) and nonwords (66.7%). The analysis of LB's reading performance is reported below. A CT scan revealed a hypodense area in the pre-and post-rolandic gyri in the left hemisphere, also extending deeply in the white matter (Plate 2, p.62).

EVALUATION OF READING ABILITIES

Screening Test

The patient was given a preliminary evaluation of his reading ability by means of a screening test. The test included 108 words and 108 nonwords. Words were matched on the following variables: part of speech (nouns, adjectives, verbs, functors), abstractness/concreteness, frequency, and letter length. Nonwords were divided into three subsets of 36 nonwords each, according to N-count (that is, the total number of words that can be derived from each nonword by changing one letter). The first subset consisted of nonwords with a low N-count (N=0=1), the second, of nonwords with a medium N-count (N=2-4), the last of nonwords with a high N-count (N=5-7). Word and nonword stimuli were presented in random order.

LB read all words promptly and correctly, but made 31/108 (28.7%) errors on nonwords (see Table 2). N-count did not exert a major effect on the number of errors (low N-count=13 errors; medium and high N-count=9 errors each). Ten errors (32.3%) on nonwords resulted in words, 21 (67.7%) in nonwords. N-count was not a relevant factor in causing word vs. nonword responses (four word responses to low N-count nonwords, one to medium N-count nonwords, five to high N-count nonwords). Twenty-one of the 31 errors bore a very close visual resemblance to the stimulus, consisting of substitutions, deletions or additions of single letters. The remaining errors were: two transpositions, five mixed, two unrelated productions, and one fragment.

It is clear from the results obtained on the Screening Test that LB, like AG, can read words of all form classes, including affixed words and functors without difficulty. By contrast, he has a marked deficit in reading nonwords. Further exploration of his reading disturbance focused on the processing of morphologically decomposable nonwords.

Reading Morphologically "Legal" and Morphologically "Illegal" Nonwords

We have proposed that if morphemes in the lexicon are accessed directly through a whole word address (i.e., not parsed morphologically), no difference should be found between reading performance of morphologically "legal" and morphologically "illegal" nonwords: LB should read both poorly, since no lexical address is available for either type of nonword. If, on the contrary, morphemes can be addressed through a parsing process, performance in reading morphologically "legal" nonwords should differ from that of morphologically "illegal" nonwords, as the two types of nonwords would be read through different mechanisms. Morphologically "legal" nonwords would be processed by a parsing mechanism that can identify orthographic segments corresponding to morphemes; morphologically "illegal" nonwords (that do not contain an orthographic segment that can be parsed as a real root) would be read by activation of the nonword reading mechanism that mediates conversion of print into sound. To explore the two alternative hypotheses, another reading test was devised.

Materials

The reading test consisted of 280 words and of 280 nonwords, presented in random order. Half of the words were verbs, half belonged to other word classes and were matched in frequency to the verbs. The 280 nonwords consisted of the following three sets:

Set A consisted of 100 morphologically "legal" nonwords. Eighty nonwords were constructed by coupling a real verb root with a verb inflection that, although appropriate for other verbs, was not permissible for that particular root, and 20 by coupling a real root with a letter string that was only visually similar to a real verb suffix. An example of the first type of nonword in Set A is *chiediva,* where *chied-* is the root of the verb *chiedere* (to ask), and *-iva* is a real verb suffix that is not permissible with *chied-*. An example of the second type of nonword in this set is *chiedova,* where *chied-* is a real verb root, but *-ova* is not a real verb suffix. (Although performance on these two types of stimuli did not differ appreciably, we will consider the difference between the two types of stimuli in our discussion of the patient's reading performance.)

Set B included 100 morphologically "illegal" nonwords. They consisted of letter strings visually similar to verb roots, coupled either with a string of letters visually similar to verb suffixed (n-80), or with verb suffixes (n=20). Thus, an example of a nonword of the first type in this set is *chiadova*, where *chiad-* and *-ova* are visually very similar to a real verb root and real verb suffix, respectively (*chied-* and *-eva*). An example of the second type of nonword in this set is *chiadiva*, where a letter string visually similar to a verb root (*chiad-*) is coupled with a verb suffix (*-iva*). (Again, no appreciable difference in reading performance was noted for the two types of stimuli but we will distinguish these two types of stimuli in discussing LB's reading performance.) Thus, stimuli in both Sets A and B are orthographically very similar to real verb forms (compare *chiedeva* (real verb, "s/he was asking") with *chiediva*, *chiedova*, and *chiadiva*, *chiadova*). However, while all stimuli in Set A could be parsed into a real verb root+real suffix/pseudo-suffix, none of the stimuli in Set B contained a real root.

Set C included 80 other nonwords not matched to verbs in orthographic structure.

Nonwords in Sets A and B were matched in letter length and N-count. They were also matched in letter length to the verb forms included in the word list. Nonwords in list C were exactly matched in letter length to the words in the word list that were not verbs. Although nonwords in Sets A and B were not exactly matched in N-count with nonwords in Set C, the difference was minimal (mean N-count: Sets A+B=.85, Set C=.80).

Results

The complete corpus of LB's errors is reported in the Appendix.

LB read correctly 272/280 (97.1%) words (see Table 2). He made 6/140 (4.3%) errors on verbs and 2/140 (1.4%) errors on other words--an adjective and a functor. His reading errors resulted in seven (88%) words and one (12%) nonword. All the errors were visually similar to the stimulus (e.g., *passavano* (they were passing) was read as "passavamo" (we were passing), *neppure* (not even) was read as "seppure" (even if), *corsero* (they ran) as "ossero" (nonword)).

By contrast, LB read correctly only 161/280 (57.7%) nonwords (see Table 3). He produced the correct response to 76/100 morphologically "legal" nonwords in Set A, to 51/100 morphologically "illegal" nonwords from Set B, and to 34/80 (42.5%) other nonwords from Set C. The difference between number of correct responses to morphologically "legal" and "illegal" nonwords is significant ($X^2=13.48$; $P<.001$). The difference between reading of morphologically "illegal" and of other nonwords is not significant ($X^2=1.29$; n.s.).

Table 2. Summary of LB's reading of words and nonwords.

	Words			Nonwords		
	Correct	Incorrect	Total	Correct	Incorrect	Total
List 1	108		108	77	31	108
%	100		100	71	29	100
List 2	272	8	280	161	119	280
%	97	3	100	58	42	100
Total	380	8	388	238	150	388
%	98	2	100	61.3	38.7	100

The results obtained on this reading test confirm that LB was able to read words of all grammatical classes almost perfectly, but has a selective difficulty reading nonwords. His reading of nonwords was even poorer on this test than on the screening test, but the most interesting result was the dissociation between his performance on morphologically "legal" and morphologically "illegal" nonwords. LB read nonwords that could be parsed into a root plus suffix or pseudo-suffix (Set A) significantly better than nonwords which could not be parsed into a root plus suffix (Set B). This dissociation supports the view that morphologically decomposed forms can be computed rather than only accessed. It also suggests that LB's morphological parsing ability is spared, relative to his ability to convert print into sounds through a non-lexical mechanism.

Table 3. Summary of LB's reading of morphologically "legal," morphologically "illegal," and other nonwords.

	Correct	Incorrect	Total
Set A: Morphologically "legal"	76	24	100
Set B: Morphologically "illegal"	51	49	100
Set C: Other	34	46	80

A more detailed analysis of LB's reading performance that focuses on the distinction between pseudo-affixed nonwords composed either of root morpheme+pseudo-suffix (e.g., *chiedova*) or pseudo-root morpheme+

suffix (e.g., *chiadiva*) further elucidates the nature of the Lexical Address Procedure in reading. Although the relevant observations are based on a small number of words (N=20 for each of the two types of nonwords) the results are suggestive. LB read correctly 16/20 (80%) nonwords composed of root morpheme+pseudo-suffix but only 9/20 (45%) nonwords composed of pseudo-root morpheme+suffix: nonwords with real word roots were treated like morphologically "legal" nonwords while nonwords with pseudo-word roots were treated like morphologically "illegal" nonwords despite the fact that they contained a real suffix. This suggests that the presence of a legal affix in a nonword *is not a necessary* condition for implicating the Lexical Address Procedure in reading nonwords, but that the presence of a real root morpheme *is a necessary* condition for implicating this system in reading nonwords.

On the hypothesis that morphologically "legal" nonwords are read by means of a mechanism different from that used in reading morphologically "illegal" nonwords we might expect not only different rates of correct performance but also different types of errors in reading the two types of nonwords.

Reading errors produced by LB when reading nonwords from Sets A, B, and C were analysed for visual similarity to the stimulus nonword. Errors were divided into two broad categories. "Simple" errors were considered to be those involving substitution, insertion, or deletion of only one letter in the stimulus: "complex" errors included all other responses involving more complex changes of the structure of the stimulus (i.e., transposition of two or more letters; multiple substitutions and/or insertions and/or deletions and/or transpositions of letters; unrelated productions; fragments). The incidence of "simple" vs. "complex" errors in the responses given to morphologically "legal" and morphologically "illegal" nonwords is shown in Table 4. "Simple" errors were produced significantly more often in response to morphologically "legal" nonwords than in response to morphologically "illegal" nonwords (X^2=9.52; P<.01). No difference was found in the comparison between morphologically "illegal" and other nonwords (X^2=.23; n.s.).

These results support the hypothesis that different mechanisms are implicated in reading morphologically "legal" and "illegal" nonwords. However, a more precise prediction can be made regarding the types of errors produced in reading the two types of nonwords under consideration. Specifically, since on our account reading morphologically "legal" nonwords implicates access of lexical (morpheme) representations, errors in this process should lead to a proportionately high rate of morphologically "legal" responses, some of which could be word responses --errors within this system should involve lexical units (morphemes)

Table 4. LB's reading errors on nonwords: Degree of similarity between stimulus and response for errors produced when attempting to read morphologically "legal," morphologically "illegal" and other nonwords.

		Simple[a]	Complex[b]	Total
Set A:	Morphologically "legal"	19(79.2%)	5(20.8%)	24(100%)
Set B:	Morphologically "illegal"	20(40.8%)	29(59.2%)	49(100%)
Set C:	Other	21(45.7%)	25(54.3%)	46(100%)

[a] Errors involving substitution, insertion or deletion of a single letter in the stimulus

[b] Errors involving transposition of two or more letters; multiple substitutions and/or deletions and/or insertions; unrelated; fragments.

resulting in incorrect morphologically "legal" nonword and word responses. By contrast, since reading morphologically "illegal" nonwords does not involve the lexical system but a non-lexical process, errors in this process should result in a relatively low rate of morphologically "legal" nonword and word responses. This latter prediction was tested by analysing the number of morphologically "legal" and "illegal" nonword errors and the number of word and nonword errors made by LB when reading morphologically "legal," "illegal" and other nonwords. The results are striking: LB produced 79%, 24%, and 4% morphologically "legal" (word and nonword) responses to morphologically "legal," morphologically "illegal" and other nonwords, respectively. Table 5 shows the number of incorrect words and nonwords produced by LB in response to morphologically "legal," morphologically "illegal" and other nonwords.

Table 5. LB's errors on reading nonwords: Incorrect word and nonword responses to morphologically "legal," morphologically "illegal" and other nonwords.

		Word Responses	Nonword Responses	Total
Set A:	Morphologically "legal"	13(54.2%)	11(45.8%)	24(100%)
Set B:	Morphologically "illegal"	8(16.3%)	41(83.7%)	49(100%)
Set C:	Other	2 (4.4%)	44(95.6%)	46(100%)

The patient produced 13 word responses out of 24 errors (54.2%) to nonwords from Set A, but only 8 word responses out of 49 errors (16.3%) to nonwords from Set B. Even fewer incorrect word responses were produced after attempts at reading other nonwords (2 word responses out of 44 errors--4.3%). The difference between incidence of incorrect word vs. nonword responses to morphologically "legal" as opposed to morphologically "illegal" nonwords is significant (X^2=11.26; P<.001). The difference between morphologically "illegal" and other nonwords is not significant (X^2=3.61; n.s.).

Discussion

The results we have reported for LB are as striking as those reported for patient AG in terms of the highly selective nature of the reading deficit: LB was able to read essentially all words (98% correct) but presented with a marked impairment in reading nonwords (70% correct). This pattern of performance confirms the dissociability of nonword and word reading mechanisms already documented for patient AG. In particular, the results show that the co-occurrence of difficulties in reading affixes and function words in conjunction with difficulties in reading nonwords is not cognitively necessary (see also Funnell, 1983) but most likely reflects accidental properties of the neuroanatomical distribution of psychologically distinct mechanisms (i.e., independent cognitive mechanisms that implicate adjacent neuroanatomical structures).

The other major issue addressed in our analysis of the reading performance of case LB concerned the nature of morphological processing. The results we have reported strongly confirm the thesis that the lexicon represents words in morphologically decomposed form and that we must postulate the existence of a mechanism that parses letter strings to recover the root form of words. The evidence in support of this contention is the fact that nonwords that could be parsed into a root morpheme plus suffix were read significantly better than nonwords that could not be parsed in this manner. Thus, LB was able to read 76% of the morphologically "legal" nonwords but only 51% of morphologically "illegal" nonwords.

The result is incompatible with the hypothesis that morphologically decomposed forms can be accessed *only* through a direct address system. That is, since neither the morphologically "legal" nor the "illegal" nonwords have lexical addresses, the "morphemes" that make up the morphologically "legal" nonwords should not be accessible through a direct address procedure. Consequently we would not expect better performance for the morphologically "legal" versus "illegal" nonwords. In contrast, if we assume that there is a mechanism devoted to parsing letter strings to recover morphemes, then morphologically decomposable nonwords should be privileged relative to morphologically "illegal" nonwords since these latter items can be processed only by assembling the phonology of non-morphological (and hence non-lexical) segments. This argument rests, of course, on the assumption that in our patient the mechanism for assembling non-lexical phonology is disrupted while the mechanism for assembling lexical phonology (roots and affixes) is spared.

Additional evidence for the interpretation we have presented comes from the analysis of LB's errors in reading nonwords (and words). If our argument about the manner in which morphologically "legal" nonwords are processed is correct, we would expect a significant proportion of the errors to be lexically based. Processing this type of nonword implicates the activation of lexical (morphemes) representations e.g., *chied-* and *-iva*) and their associated phonological forms which are subsequently assembled for output. Errors that occur *within* this system of processing will necessarily involve the misselection of morphological units, either root morphemes (e.g., *chied-* → *chiar-*) or affixes (e.g., *-iva* → *-ete*), since these are the units of analysis in this system. Errors in this system, then, should result in morphologically "legal" responses including words (e.g., *chiediva* → *chiedete; chiediva* → *chiariva*). By a similar logic, our expectation is that errors in reading words should result in a proportionately high rate of word errors.

In contrast, reading errors for morphologically "illegal" nonwords should not follow this pattern: Reading this type of nonword does not implicate the activation of morphemes but depends exclusively on the activation and assembly of sub-morphemic phonological segments. Errors in the functioning of the latter mechanism should not be biased in the direction of word responses. The results we have reported confirm these expectations. LB's few word reading errors almost always resulted in other words (7/8) and the proportion of word responses to morphologically "legal" nonwords was also quite high (54%). The proportion of word errors for morphologically "illegal" nonwords, on the other hand, was very low (16%).

While the results we have reported are generally in agreement with the postulation of a morphological parsing device, there remains the question of why LB makes any errors at all in reading morphologically "legal" nonwords. We have argued that these nonwords can be parsed and that appropriate morphemic representations can be activated in the lexicon. Why, then, should there be a difference in reading performance between these nonwords and words? Several possibilities come to mind. We will consider two.

One possibility is that the parsing device does not function perfectly normally in this patient. We could assume, then, that on those reading attempts in which the parsing process fails, the morphologically "legal" nonword is read through the nonword reading mechanism leading to errors. However, this hypothesis is not consistent with the pattern of error data reported for LB. On this account of the source of errors in reading "legal" nonwords, the pattern of errors for this type of stimulus should not be different from that obtained with the "illegal" nonwords since the same mechanism is responsible for errors in reading "legal" and "illegal" nonwords--a prediction disconfirmed by our results.

Another possibility is that the parsing device functions relatively normally but that there is an impairment in the assembly procedure for the activated morphological representations. This account is consistent with the reported error data but forces us to draw a distinction between the procedure for the "assembly" of morphemes of words and the assembly procedure for "morphemes" of nonwords. Drawing a distinction of this type is not unreasonable, however. Although words are represented in the lexicon in morphologically decomposed form, the lexicon must specify which combinations of roots and affixes are permissible (i.e., truly legal) in the language. In other words, the lexicon specifies, for example, that *chied-* plus *-eva* is a word but not *chied-* plus *-iva*. Furthermore, we can make the plausible assumption that the output procedure for *word* entries (e.g., *chiedeva*) may involve the activation of preassembled lexical forms in an output lexicon while a pseudolegal form (e.g., *chiediva*) will involve an assembly process similar to one used for any nonword: that is, by assembling phonological segments of different sizes--phonemes, syllables, and morphemes. A disruption of this nonlexical assembly process will result in errors reading morphologically "legal" nonwords.

This latter hypothesis allows an elegant explanation of the difference in the overall rate of errors and the rate of "simple" and "complex" errors for morphologically "legal" and "illegal" nonwords. Specifically, if we assume that the probability of an error in assembling phonological segments is independent of their size, the expectation is that more errors should be made in reading nonwords that involve assembling "many" phonological segments (morphologically "illegal" nonwords) than in reading nonwords that involve "few" phonological segments (morphologically "legal" nonwords). Furthermore, since, by assumption, reading morphologically "illegal" nonwords involves the assembly of "many," small phonological segments, independent errors on these segments will lead to "complex" errors relative to the process of reading "legal" nonwords which involves the assembly of "few," large phonological segments.

CONCLUSIONS

Taken together, the results we have reported for patients AG and LB allow us to draw firm conclusions about some aspects of the structure of the normal reading system and the nature of the mechanisms disrupted in the "phonological" dyslexics we have described as well as other cases in the literature.

One conclusion concerns the processes involved in nonword reading. The striking dissociation in our patients between their ability to read all types of words and their marked deficit in reading nonwords strongly suggests that different mechanisms are implicated in word and nonword reading. We assume that nonword reading involves a system of processing that converts letters and letter clusters into phonological segments and assembles these submorphemic segments for speech output. This system can be disrupted independently of the word reading system which involves the access of morphologically decomposed lexical representations (root+affix; e.g., *chied-* + *-ete*) and associated phonological forms.

Another conclusion strongly indicated by the contrast in reading performance of affixes and functors between our two patients (and Funnell's case WB) and patients RG (Beauvois & Dérouesné, 1979), AM (Patterson, 1982) and AMM (DeBastiani et al., Note 1.) concerns aspects of the representation and organisation of the lexicon. The fact that some patients (RG, AM, AMM) present with a selective difficulty in reading function words, affixes, and nonwords, and the fact that the nonword reading deficit can occur in complete isolation (AG, LB, and WB) suggest that the nonword reading process is not implicated in reading affixes and function words. More importantly, however, the dissociations described argue for an organisation of the lexicon along a morphological principle which distinguishes between root morphemes, on the one hand, and affixes and function words, on the other (Garrett, 1980; Caramazza & Berndt, 1985).

A third conclusion concerns the process by which lexical information is addressed. The analysis of LB's reading performance for morphologically "legal" and "illegal" nonwords suggests that morphemic representations in the lexicon can be addressed through the application of a parsing procedure to a written stimulus. Specifically, we have interpreted the fact that LB performed better in reading morphologically "legal" than "illegal" nonwords and that the reading errors for morphologically "legal" nonwords often resulted in words while those for morphologically "illegal" nonwords were predominantly nonwords, as evidence that the patient was able to address lexical information with the "legal" but not the "illegal" nonwords. Furthermore, since LB's reading performance was considerably better for nonwords composed of root morpheme+pseudo-suffix (e.g., *chiedova*) than for nonwords composed of pseudo-root morpheme+suffix (e.g., *chiediva*) (80% and 45% correct, respectively), it would appear that the presence of a real word root is a necessary condition for implicating the lexical system in reading a nonword. An implication of this latter conclusion is that the "lexical status" of root morphemes and affixes is not quite the same. This issue obviously needs further exploration at both the theoretical and empirical levels.

That we must postulate the existence of a morphological parsing device for unfamiliar letter strings should not be controversial. For, how else could we "know" that a first-time-seen inflected form of a known word is a word of the language? The compelling force ("compellingness") of this argument is easily appreciated, especially when considering richly inflected languages where there are statistically many more opportunities than in a language like English for encountering immediately recognisable, new, inflected forms of words of the language.[7] In such situations it must be the case that we recognise the root morpheme of the new word as a known morpheme and, furthermore, that we recognise the inflection of this word as an appropriate one for the identified root. This process clearly presupposes a parsing procedure that generates the correct segmentation of the presented word.

The postulation of the existence of a morphological parsing procedure does not necessarily imply that access of known words proceeds by means of an active, morphological parsing process. That is, it is not necessarily the case that to recognise the known letter string *chiedete* as a word involves parsing the string into *chied-* plus *-ete* in order to address the corresponding morphemes in the lexicon. Instead, we could assume that the functioning of the parsing procedure is only revealed when we encounter letter strings that do not have a whole word address in the Lexical Address System. Known words could be processed by activating a whole word entry in a logogen-like system (e.g., Morton, 1979; Gordon, 1983) which serves as an address to a morphologically decomposed lexicon that represents separately the root morpheme and affix of a word (Addressed Morphology Model): The logogen-like entry, corresponding to a whole word, in the Lexical Address System will access both the root morpheme and affix of the activated word entry.

In conclusion, the general architecture of the lexical processing system proposed distinguishes among three different procedures for processing letter strings. Known words are processed by activating entries in a logogen-like system which serve as addresses to morphologically decomposed representations in the lexicon. Letter strings that do not find an entry in the Word Recognition System may, if the parsing process is successful, permit access to morphemes in the lexicon. If the parsing process fails the only possibility for reading the presented letter string is through a processing procedure that converts sub-morphemic orthographic segments (letters and letter clusters) into phonological segments. Brain damage can disrupt each of the three systems independently. The two patients we have described represent the case of a selective disruption of the nonword reading process based on the conversion of sub-morphemic orthographic segments into phonological sequences.

ACKNOWLEDGEMENTS

The research reported in this paper was supported in part by a grant from the CNR (Italy) and by NIH grant NS14099 to The Johns Hopkins University. The authors thank Michael McCloskey, Howard Egeth, Max Coltheart, Bepi Sartori, Remo Job, Bobbi Goodman, and an anonymous reviewer for their very helpful comments on an earlier version of this paper. We also thank Kathy Sporney for patiently typing various versions of this paper.

REFERENCES

Beauvois, M. F. & Dérouesné, J. (1979). Phonological alexia: Three dissociations. Journal of Neurology, Neurosurgery & Psychiatry, 42, 1115-1124.

Bortolini, N., Tagliavini, C. & Zampolli, A. (1979). Lessico di frequenza della lingua Italiana contemporanea. Milano: Garzanti.

Butterworth, B. (1983). Lexical representation. In B. Butterworth (Ed.), Language production (Vol. 2). London: Academic Press.

Caramazza, A. & Berndt, R. S. (1985). A multi-component deficit view of agrammatic Broca's aphasia. In M.L. Kean (Ed.), Agrammatism, 27-63. New York, NY: Academic Press.

Coltheart, M. (1981). Disorders of reading and their implications for models of normal reading. Visible Language, 15, 245-286.

Funnell, E. (1983). Phonological processes in reading: New evidence from acquired dyslexia. British Journal of Psychology, 74, 159-180.

Garrett, M. F. (1980). Levels of processing in sentence production. In B. Butterworth (Ed.), Language Production. New York, NY: Academic Press.

Gordon, B. (1983). Lexical access and lexical decision: Mechanisms of frequency sensitivity. Journal of Verbal Learning and Verbal Behavior, 22, 146-160.

Henderson, L., Wallis, J. & Knight, D. (1984). Morphemic structure and lexical access. In H. Bouma & D. G. Bouwhuis (Eds.), Attention and Performance X: Control of Language Processes. Hillsdale, NJ: Lawrence Erlbaum Associates.

Job, R. & Sartori, G. (1982). Prelexical decomposition: Evidence from acquired dyslexia. British Journal of Psychology, 74, 159-180.

Kempley, S. T. & Morton, J. (1982). The effects of priming with regularly and irregularly related words in auditory word recognition. British Journal of Psychology, 73, 441-454.

MacKay, D. G. (1978). Derivational rules and the internal lexicon. Journal of Verbal Learning and Verbal Behaviour, 17, 61-71.

Manelis, L. & Tharp, D. A. (1977). The processing of affixed words. Memory & Cognition, 5, 690-695.

Marcel, T. (1980). Surface dyslexia and beginning reading: A revised hypothesis of the pronunciation of print and its impairments. In M. Coltheart, K. E. Patterson & J. C. Marshall (Eds.), Deep dyslexia. London: Routledge & Kegan Paul.

Marshall, J. C. & Newcombe, F. (1973). Patterns of paralexia: A psycholinguistic approach. Journal of Psycholinguistic Research, 2, 175-199.

Martin, R. & Caramazza, A. (1986). Theory and method in cognitive neuropsychology: The case of acquired dyslexia. In H. Julia Hannay (Ed.), Experimental Techniques in Human Neuropsychology, 363-385. New York, NY: Oxford University Press.

Morton, J. (1979). Word recognition. In J. Morton & J. Marshall (Eds.), Psycholinguistics 2: Structure and processes. Cambridge, MA: MIT Press.

Morton, J. & Patterson, K. E. (1980). A new attempt at an interpretation, or, an attempt at a new interpretation. In M. Coltheart, K. E. Patterson & J. C. Marshall (Eds.), Deep dyslexia. London: Routledge & Kegan Paul.

Murrell, G. A. & Morton, J. (1974). Word recognition and morphemic structure. Journal of Experimental Psychology, 102, 963-968.

Nolan, K. & Caramazza, A. (1982). Modality independent impairments in processing in a deep dyslexia patient. Brain and Language, 16, 237-266.

Patterson, K. (1981). Neuropsychological approaches to the study of reading. British Journal of Psychology, 72, 151-174.

Patterson, K. (1982). The relation between reading and phonological coding: Further neuropsychological observations. In A. W. Ellis (Ed.), Normality and pathology in cognitive functions. London: Academic Press.

Rubin, G. S., Becker, C. A. & Freeman, R. H. (1979). Morphological structure and its effects on visual word recognition. Journal of Verbal Learning and Verbal Behavior, 18, 757-767.

Saffran, E. M. (in press). Acquired dyslexia: Implications for models of reading. In G. MacKinnon & T. G. Waller (Eds.), Reading research: Advances in theory and practice (Vol. 4). New York, NY: Academic Press.

Sartori, G., Barry, C. & Job, R. (1984). Phonological dyslexia: A review. In R. Malatesha & H. Whitaker (Eds.), Dyslexia: A global issue. The Hague: Nijhoff.

Shallice, T. (1981). Neurological impairment of cognitive processes. British Medical Bulletin, 37, 187-192.

Shallice, T. & Warrington, E. K. (1980). Single and multiple component central dyslexic syndromes. In M. Coltheart, K. E. Patterson, & J. C. Marshall (Eds.), Deep dyslexia. London: Routledge & Kegan Paul.

Stanners, R. F., Neiser, J. J., Hernon, W. P. & Hall, R. (1979). Memory representation for morphologically related words. Journal of Verbal Learning and Verbal Behavior, 8, 399-412.

Taft, M. (1979). Recognition of affixed words and the word frequency effect. Memory and Cognition, 7, 263-272.

Taft, M. & Forster, K. I. (1975). Lexical storage and retrieval of prefixed words. Journal of Verbal Learning and Verbal Behavior, 14, 638-647.

REFERENCE NOTES

1. DeBastiani, P., Barry, C. & Carreras, M. (1983). Mechanisms for reading nonwords: Evidence from a case of phonological dyslexia in an Italian reader. Paper presented at the First European Workshop on Cognitive Neuropsychology, Bressanone, Italy.

2. Laudanna, A. & Caramazza, A. (1984). Morphological parsing and lexical access. Unpublished manuscript. The Johns Hopkins University.

3. Martin, R. C., Caramazza, A. & Berndt, R. S. (1982). The relationship between oral reading and writing and speech production in aphasia. Unpublished manuscript. The Johns Hopkins University.

APPENDIX

Errors made by LB on words and nonwords in the Reading Test of Morphologically "Legal" vs. Morphologically "Illegal" Nonwords. Word stimuli and responses are indicated by the translation in parentheses.

a) Errors on Words

molta (many, Fem. Sing.)	"molto" (many, Masc. Sing.)
neppure (not even)	"seppure" (even if)
sposava (s/he was getting married)	"posava" (s/he was putting)
sperasti (you hoped)	"separasti" (you separated)
contata (counted)	"contrata" (countered)
passavano (they were passing)	"passavamo" (we were passing)

entrano (they enter)   "entrando" (entering)
corsero (they ran)   "ossero"

b) *Errors on Nonwords*
  1. *Morphologically "Legal" Nonwords*
chiediva   "chiedeva" (s/he was asking)
scrivate   "schivate" (avoided)
spieghirei   "spiegherei" (I would explain)
occupesti   "occuperesti" (you would occupy)
legimi   "leggemi" ((you) read to me)
disperendo   "disperdendo" (scattering)
inventire   "invertire" (to invert)
andrasti   "andasti" (you went)
partesti   "partesti" (you looked like)
guardessaro   "guardessero" (they looked--Past
                                            Subject)
mordare   "mondare" (to cleanse)
nuotuto   "nuociuto" (harmed)
tirarei   "tireo" (I will throw)
giovirai   "giovinai"
sollevivano   "solleviano"
sentando   "setando"
scansessi   "cansessi"
cantevi   "cantievi"
legiti   "leggiti"
bastivi   "stivi"
fermida   "fremida"
occulesti   "occludeste" (you occluded--2
                                            Plur.)
roreda   "rodeva" (it was gnawing)
nemerbi   "imberbi" (callow, Masc.Pl.)
voncerono   "vinceranno" (they will win)
rimpovono   "rimponevano" (they were
                                            reimposing)
cintundo   "cinturo" (I grab s.o. at waist
                                            level)
spiegorei   "fiegorei"
cuocire   "chiucire"
aiutette   "anghette

2. Morphologically "Illegal" Nonwords

roreva	"rodeva" (it was gnawing)
occuliati	"occultati" (concealed)"

letiti	"letimi"	*dovenussi*	"dovessuvi"
refluto	"tufluto"	*sporote*	"postore"
selolo	"selovo"	*spienirei*	"spighetemi, spinitei"
cardune	"cardume"		
velutindo	"velutendo"	*femmida*	"fremida"
betaroste	"betatoste"	*geriroi*	"gerorio"
vontiemo	"voltiemo"	*riccogliovo*	"riccioglivo"
prindore	"prindone"	*appiutote*	"appitoto"
mansete	"masete"	*ponsote*	"posoto"
grottemo	"gottemo"	*ripasote*	"risposote"
centeroi	"centoi"	*adiavo*	"andiovo"
vesitiemo	"vestiemo"	*troccindo*	"tocchindo"
ricomuvo	"ricuvo"	*screvovo*	"schievelovo"
arrasti	"arriasti"	*svonendo*	"spolindo"
strivate	"strivante"	*suocideto*	"sciocito"
letimi	"lietimi"	*accagliuvo*	"acchialuglio"
getruva	"gertruva"	*cemminoi*	"cauninoi"
strippore	"stripporze"	*aiupette*	"oopatte"
vestote	"vestono"	*aiupotte*	"antipuote"
sceluvo	"scevulo"	*spienorei*	"spie..."
recordoi	"recordio"	*asfoltovo*	"ostol...fo..."

3. Other Nonwords

ettico	"ittico" (fishing-adj.)
achirsa	"acquista" (s/he purchases)

nopago	"ropago"	*canquirpa*	"campirqua"
drugga	"druzza"	*sfuppa*	"stuffa"
onupio	"ocupio"	*pruso*	"frusso"
cevini	"cevimi"	*salcoti*	"santoti"
libongi	"gibongi"	*ghennia*	"chemmia"
cabissa	"gabissa"	*chiagico*	"chiaccico"
arotipa	"atotipa"	*leruceso*	"leducedo"
garnace	"garcace"	*fributeggia*	"fribucella"

voscale	"vosciale"	*sfergande*	"sferragrande"
antruspo	"astruspo"	*dregupo*	"gebupo"
nurzioche	"nunzioche"	*renuzlo*	"renuncio"
gilino	"giglino"	*ulebbia*	"ubelba"
zimbia	"zimbria"	*acrumba*	"acubai"
frapio	"fapio"	*fistrelo*	"fistello"
sisso	"isso"	*scampotte*	"scamozze"
cisbustri	"cisbutri"	*slazonitino*	"salitino"
prelumone	"pelumone"	*clirco*	"ortico"
slomba	"somlba"	*bilotro*	"fribiatro, biostio"
crobo	"cobro"	*crastulpa*	"castope"
mantuvia	"mantiuva"	*statepanze*	"stapamena"
pognilde	"polginde"	*surmile*	"sul...sulmi..."

NOTES

[1] It is unclear how the correct pronunciation of irregular function words (e.g., "of") would be obtained in this model of reading. In its present form Patterson's proposal leads to the prediction that irregular function words should be mispronounced by *normal* readers of the language--a strange prediction.

[2] It is possible that we may have to distinguish further between mechanisms implicated in processing bound and free-standing grammatical morphemes. Sartori et al. (1984) have reported a case (Beatrice) who presents with difficulties in processing the latter but not the former. This dissociation suggests that the two forms of grammatical morphemes may, after all, be represented in separate subcomponents of the lexicon.

[3] This argument is based on two implicit assumptions. First, it is assumed that an address for a lexical entry can be activated by nonwords in proportion to their visual similarity to the word represented in the lexicon. Second, it is assumed that the criterion for making a response available on the basis of lower-than-normal levels of activation of lexical addresses can be relaxed in the pathological state.

[4] This expectation is motivated by the assumption that negative decisions in cases in which a root address has been found in the lexical system are more time consuming than negative decisions in cases in which no address has been found.

[5] In this context, it is interesting to note that Funnell's case WB could not read isolated affixes that he could read when bound to a word root. This result supports the view that access of bound morphemes in the

lexicon requires that the condition of "boundness" of affixes be respected in order for these items to be processed normally by the Lexical Address System.

[6] By morphologically "legal" we mean that there is a parsing of the nonword which results in an orthographic segment that corresponds to a real word root. Morphologically "illegal" nonwords do not permit such parsing. "Parsing" is used here strictly in the sense of morphological parsing. Other forms of parsing processes (e.g., perceptual and graphemic) must be assumed to be involved *both* in the case of addressed and computed morphological access procedures.

[7] For example, consider the case where a speaker of Italian knows the verb *chiamare* (to call) but has never encountered the form *chiameranno*. When this latter form is presented, the parsing of the string into the root *chiam-* plus *-eranno* allows the individual to recognise it as the future, third person, plural form of the verb *chiamare*.

CHAPTER THREE

THE ROLE OF THE (OUTPUT) PHONOLOGICAL BUFFER IN READING, WRITING, AND REPETITION

INTRODUCTION

Recent efforts directed at understanding the nature of cognitive disorders have been guided by the assumption that the analysis and interpretation of cognitive impairments cannot proceed independently of a clearly formulated model of the cognitive systems assumed to be disrupted. In other words, the approach that is used increasingly in the analysis of cognitive disorders is to formulate a detailed model of the component structure of a particular cognitive system which, when "lesioned" appropriately, functions in such a way as to generate the patterns of cognitive impairments observed in brain-damaged patients. Research within this framework has already contributed to a general characterisation of the architecture of various cognitive systems; it has helped raise a number of important questions about the structure of specific components of these systems; and it has contributed to the formulation of specific hypotheses about the locus of functional lesions that underlie particular forms of cognitive impairment.

Especially active areas of research within this framework have been the areas of reading, writing, and repetition. A rich database now exists on patterns of selective impairments in each of these areas. These data have played an important role in the formulation of models of reading (e.g., Coltheart, in press), writing (e.g., Ellis, in press; Patterson, in press), and repetition (e.g., McCarthy & Warrington, 1984). The emphasis in this research has been on the characterisation of specific processing components implicated in each of these tasks. Considerably less attention has been directed to those components of processing that subserve *all* three tasks--perhaps because a deficit to some such component would be reflected in a pattern of association of symptoms whose analysis is (inappropriately) considered methodologically problematic (see Caramazza, 1986, for discussion). However, the development of complete models of each of these tasks may require the postulation and, therefore, the analysis of these shared components. The role played by components of processing that subserve several different cognitive abilities may be revealed by considering in some detail a specific cognitive performance.

Reproduced, with permission, from Cognitive Neuropsychology, Vol. 3. Copyright 1986 by Lawrence Erlbaum Associates Ltd.

Consider, in this regard, the functional architecture of the writing system (but we could just as easily take the reading system as an example) that has emerged from theoretical analysis of the writing process and the analysis of patterns of writing impairment that have been reported. A major distinction is drawn between a lexically-based processing system and a non-lexical processing system in writing. The lexically-based (lexical route) system essentially involves the activation of graphemic representations in the graphemic output lexicon. Representations in this lexical system are addressed from the lexical-semantic system. The activated, graphemic representations are then placed in a graphemic buffer in preparation for the application of procedures for converting graphemes to specific letter forms (allographic conversion). This system is used in writing words.

Writing unfamiliar words and nonwords involves converting phonological representations stored in a phonological buffer into graphemic representations, by the application of a "phoneme/grapheme" conversion procedure. The phoneme/grapheme conversion process consists of a system of rules that transcode phonemes or syllables into graphemic representations in order to derive a plausible spelling (e.g., /kif/ could be written as keef, keaf, keeph, kefe, etc).[1] The graphemic representation computed through the application of the conversion procedure is then placed in the graphemic buffer, as in the case of lexically activated graphemic representations. A schematic representation of the proposed architecture for the writing system, focusing on the output side of the system, is shown in Figure 1 as a graphic aid for discussion (see Ellis, 1982, for a more detailed account of the writing system, and Morton, 1980, for a model of reading, writing, and repetition). Figure 1 also shows processing components that form part of the functional architecture of the reading and repetition processes. The empirical and theoretical justification for the proposed functional architecture for reading and repetition follows a parallel logic to that presented here for writing (see Coltheart, in press, for discussion on reading).

The architecture of the writing system proposed here provides a motivated basis for the explication of various patterns of writing impairment reported in the neuropsychological literature and, in turn, has received empirical support from this literature. Two patterns of writing impairment are especially relevant to the proposed functional architecture. One pattern of impairment is characterised by the inability to write nonwords in the face of relatively intact word-writing ability (Shallice, 1981). The other pattern of impairment is characterised by phonologically plausible spelling errors in writing words (e.g., writing CHARE for CHAIR) and intact nonword writing (Beauvois & Dérouesné, 1981;

Hatfield & Patterson, 1983). The double dissociation between word and nonword writing abilities indicates that accurate writing of each type of stimulus relies on different processing components: nonword writing depends on a transcoding process that converts phonemes to graphemes (i.e., procedures applied to derive plausible candidate spellings) without recourse to lexical information; word writing, instead, depends on processes that access whole-word spelling patterns (i.e., addressed spelling) without recourse to use of phoneme/grapheme conversion processes.

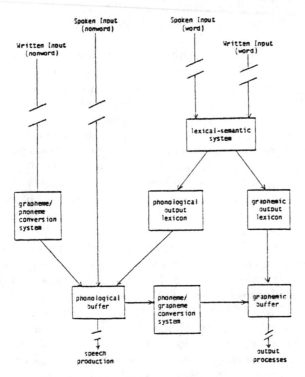

Figure 1. Schematic representation of the functional architecture for reading, writing, and repetition.

While these reported fractionations of skills necessary for accurate writing support the general architecture of the writing system proposed, there is an obvious need to articulate further the structure of the cognitive/linguistic mechanisms implicated in writing in order to explicate the bases for other patterns of writing impairment. Thus, for example, apart from the unambiguous prediction regarding the pattern of spelling errors in patients with a disruption of the lexical route (i.e., access of lexical-graphemic representations) in writing, where the expectation is that spelling errors should consist of phonologically appropriate responses (e.g. table → taybel), the proposed model is silent with respect to other forms of spelling errors. This situation reflects the relatively underspecified nature of the proposed model and, hence, the lack of an explicitly specified relationship between the type of spelling error and the cognitive mechanisms that give rise to these error patterns. There have certainly been attempts to deal with the issue of the bases for nonphonological spelling errors (e.g., Ellis, 1982; Nolan & Caramazza, 1983; Miceli, Silveri, & Caramazza, 1986), but these have been less than successful.

Spelling errors have been subdivided into two major types--phonological and non-phonological spelling errors. Phonological spelling errors consist of phonologically plausible spellings of words (e.g. sleek → sleak, sleake); non-phonological spelling errors represent phonologically implausible renditions of a stimulus word (e.g., language → languate). Phonological spelling errors are assumed to result from the "correct" application of phoneme/grapheme conversion rules to phonological representations when lexical-graphemic representations are inaccessible for some reason (perhaps a disruption of the graphemic output lexicon). These spelling errors constitute a homogeneous set in the sense that observed spelling patterns are explicable in terms of a well-defined set of sound-to-print conversion procedures.

By contrast, non-phonological spelling errors represent a heterogeneous group. Some errors are close approximations of the target response (e.g., language → languate--patient VS, Nolan & Caramazza, 1983) others bear a complex relationship to the target response (e.g., giraffe → garfara--patient RD, Ellis, Miller, & Sin, 1983). Spelling errors in writing nonwords also vary in degree of approximation to target responses: Some are recognisable approximations while others bear no recognisable relationship to target responses. Various hypotheses about the functional locus of deficit underlying these types of errors are possible.

One hypothesis places the locus of deficit responsible for non-phonological spelling errors in word writing in the graphemic output lexicon. In this view it is assumed that the patient has "...access to some word-specific spelling information but not enough to permit the word to be spelled correctly" (Miller & Ellis, in press). Another hypotheses that has been entertained is that the locus of deficit for non-phonological spelling errors is in the graphemic buffer (Miceli, Silveri, & Caramazza, 1986). Obviously, these hypotheses are not mutually exclusive. Damage to any of these functional loci or damage to combinations of these cognitive mechanisms could be responsible for different types of spelling errors. It seems unlikely that an explanation in terms of a disruption to *only* one of these cognitive mechanisms can explain the different patterns of non-phonological spelling errors that have been reported. A more reasonable expectation is that various functional loci contribute to different patterns of spelling errors.

Consider the following examples of the type of predictions we could make about patterns of writing impairments on the basis of the functional architecture of the writing system proposed here. If we were to assume that a patient has a functional lesion to the phoneme/grapheme conversion system, we would predict that s/he should be able to write words normally, but show an impairment in writing nonwords. However, we are unable to specify the nature of errors in writing nonwords unless we specify in some detail the computational structure of the phoneme/ grapheme conversion system. Similarly, if we assumed that the graphemic buffer was damaged in a patient, we would predict that s/he would show an impairment in writing and normal spelling of both words and nonwords. Again, however, the specific nature of spelling errors depends on the kinds of assumptions we make about the hypothesised structure of the graphemic buffer. Finally, consider the case where we might hypothesise a deficit to the allographic conversion system--the system that converts abstract graphemic representation into specific letter patterns. In this case, we would be able to predict that the patient should make spelling errors in writing both words and nonwords but should show normal performance in oral spelling (Goodman & Caramazza, 1986). In this case too, however, the exact nature of the spelling errors we expect can only be specified by articulating the computational structure of the allographic conversion system. These examples clearly demonstrate that spelling errors can result from damage to different processing components but that the relationship between type of spelling error and mechanism contributing to type of error cannot be specified without an explicit account of the internal structure of these components of processing. Fortunately, there are cases where converging evidence allows us to be relatively certain of the locus of damage responsible for a particular pattern of spelling errors. These cases can serve as the basis for the development of a taxonomy of spelling errors which in turn, can guide theoretical developments in specifying the internal structure of the proposed cognitive components. A case in point is the expected pattern of performance in patients with damage to the phonological buffer.

Consider the asymmetry in functional roles played by the graphemic buffer and the phonological buffer in the proposed cognitive architecture of the writing, reading, and repetition systems (Figure 1). The graphemic buffer is a system-specific cognitive component--it has a functional role only in the writing system (and oral spelling, but this is a "derivative" form of writing). Damage to this cognitive component should affect only writing performance, both in writing words and nonwords. In contrast, the phonological buffer forms part of the functional architecture of the reading, writing, and repetition system. Damage to this component should affect performance in all three tasks. In other words, acceptance of the proposed functional architecture entails the prediction of a necessary co-occurrence of deficits in writing, reading, and repetition, if the phonological buffer is damaged. The expected pattern of impairments across tasks is the following: writing--nonword writing should be impaired while word writing should be spared since only the former task implicates the phonological buffer in its processing configuration: reading and repetition--non-word reading and repetition should be impaired as *may* word reading and repetition, since the phonological buffer is implicated in the processing configuration for both classes of stimuli. The reason for the uncertainty concerning the prediction of performance in reading and repeating words stems from the fact that the interaction between the phonological buffer and subsequent production mechanisms in the proposed model is not fully specified. Thus, if we were to assume that oral production of words involved processing phonologically and articulatorily preassembled lexical representations (Caramazza, Miceli, Silveri, & Laudanna, 1985), we would expect a minimal or even totally absent role for the phonological buffer in this task. By contrast, the oral production of nonwords entails the assembly of phonological segments in the phonological buffer in preparation for transformation into articulatory programs and, thus, requires an intact phonological buffer for the normal production of nonwords.

There is a second type of prediction we can make concerning the effects of damage to the phonological buffer. This prediction is motivated by assumptions about the nature of the internal structure of the damaged component. Although we are far from being able to give a detailed description of the structural characteristics of the phonological buffer, we are obviously committed to the position that the representations held in the buffer are specified in a phonological code. This fact places a strong predictive constraint on the type of errors in performance that can result from damage to the phonological buffer. Specifically, if the error performance assumed to result from malfunctioning of the phonological buffer has *any* interpretable structure (or pattern), then it must be explicable in terms of phonological principles, and not, say, in terms of visual similarity.

We have suggested that a set of observations (a particular pattern of co-occurring deficits in reading, writing, and repetition in conjunction with a pattern of errors in these tasks explicable in terms of phonological principles) converge to specify uniquely damage to the phonological buffer in the proposed functional architecture for reading, writing, and repetition. Furthermore, implicit in this discussion is the claim that we can interpret a pattern of writing performance, characterised by phonologically related spelling errors, to result from damage to the phonological buffer (as opposed to the phoneme/grapheme conversion system or the graphemic buffer to other cognitive mechanisms) when this pattern of errors is found in the context of similar errors in reading and repetition. We are thus able to begin to formulate a taxonomy of spelling errors which can be used to address questions concerning the source of different patterns of spelling dysgraphia and the internal structure of various cognitive components involved in the writing process (but, also, *mutatis mutandis*, for reading).

In this paper, we report an analysis of a patient presenting a pattern of deficits in reading, writing, and repetition that conforms to the constellation of features we have assumed to characterise damage to the phonological buffer in the proposed functional architecture of the reading, writing, and repetition processes.

CASE HISTORY

IGR is a 40-year old right-handed Italian male with a degree in engineering. On August 6, 1981, he was admitted to a hospital because of a right-hemisphere stroke that caused a left hemiplegia and global aphasia. A CT scan performed on the same day was negative, but a right carotid angiography showed an occlusion of the right internal carotid artery at the syphon. During the following months the patient made a quick, though incomplete, recovery. He remained in good health until July 1983, when he was admitted to the Neurology ward of the Catholic University, because of a generalised seizure.

The neurological exam, given immediately after the seizure had been treated, was unchanged relative to a routine neurological check-up executed two months before. IGR showed a very mild left hemiparesis, more marked in the upper limb, with slightly increased muscle tone. No obvious sensory deficit was demonstrable, but on simultaneous tactile double stimulation the patient sometimes failed to report stimuli on the left side of the body. No visual field defect was demonstrated.

A CT-scan (Figure 2) showed a large old lesion in the right hemisphere, involving the superior and the inferior parietal lobule, the superior and middle temporal gyri, the angular gyrus, and the supramarginal gyrus.

A. Caramazza

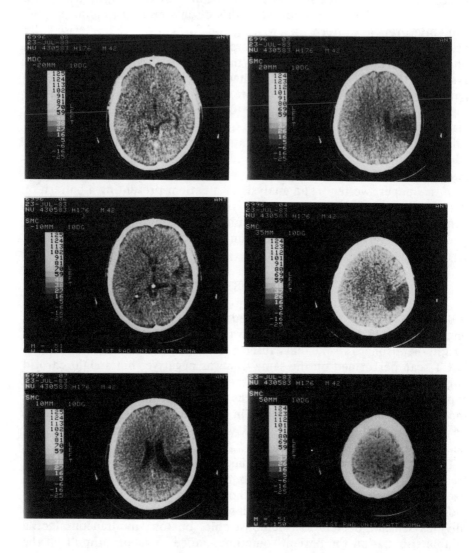

FIG. 2   CT scan showing a lesion in the right hemisphere, involving the superior and inferior parietal lobule, the superior and middle temporal gyri, the angular gyrus, and the supramarginal gyrus.

The underlying white matter was also extensively involved. No signs of recent lesions were present.

The results reported in the present study were collected between August, 1983 and June, 1984. During this period, IGR was followed as an out-patient in the Neuropsychology Service of the Catholic University, Rome.

LANGUAGE EVALUATION

The patient's speech was mostly fluent and without articulatory or prosodic difficulty. Occasionally, however, his speech had a stuttering-like quality, with pauses and false starts at the beginning of words, which only very infrequently resulted in phonemic paraphasias. Occasional word-finding problems and even less frequent semantic substitutions were present. IGR displayed a normal use of morphological and syntactic structures.

Oral naming from auditory description and oral and written naming of objects of high frequency and familiarity were error-free (N=20 for each test). On tests of oral naming of pictured objects and of actions which included low-frequency, low-familiarity items, mild difficulties were noted: IGR made 12/70 errors in naming objects (2 semantic substitutions, 6 circumlocutions, 4 failures to produce a response) and 7/44 in naming actions (4 semantic substitutions, 1 phonemic substitution, 1 circumlocution, 1 failure to produce a response).

Word repetition was flawless (108/108) correct, but at times the patient exhibited difficulty on the initial syllable). Repetition of sentences was essentially normal, as IGR made 2 single-word errors in 30 sentences (Il cane e'dentro la casa (The dog is inside the house) → il cane e' dentro *nella* casa (The dog is inside in the house; Il gatto e' sul tavolo (The cat is on the table) → Il gatto e' *sopra* il tavolo (The cat is above the table)).

Single-word comprehension was normal both for auditory and for visual input. Comprehension of reversible sentences of a variety of types (active and passive declaratives, active and passive relatives, sentences expressing temporal relations) was normal both for auditory and for visual input. On the auditory shortened version of the Token Test (DeRenzi & Faglioni, 1978), the patient produced 23/36 correct responses, reflecting a mild comprehension disorder.

NEUROPSYCHOLOGICAL EVALUATION

The patient had been fully right-handed since childhood. None of the members of his family (from his grandparents to his children) were known to be left-handers or ambidextrous.

Immediate memory of meaningless patterns was normal; immediate and delayed memory of pictures were entirely normal. Scores on Corsi's block tapping test were 6 forward, 5 backward. Recall of a list of 15 words was very poor (3/15). After 5 presentations of the list, IGR was able to report 12/15 stimuli, and 15 minutes later he recalled 9/15; these scores correspond to lower normal levels. Very poor results were obtained on the digit span test (3 digits forward, 3 digits backward).

Buccofacial and limb praxis were moderately impaired on verbal instructions (6/10 and 9/12 correct, respectively) but were normal on imitation. Performance on limb praxis was comparable for the two hands. Tasks of verbal and non-verbal buccofacial agility were executed somewhat slowly but always accurately. Constructional praxis was normal. On clinical testing, no relevant disorders of spatial exploration nor signs of visual hemi-inattention were discovered. IGR obtained normal scores on the Raven's Coloured Matrices (33/36 correct).

EXPERIMENTAL STUDY

1. *Letter naming*
IGR named isolated letters promptly and easily.
2. *CV syllables*
Two hundred and eighty syllables--20 presentations of each of 14 syllables (pa, ta, ca, ba, da, ga, ma, na, la, ra, sa, za, fa, va) were presented for oral reading. The patient read all the stimuli correctly.
3. *Reading text*
IGR was asked to read aloud a 400-word written narrative of the Little Red Riding Hood story. The task was executed with a few self-corrections, but without errors.
4. *Reading words and nonwords*
IGR was required, over several sessions, to read 550 words and 505 nonwords. Several factors were varied systematically in the word list: word length, frequency, and grammatical category. In the nonword list, the factors varied systematically were: length, N-count (where N indicates the number of real words that can be obtained by substituting one letter of the stimulus at a time) and morphological decomposability (whether a nonword could be parsed "morphologically" into a real word root-morpheme and a real affix, inappropriate for that root, or whether no such parsing was possible for the nonword, e.g., cantevi and canzovi, respectively).

IGR made 10 errors in reading words (1.8%) and 78 errors in reading nonwords (15.5%). Of the errors on words, 6 resulted in the production of other words (60%); of these, 3 could be interpreted as visual and/or inflectional errors (macchine (cars) → macchina (car); contento (happy; masculine, singular) → contenta (happy; feminine, singular); rimarrai (you will remain) → rimarrei (I would remain)) two as visual/phonological errors (saluti (wishes) → salute (health) toglievo (I was taking away) → coglievo (I was picking)); and one as a function word substitution or as a visual error (stavolta (this time) → talvolta (sometimes)). The 4 nonwords incorrectly produced as responses to words resulted from incorrect stress assignment (N=2) and from visual errors (N=2).

Of the errors on nonwords, only 11 resulted in words (13.7%). Length, N-count, and whether or not a nonword could be parsed morphologically did not influence IGR's performance appreciably. Length of nonword had only a mild effect on this reading performance: the patient made 12.2% errors on 4-5 letter nonwords, 18% on 6-7 letter nonwords, and 14.8% on 8-9 letter nonwords. On a subset of 108 nonwords controlled for similarity to real words and matched for length, he made 6/36 errors on low N-count items, 2/36 errors on medium N-count items, and 4/36 errors on high N-count items. Finally, on a subset of the nonwords, including 40 morphologically-decomposable and 40 morphologically non-decomposable items matched for length and N-count, he made the same number of errors in morphologically-decomposable and morphologically non-decomposable nonwords (6/40 in each case, 15%).

The distribution of incorrect responses in terms of error types is shown in Table 1. It is clear that the vast majority of the errors are off-target by only one letter and that, within errors types, substitution of a single letter is by far the most frequent error type.

Table 1. Errors in reading words and nonwords: Distribution of error types.

	Error Types	Words	Nonwords	Total
Single letter errors	Substitutions	5(50%)	57(67.9%)	62(66.0%)
	Insertions	1(10%)	9(10.7%)	10(10.6%)
	Deletions		4 (4.8%)	4 (4.3%)
Multiple letter errors	Multiple Substitutions		8 (9.5%)	8 (9.1%)
	Multiple Deletions		1 (1.2%)	1 (1.1%)
	Substitution & Insertion		4 (4.8%)	4 (4.3%)
	Substitution & Deletion	1(10%)		1 (1.2%)
	Substitution & Transposition	1(10%)	1 (1.2%)	2 (2.1%)
	Accent	2(20%)		2 (2.1%)
	Total	10	84	94

Inspection of error responses (see Appendix 1) revealed a striking pattern: Error responses have a systematic phonological relationship to the target response. A more detailed analysis of reading errors was carried out in order to assess the stimulus/error relationship in terms of phonological relatedness. In order to work on a homogeneous corpus of errors (i.e., of errors that could be attributed to the disruption of the same mechanisms), incorrect responses to words were excluded from this analysis, as it was clear that they could very well derive from more than one source (see Introduction). If more than one error was present in any item, each error was counted separately. The analysis was carried out on 83 target letters incorrectly produced by IGR when reading nonwords. Of these errors, six insertion errors and two deletion errors were excluded because no relationship between the error and the target could be identified. The remaining three insertions and two deletions were included, as they involved double consonants which in Italian are marked phonologically (e.g. dochio → docchio; ebbiomo → ebiomo). The confusion matrix displaying the phonological relationship between stimuli and errors is shown in Table 2. The vertical axis represents the stimulus letter and the horizontal axis gives the corresponding phonological response.

The pattern of results shown in Table 2 reflects a clear phonological relationship between stimulus (letter) and error response (phoneme). Thus, for example, 41/49 (83.7%) errors on occlusive consonants (stops and nasals) were incorrectly produced as other occlusive consonants. Overall, 56/71 (78.9%) consonants produced incorrectly belonged to the same phonological category, defined by manner of articulation (e.g., occlusives, fricatives, etc.), as the stimulus, and 11/12 vowels (91.7%) were substituted for other vowels.

To summarise, IGR reads words essentially normally but is much less proficient in reading nonwords. It is striking that most of his incorrect responses to nonwords are off-target by one or two letters, and the phonemes produced incorrectly bear a close phonological relationship to the target.

Evaluation of Writing Abilities

1. *Written naming*
The patient wrote correctly the names of 60 objects of high and medium familiarity. Two self-corrections were observed: anello (ring) → annello → anello; cappello (hat) → capello (hair) → cappello.

TABLE 2

Stimulus (Letter)/Response (Phoneme) Confusion Matrix for Reading Errors

Error / Stimulus	p	t	k	b	d	g	m	n	l	r	f	v	dჳ	č	s	p	ʎ	SCᵃ	DCᵇ	z	a	e	i	o	u
p	1														2										
t	1		1		3																				
k	9				1	2																			
b	7		1	2	3																				
d	1		6	1	3																				
g	1					1	1	1	1																
m							1	2																	
n							2																		
l	1								1																
r			1							1					1										
f											3				1										
v												2													
dჳ						1							1												
č														1	1										
s			1												1										
p																	3								
ʎ																		2	3						
SCᵃ																									
DCᵇ																									
z					1																2		3	2	
a																						2		2	
e																					1		3	1	
i																									
o																								1	
u																									2

ᵃSC = single consonant   ᵇDC = double consonant

2. *Writing to dictation*

a) *Letters.* The patient wrote quickly and correctly letter names pronounced by the examiner.

b) *Syllables.* Fourteen CV syllables (/pa/, /ta/, /ka/, /ba/, /da/, /ga/, /ma/, /na/, /ra/, /la/, /fa/, /va/, /sa/, /dza/) were dictated, 20 times each, in random order. The patient made 4 errors (1.4%). He wrote incorrectly: /pa/ as /ta/ (twice), /da/ as /ba/ and /fa/ as /va/.

c) *Sentences.* Thirty sentences were dictated to IGR. He made only one error (La camicia e' nel cassetto nel como' [The shirt is in the drawer of the chest of drawers] → La camicia e' nel cassetto nel como' [The shirt is in the drawer in the chest of drawers]).

d) *Words and nonwords.*

(i)Immediate writing--IGR was asked to write to dictation 628 words and 514 nonwords, presented in random order. Because of the large number of stimuli to be written, the task was administered over several sessions. Words of different length, frequency, grammatical class, and abstractness/concreteness were used. Nonwords ranged in length from four to nine letters. A subset of nonwords included items that could be parsed morphologically into a real root and affix, inappropriate for that root morpheme; for example, one such stimulus was "amevi," where the root "am-" (from the verb "amare"--to love) is combined with an inappropriate inflection (in this case, "evi," that is correct for other verbs in Italian).

IGR made 17 errors on words (2.7%) and 149 on nonwords (29%). Four errors on words resulted in the production of an incorrect word (23.5%). Errors were not influenced by any of the variables listed above (e.g. grammatical class, frequency, etc.).

Of the nonword errors, only 3 (2%) resulted in the production of words. A clear effect of length was present: 19.5% errors for 4-5 letter nonwords, 26.4% errors for 6-7 letter nonwords, and 38.1% errors for 8-9 letter nonwords. Whether or not a to-be-written string could be parsed into a word root plus affix, inappropriate for that root, did not influence IGR's performance. On a subset of 146 nonwords matched for length and similarity (N-count) to words, of which half were morphologically-decomposable and half were not, the patient made 13 (17.8%) errors in writing items from the first subgroup and 16 (21.9%) in writing items from the second subgroup.

In order to determine whether the mild length effect observed in nonword writing could be attributed to the rapid decay of the phonological representation of the dictated nonword, two tests were administered.

(ii) Delayed writing--Fifty words and fifty nonwords matched for length were dictated in random order. After each stimulus had been presented, the patient had to wait for 3 to 10 seconds (at random) before the examiner allowed him to write. Half of the stimuli were written after 3, half after 10 seconds. The patient wrote correctly all words but made 3 errors (12%) on nonwords in the 3-seconds delay condition, and 1 error (4%) on words and 3 errors (12%) on nonwords in the 10-seconds delay condition. The discrepancy in performance in writing nonwords in this task (12 % errors) versus the immediate writing task (29% errors) is probably due to the fact that the mean length of the nonwords in the delayed writing condition was shorter (6.5 letters) than that of the nonwords in the immediate writing condition (7.1 letters). (The small sample size of nonwords used in the delayed writing condition precludes meaningful analysis of the discrepancy in overall performance obtained between immediate and delayed writing tasks.)

(iii)Repetition of stimuli after writing to dictation--Fifty-four words and fifty-four nonwords matched for length were presented in random order. After writing the stimulus the patient was asked to repeat it. IGR wrote incorrectly 2 words (3.7%) and 11 nonwords (20.4%). He repeated correctly all words and made 2 errors when repeating nonwords (3.7%). Only one of the nonwords repeated incorrectly was also written incorrectly. The results from these last two tasks suggest that the patient's difficulty in writing nonwords is not due just to a rapidly decaying phonological memory.

Qualitative Analysis of Errors Made in Writing Words and Nonwords to Dictation

The Distribution of error types is shown in Table 3. As in the case of the results obtained for reading, most writing errors (76.5% on both words and nonwords) differed from the stimulus by only one letter, and were for the most part substitutions. (A complete list of writing errors is given in Appendix 2.)

A more detailed analysis was also undertaken, aimed at ascertaining whether the errors in writing, like those in reading, maintained a phonological relationship to the stimulus. If more than one error occurred in the same item, each incorrect production was counted separately.

Out of 21 scorable errors in words (19 substitutions and 2 insertions, involving the production of a double "l" instead of a single "l"), 13 (61.9%) were closely related to the stimulus phonologically, and 2 consisted of producing "n" as "l" and "l" as "n" before "z" (anzi → alzi; alzare → anzare).

A. Caramazza

A much larger error corpus was collected from tests of nonword writing. One hundred and sixty-four scorable errors were counted in one hundred and forty-one nonwords written incorrectly (a stress assignment error, six fragments, and a neologism were not included in this analysis). Only those cases where both a phoneme in the stimulus and the corresponding incorrect grapheme in the response could be identified were included in the confusion matrix analysis. Thus, all transpositions, 10/9 insertions, and 13/29 deletions, were excluded. The remaining 9 insertions and 16 deletions were included, as a clear relationship between the dictated stimulus and the written production was evident--all these errors involved duplication of a single consonant or omission of a consonant in a double-consonant group (e.g., nafo → naffo; izzi → izi). Overall, 130 errors were included in the confusion matrix relating stimulus to error in terms of phonological proximity (Table 4).

Table 3. Errors in writing words and nonwords to dictation: Distribution of error types.

	Errors types	Words	Nonwords	Total
Single letter errors	Substitutions	13(76.5%)	78(52.3%)	91(54.8%)
	Insertions		15(10.1%)	15(9.0%)
	Deletions		19(12.8%)	19(11.4%)
	Transpositions		2(1.3%)	2 (1.2%)
Multiple letter errors	Multiple substitutions	2(11.8%)	15(10.1%)	17(10.2%)
	Multiple Insertions		1(0.7%)	1(0.6%)
	Substitution & Insertion	2(11.8%)	3(2.0%)	5(3.0%)
	Substitution & Deletion		2(1.3%)	2(1.2%)
	Deletion & Insertion		2(1.3%)	2(1.2%)
	Deletion & Transposition		3(2.0%)	3(1.8%)
	Subst. & Delet. & Transp.		1(0.7%)	1(0.6%)
	Stress Assignment		1(0.7%)	1(0.6%)
	Fragment		6(4.0%)	6(3.6%)
	Neologism		1(0.7%)	1(0.6%)
	Total	17	149	166

The data reported in the confusion matrix are striking, as 122 (93.8%) incorrectly-produced graphemes were members of the same phonological category (defined by manner of articulation) as the target grapheme determined by the stimulus. Thus, for example, 83/85 (97.6%) errors on occlusive consonants (stops and nasals) and 10/10 errors on fricatives were occlusive and fricative consonants, respectively. All vowels were substituted for by other vowels.

TABLE 4

Stimulus (Phoneme)/Error (Letter) Confusion Matrix for Writing Errors

Stimulus \ Error	p	t	k	b	d	g	m	n	l	r	f	v	dʒ	č	s	ɲ	ʎ	SC[a]	DC[b]	z	a	e	i	o	u
p		2	4	4																					
t	3				4							1													
k		4			1	2																			
b	2	1			1	1																			
d		17		1																					
g		2	2																						
m	1							4																	
n							9																		
l										2		1													
r								1	1			4													
f												5													
v											1														
dʒ														1											
č													1												
s													1	1											
ɲ																	1								
ʎ																									
SC[a]																			5						
DC[b]																		14							
z																									
a																						1			
e																							1		
i																					1	2			
o																					2	1			
u																							1		

[a]SC = single consonant [b]DC = double consonant

To summarise the results of IGR's writing performance, he wrote words of all grammatical classes and frequencies almost without error, but made many errors in writing nonwords. Of the various variables considered in list construction (e.g., frequency, length, etc.), the only factor that influenced nonword writing was length. Most errors involved only one letter of the dictated item, and bore a clear phonological relationship to the stimulus.

The results reported thus far, obtained from an extensive exploration of IGR's reading and writing performance, show that his ability to read and write words is excellent (98.2% and 97.3% correct responses, respectively); performance on nonwords is much poorer, more so in writing (71% correct) than in reading (84.4% correct). The error pattern between reading and writing, however, is remarkably similar: in both tasks, approximately 76% of the errors involve single letters of the stimulus, of which 52-75% are substitutions. Furthermore, there was a striking phonological relationship between stimulus and error: 78.9% incorrect phonemes in reading and 93.8% incorrect graphemes in writing belonged to the same phonological category (i.e., manner of articulation) as the correct target. These data strongly implicate a phonological processing disorder as the most likely source of IGR's difficulties. To explore the possibility further, we administered to IGR other tasks involving phonological processing, including repetition tasks.

Evaluation of Repetition Performance

In the clinical language-evaluation section of this paper, we reported that IGR showed no difficulties in repeating words and sentences. In this section, we report his performance in *repetition of nonwords*.

The patient was asked to repeat 426 auditorily presented nonwords. The examiner produced each nonword once and the patient was required to repeat the nonword immediately after the examiner had presented the stimulus. The nonword stimuli ranged in length from four to ten letters (letter length instead of syllable length is used, for comparison to stimuli used in the reading and writing tasks.).

IGR repeated 103 nonwords (24.2%) incorrectly. Stimulus length was a significant factor in nonword repetition, as the patient made 10.4% errors on 4-5 letter nonwords, 21.5% on 6-7 letter nonwords, and 32.9% on 8-10 letter nonwords. All the errors were very closely related phonologically to the stimulus, as in the results obtained in the reading and writing tasks.

Qualitative Analysis of Errors Made in Repetition of Nonwords

The distribution of error types made by IGR in repeating nonwords is shown in Table 5. (A complete list of the repetition errors included in this analysis is presented in Appendix 3.) As in the case of errors in reading and writing nonwords, the majority of errors were phoneme substitutions (66/104, 63%) and 51/104 (49%) errors involved a single phoneme error. Furthermore, there was a striking phonological relationship between stimulus and errors with 82% of scorable errors falling in the same phonological category (defined by manner of articulation) as the stimulus. The confusion matrix displaying the phonological relationship between stimuli and errors is shown in Table 6.

Table 5. Errors in repetition of nonwords: Distribution of error types.[a]

	Error types	
Single	Substitutions	51(49.0%)
phoneme	Insertions	7(6.7%)
errors	Deletions	2(1.9%)
	Transpositions	3(2.9%)
Multiple	Multiple Substitutions	15(14.4%)
phoneme	Multiple Insertions	1(1.0%)
errors	Substitution & Insertion	2(1.9%)
	Substitution & Deletion	1(1.0%)
	Fragments	22(21.2%)
	Total	104

[a] A total of 104 scorable errors are reported even though only 103 words were written correctly. The reason for the discrepancy is that the patient produced two incorrect responses for one of the stimulus nonwords (see Appendix 3).

Evaluation of Input Phonological Processing

The results we have reported thus far suggest that a disruption of the phonological system may be responsible for the pattern of impairment displayed by IGR in nonword writing, reading, and repetition. We have argued that this pattern of performance is consistent with the hypothesis that damage to the phonological buffer is the underlying cause for the reported co-occurrence of deficits in reading, writing, and repeating nonwords and for the specific pattern of errors in the performance of these tasks. It is possible, however, to entertain an alternative, multi-deficit hypothesis for the underlying cause for the reported pattern of impairment. This alternative account includes a hypothesis of damage to

A. Caramazza

TABLE 6
Stimulus (Phoneme)/Error (Phoneme) Confusion Matrix for Repetition Errors

Error → Stimulus ↓	p	t	k	b	d	g	m	n	l	r	f	v	dʒ	č	s	ʃ	ʎ	SC[a]	DC[b]	z	a	e	i	o	u
p	1		1	2	1																				
t		5	2		1																				
k	3		1			6		1	1					1	1	1							1		
b	3		1		1	1									1										
d	2	9	2	2	3	2		2																	
g												1													
m				2			3	2																	
n								1	1																
l								1	1	3					1		1	1							
r									1	1	1	3													
f						2			1		1	1													
v								1	1																
dʒ													2												
č														1											
s	1							1					2							1					
ʃ																									
ʎ																									
SC[a]																		1							
DC[b]																			2						
z														1											
a																									
e																									
i																					1				1
o																									
u																									

[a]SC = single consonant [b]DC = double consonant

auditory perceptual mechanisms. Damage to auditory perceptual processing could account for IGR's pattern of impairment in writing to dictation and repetition (but not reading). While we think that there are reasonable arguments against a multi-component deficit hypotheses for IGR's pattern of impaired performance, we can obtain empirical evidence that speaks directly to this issue, undermining further the credibility of this hypothesis. Specifically, we can assess directly whether IGR presents with difficulties in auditory perception.

1. *Auditory discrimination of phonemes*
A "same-different" test of auditory phoneme discrimination was prepared, using the six stop consonants. The members of this phonological category can be contrasted for voice (/p/, /t/, /k/ are voiceless; /b/, /d/, /g/ are voiced), place of articulation (/p/ and /b/ are labials; /t/ and /d/ are alveolars; /k/ and /g/ are velars) or both. Each stop was the first phoneme in six meaningless CCVC syllables (/prIn/, /trIn/, /krIn/, /brIn/, /drIn/, /grIn/). IGR's ability to discriminate all possible contrasts was explored by having him judge whether the members of each of 120 pairs of CCVC syllables were same or different. Half of the pairs contained the same syllable repeated twice (e.g., /brIn/, /brIn/); the remaining 60 pairs contained 2 different syllables, so that voice, place, and place + voice contrasts were presented 20 times each. Pairs were presented in random order with a very short pause between syllables (approximately 500 msec). The patient had to indicate whether the two syllables were the same or different. IGR responded incorrectly to 2/120 stimuli (1.7%), well within normal limits for his age and education (errors in a group of 50 normal speakers range from 0-10). He failed to recognise as identical two pairs of syllables.

2. *Auditory/visual matching*
Performance on the auditory discrimination task is a good indicator of gross phonetic processing ability. However, good performance on this task does not necessarily reflect normal ability to process an auditory stimulus in terms of its phonological properties--the task could be performed at an auditory as opposed to a phonemic discrimination level (see Caramazza, Berndt, & Basili, 1983, for discussion). A more sensitive task of phonological perceptual processing is the auditory/visual matching task. In this task, the subject is required to decide whether a spoken stimulus (/brIn/) and a written stimulus (brin) are the same or different (more precisely, to be labelled by the initial letter in the written stimulus). To assess further IGR's phonological perceptual abilities, we tested him in an auditory/visual matching task.

The test material used in this task is essentially identical to that used in the auditory discrimination test, except that the second member of each pair was replaced by its corresponding written form (e.g./brIn/ → brin). Thus, the task consisted of judging whether an aurally presented stimulus and a written stimulus were the same or different (e.g./prIn/, "prin"--same; /prIn/, "drin"--different). The examiner presented one syllable auditorily while showing at the same time a card portraying the other syllable of the pair in written form.

IGR's performance on this test was again very good. He responded incorrectly in only 5/120 (4.2%) trials, well within normal limits (errors in a group of 50 normal speakers range from 0-10); he failed to recognise 2 pairs as identical and 3 as different.

The results in these two tasks--the auditory discrimination and the auditory/visual matching tasks--demonstrate that IGR is not impaired in perceptual processing of speech sounds, certainly not to a level that would serve as a basis for explaining the relatively major difficulties he shows in writing nonwords to dictation.

Comparison Across Tasks

There are several features of IGR's performance in reading, writing, and repetition that warrant a comparative analysis. One concerns the overall performance level in nonword processing across tasks. The percentage of errors in reading, writing, and repetition were: 15.5%, 29.0%, and 24.2% respectively. The difference in performance across tasks is statistically reliable ($X^2(2) = 27.0; P < 0.001$). A factor that may have contributed to the obtained difference in overall performance is stimulus length, which was not controlled across tasks--mean length of nonwords in reading, writing, and repetition was 6.7, 7.1, and 7.5, respectively. Alternatively, and more reasonably in our view, the difference in performance may reflect different processing characteristics across tasks. Thus, while writing and repetition involve the processing of a temporally labile auditory stimulus which must be held as a whole in a phonological buffer for output processes, reading presents radically different processing opportunities--the visual stimulus is temporally stable and available to the subject for multiple glances and the application of diverse processing strategies (e.g., encoding of the whole stimulus or the iterative encoding of successive parts of the stimulus). Other aspects of IGR's performance support this latter interpretation of the differences in overall performance in reading, writing, and repetition of nonwords--the effect of stimulus length on performance is highly suggestive in this regard.

The percentage of errors made by IGR for stimuli of different length in reading, writing, and repetition is shown in Table 7. As already noted, both writing and repetition show a strong effect of length on performance. But there is no effect of length in reading performance for stimuli of length four to nine letters. However, if we include the reading performance for CV syllables, which the patient read correctly, then there is an effect of length also for reading, but it seems to reach a plateau at about four or five letters. The differential effect of stimulus length in reading vs. writing and repetition reveals the contribution of different processing mechanisms in these tasks. Specifically, the fact that reading performance remained relatively stable for stimuli ranging in length from four to nine letters, but that there is a major effect between two and four or five letters, could reflect the application of a part-by-part processing strategy which is possible in this task but not in writing and repetition. In other words, in the reading task the patient could be encoding the input (or "checking" the information encoded) in letter clusters of four or five letters, leading to a reduced effect of stimulus length on performance.

Table 7. Percentage errors in reading, writing, and repetition as a function of stimulus length.

Task Type	Stimulus Length (in letters)		
	4-5	6-7	8-9
Reading	12.2	18.0	14.8
Writing	19.5	26.4	38.1
Repetition	10.4	21.5	32.9[a]

[a] The repetition task contained 10-letter stimuli which have been included with the 8-9 letter stimuli.

Another aspect of IGR's performance that may be worth considering is the pattern of the ordinal position of errors made in the different tasks. That is, under consideration here is the place in a stimulus--first letter, second letter, third letter, and so forth--where the patient made an error. For this analysis we used a procedure proposed by Wing and Baddeley (1980) which allows us to collapse performance across letter strings of different lengths. We chose to consider a minimum length of 5 positions for this analysis; thus, only, 5-, 6-, 7-, 8-, 9-, and 10-letter-long stimuli were included for analysis (see Wing & Baddeley, 1980, for details of the scoring procedure). Table 8 presents the percentage of errors in reading, writing, and repetition for each of the five stimulus positions: errors are

A. Caramazza

not distributed homogeneously across the five positions in the three tasks $(X^2 (8) = 19.05; P < 0.05)$. The most striking effect concerns the distribution of errors in the reading task where the errors in the initial position are compared to their respective positions in the other tasks. It is unclear, however, what may be contributing to this particular distribution of errors. One possibility that could be entertained is that the relatively elevated level of errors for stimulus initial position in the reading task is due to some type of input deficit. This possibility is suggested by the fact that IGR has a right-hemisphere lesion which could conceivably give rise to some form of impoverished perceptual processing of the left-hand part of the stimulus.

Table 8. Frequency and (percentage) of error position in reading, writing, and repetition (for nonwords of five or more letters).

Task Type	Position				
	1	2	3	4	5
Reading	23(26.7)	19(22.1)	21(24.4)	20(23.2)	3(3.4)
Writing	23(18.2)	39(30.7)	33(25.9)	19(14.9)	13(10.2)
Repetition	11(13.3)	16(19.3)	20(24.1)	21(25.3)	15(18.1)

The analyses reported in this section have revealed differences in IGR's performance in reading, writing and repetition. These differences reflect the contribution of task-specific mechanisms needed for normal processing in one system (e.g., visual-perceptual analysis in reading) or they may reflect the effects of particular processing opportunities in one task or another (e.g., multiple glances at the visual stimulus in reading). It must be stressed, however, that these differences in performance across task types do not diminish the importance of the co-occurrence of a systematic, phonologically-specifiable relationship between errors and target responses in reading, writing, and repetition.

DISCUSSION

In the Introduction we proposed a model of the processing components assumed to underlie the performance of oral reading, writing, and repetition. This model assigned a precise role to the (output)[2] phonological buffer in the execution of these tasks. Specifically, the phonological buffer was assumed to be a working memory space in which are stored phonological representations in preparation for the application of various output processes such as phoneme/grapheme conversion procedures implicated in writing nonwords, and phonological/articulatory mapping procedures needed in producing speech. Given the role of the phonological buffer in oral reading, writing, and repetition, it was hypothesised that damage to this cognitive component should result in a pattern of co-occurring deficits affecting all three tasks and, furthermore, that if any structure was present in the pattern of errors in each of these tasks, it should be explicable in terms of phonological principles. The results we have reported are generally consistent with this hypothesis, although there are features of IGR's performance that invite a more detailed characterisation of the role of the phonological buffer and its relationship to other components of the proposed functional architecture. Indeed, there is the issue of why (given our hypothesis of the locus of functional damage in IGR) there is such a large discrepancy between his performance in reading and repeating words and nonwords. In what follows, we propose a specific elaboration of the hypothesised functional architecture so as to be able to account for the observed discrepancy in processing words and nonwords. We also attempt to explicate in greater detail the nature of the hypothesised damage to the phonological buffer so as to provide a motivated explanation for the pattern of observed errors in reading, writing, and repetition of nonwords.

In the proposed functional architecture for the reading, writing, and repetition processes, the phonological buffer has a relatively transparent and unambiguous role in the writing process. It has been assumed that the phonological buffer is implicated in writing nonwords (and unfamiliar words), but is not needed in writing familiar words. This distinction is easily motivated on theoretical grounds for orthographically opaque languages such as English and French (but we also assume it for Italian, which is an orthographically transparent language). Writing in an orthographically opaque language requires knowledge of word-specific spelling patterns which must be specified in a graphemic code in a graphemic output lexicon. Thus, in writing words, the assumption is that we access representations in the graphemic output lexicon and place these representations directly in a graphemic buffer for subsequent output processes. Nonwords do not have stored graphemic representations in the lexicon and, therefore, writing nonwords to dictation requires that their graphemic representations be computed from the available phonological code. It is assumed that the to-be-written phonological representation is held in the phonological buffer for the application of a procedure that converts phonological segments into graphemic representations. As we pointed out in the Introduction, this processing distinction between writing words and nonwords receives empirical support from patterns of selective writing impairments in brain-damaged patients (e.g., Shallice, 1981; Beauvois & Dérouesné, 1981).

The specific role of the phonological buffer in oral reading and repetition is considerably less clear than its role in writing. In the functional architecture presented in the Introduction, it was assumed that both lexical and non-lexical phonological representations are stored in the phonological buffer in preparation for the application of articulatory processes for speech production. The decision to store both words and nonwords in the phonological buffer prior to the application of articulatory procedures was motivated not so much by specific theoretical considerations as much as by the absence of arguments for distinguishing between the speech production procedures for words and nonwords. This decision has a rather negative consequence, as we will see below.

On the assumption that the phonological buffer is implicated in reading both words and nonwords, our expectation is that damage to this processing component would result in impairment to reading both. The results we have reported for IGR's reading performance do not confirm this expectation--word reading was essentially spared while nonword reading was impaired. These results, then, do not confirm the stated hypothesis of the underlying cause of IGR's pattern of performance. The lack of confirmation concerns a complex hypothesis, however. The hypothesis could be false because, even though the proposed functional architecture for the reading system is correct, it could be that IGR does not have damage to the phonological buffer (but to some other component or components of processing). Alternatively, the hypothesis could be false because, even though the patient does have damage to the phonological buffer, the proposed functional architecture, which assumes that reading words and nonwords implicates the phonological buffer, is wrong. Of course, the hypothesis could also be false because both the assumption that IGR has damage to the phonological buffer is false and the proposed function architecture is wrong. We will be concerned here with evaluating only the first two possibilities.

Unfortunately, we do not have a simple, direct procedure for evaluating whether it is the assumption of damage to the phonological buffer or the hypothesis concerning the role of the phonological buffer in the proposed architecture that is false. Nonetheless, there is a relatively compelling argument that can be offered as a basis for choosing between the two. The argument has two parts. The first part consists of a justification for the claim that the co-occurrence of the specific pattern of nonword processing impairments in IGR is not accidental, but is a reflection of damage to a processing component necessary for normal performance in reading, writing, and repetition of nonwords. The second part of the argument consists of an effort to provide a principled motivation for the assumed role of the phonological buffer in word and nonword output processing.

What characteristics of a patient's performance in different tasks would provide *prima facie* evidence for the hypothesis that damage to a single mechanism is responsible for the impairment in tasks? We would like to propose that, if the pattern of errors across a set of tasks is the same, then we have reasonable grounds for entertaining the possibility that the co-occurring symptoms are functionally related; that is, that the co-occurrence of symptoms results from damage to a common processing mechanism implicated in the performance of those tasks. The pattern of performance in our patient IGR satisfies this criterion: The errors he produced in reading, in writing, and in repetition were very similar and in each case explicable in terms of phonological principles, inviting the assumption that a common mechanism is responsible for the impaired performance in all three types of processes. Thus, there is a clear empirical basis for supposing that damage to a single processing component--the phonological buffer--underlies IGR's pattern of impairment in reading, writing, and repetition. It is equally clear that satisfaction of the criterion of similarity of errors across symptoms *only* establishes that there is an empirical basis for supporting a hypothesis of damage to a common mechanism (it is necessary but not sufficient). Ultimately, however, our confidence in a hypothesis depends on whether we are successful in articulating a motivated functional architecture which when appropriately "lesioned" results in the observed patterns of impairment. In the present case, the issue is whether we can motivate a model for reading, writing, and repetition which assigns to the phonological buffer a critical role in processing nonwords but not in processing words. If we succeed in this task, then the hypothesis that damage to the phonological buffer is the underlying cause for IGR's pattern of impairment would be consistent with the reported results.

In the Introduction we attributed a specific role to the phonological buffer in the proposed model without providing a clear motivation for the assigned role. An analysis of the motivation for this proposal can serve to clarify the role of the phonological buffer in processing words and nonwords.

Two types of mechanisms are included in the proposed functional architecture: computational components that take as input one type of representation and give as output a different type of representation, and buffer systems that hold representations of a particular type of further processing. Examples of the former type of mechanisms are the phonological output lexicon and the phoneme/grapheme conversion system; examples of the latter are the phonological buffer and the graphemic buffer. While the computational components included in the model all have the same formal structure (they serve to convert one type of representation into another), they differ among themselves in two important respects: the computational components differ in the type of representations (e.g., graphemic, phonological, etc.) they compute and in the unit (i.e., the span) of analysis over which they operate. Thus, the output phonological lexicon takes as input lexical-semantic representations and gives as output word- or morpheme-phonological representations. By contrast, the phoneme/grapheme conversion system takes as input phonemic representations (phoneme or syllable units) and gives as output graphemic representations. For present purposes, the difference between these two systems to which we wish to draw attention is the size of units over which computations are carried out. In the case of the phonological lexicon, the units of conversion are words (or morphemes), while in the case of the phoneme/grapheme conversion system, the units of conversion are submorphemic segments (either phonemes or syllables).

The reason for drawing attention to the units of analysis that characterise the components of processing specified in a particular functional architecture is that this feature of components of processing could be the determining factor in decisions regarding whether and where a temporary storage space (buffer) must be included in a processing system. Specifically, the assumption could be made that a buffer must be included in a functional architecture whenever a component of processing operates over a representation that is larger than the units of analysis that characterise that component of processing. Thus for example, since it is assumed that in writing nonwords (to dictation) we transform the phonological representation of the nonword into a graphemic representation through a conversion process that operates over a phonological string longer than the units of conversion, we must postulate the existence of a phonological buffer that holds the to-be-transformed phonological representation while the conversion procedure is being applied. By contrast, in the cognitive systems under consideration here, there is no need to postulate a buffer between the lexical-semantic system and the phonological lexicon since the units of analysis of the two components are equivalent--a lexical-semantic representation maps onto a lexical-phonological representation.

Given this characterisation of the motivation for postulating a buffer in a particular functional architecture, there follows a precise definition of the role of a buffer in a cognitive system: the role of a buffer is to hold temporarily representations that do not correspond to the units of analysis at some point in the flow of information processing. With this definition in hand, we are ready to address the issue of whether both nonwords and words must be held in a phonological buffer at a point where phonological representations are to be converted into articulatory representations for speech production.

By a logic analogous to that used in dealing with the problem of converting phonological representations of nonwords into graphemic representations, we are forced to conclude that the oral production of a nonword (e.g., in reading and repetition) requires that we hold its phonological representation in the phonological buffer while phonological segments are converted into articulatory patterns. This conclusion is motivated by the assumption that phonological/articulatory mapping procedures operate over phonological representations (nonwords) that are larger than the units (phonemes or syllables) that characterise the phonological/articulatory mapping procedures. Thus, on the basis of the assumptions we have made about the role of a buffer, we are led to conclude that the phonological buffer is not only needed in writing nonwords, but also in reading and repeating nonwords.

The important issue to be addressed next is whether the phonological buffer is also needed in reading, writing, and repeating words. We have already presented arguments in favour of the view that the word-writing process need not implicate the phonological buffer; to be decided next is whether word reading and word repetition implicate the phonological buffer. This issue can be decided by determining whether the phonological representation of a word is converted into an articulatory representation through the phonological/articulatory mapping system, as is the case in nonword reading and repetition, or through some other mechanism. If the former, then the phonological buffer is implicated in word reading and repetition. Alternatively, we could assume that the articulatory representations of words are not computed through the application of the phonological/articulatory mapping system, but instead, are addressed directly as preassembled articulatory representations in an articulatory lexicon; that is, the units of analysis involved in computing articulatory representations for words correspond to lexical-phonological representations. In this account of how we compute the articulatory representations of words, there is no need to assume that the phonological representations of words are held in the phonological buffer while they are being converted to articulatory representations, since the input representation corresponds to the unit of analysis of the conversion device. In short, then, rejection of the claim that the phonological buffer is implicated in oral reading and repetition entails that we postulate a lexical-level articulatory representational system which can be addressed directly by lexical-phonological representations. It is important to note here that the claim that single-word production does not implicate the phonological buffer does not mean that this buffer plays no role in lexical processing more generally. Thus, in sentence production we assume that there is a phonological level of representation which must be held in the phonological buffer in the process of computing articulatory representations for speech production. In this account, the issue to be resolved is whether the articulatory representations computed from the sentence- (or clause-) level representation held in the phonological buffer are computed through the phonological/articulatory mapping system or whether articulatory representations are computed through the lexical-articulatory system. This issue is too complex to be addressed here, but there are indications that at least on some occasions sentence production involves the phonological/articulatory mapping system. This latter conclusion is motivated by the existence of phoneme exchange errors in spontaneous speech (e.g., Garrett, 1980). The existence of these errors suggests two conclusions. One conclusion is that the phonological segments of the words that enter in the exchange must be represented simultaneously at some level of processing, and that this level must represent information in a phonological code, since the errors are defined phonologically. We assume that the simultaneous availability of several lexical-phonological representations that can enter in exchange errors implies the existence of a phonological buffer in which lexical forms are held. The other conclusion suggested by phoneme exchange errors is that, at least on some occasions, the articulatory representations for sentence production implicate the phonological/articulatory mapping system. This conclusion is based on the observation that the neologisms that result from exchange errors do not have entries in the lexical-articulatory system and that, therefore, they must be computed through the phonological/ articulatory mapping system. This conclusion is based on the observation that the neologisms that result from exchange errors do not have entries in the lexical-articulatory system and that, therefore, they must be computed through the phonological/articulatory mapping system. In short, then, there is evidence that the phonological buffer and the phonological/articulatory mapping system are implicated in sentence production, but it remains unclear what factors determine the use of the lexical-articulatory and the phonological/articulatory mapping systems in sentence production.

The modified functional architecture incorporating this lexical-articulatory system is represented schematically in Figure 3. The model proposed here offers the basis for a principled account of IGR's pattern of performance. There are three features of IGR's performance we wish to focus attention on:

1. the co-occurrence of selective impairments in reading, writing and repetition of nonwords but not words;
2. the pattern of errors in reading, writing, and repetition of nonwords; and
3. the absence of errors in sentence processing.

The Co-occurrence of selective impairments in reading, writing, and repetition of nonwords receives a ready account in the proposed model--after all, the model was elaborated to serve as the basis for an explanation

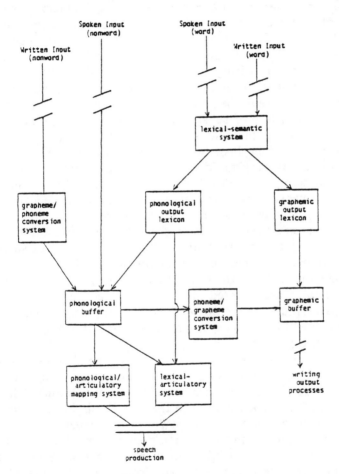

Figure 3. Schematic representation of the functional architecture that includes a computational unit for processing lexical-articulatory representations.

of the obtained pattern of performance by assuming that the patient has damage to the phonological buffer. The interesting issue now is whether the hypothesis of damage to the phonological buffer in this functional architecture can be articulated further so as to provide a reasonable account for other features of IGR's performance. We will consider first the pattern of errors in reading, writing, and repetition.

Almost all of the errors produced by IGR in reading, writing, and repeating nonwords consisted of letter or phoneme substitutions. It is important that the pattern of substitutions was not random; instead, for each task, the substitution errors were clearly explicable in terms of a specific phonological principle: Substitutions were constrained by the feature "manner of articulation." Thus, 81% of the substitutions in reading errors, 82% of the substitutions in repetition errors, and 94% of the substitutions in writing errors, remained within the same category (manner of articulation) as the target response (see Tables 2, 4, and 6). What kind of damage to the phonological buffer must we assume in order to explain this pattern of substitution errors? The hypothesis we would like to propose is that information in the phonological buffer is underspecified, either because of damage which makes phonological information decay very rapidly, or because of damage which results in information being "written in" the system incorrectly to begin with. In either case, however, there is a hierarchy of feature specification such that the phonological information relevant to specifying the manner of articulation is most resistant to loss, while the information relevant to specifying the place of articulation and voicing are most susceptible to loss. The hypothesis, then, is that the phonological buffer is damaged in such a way that the information that specifies place of articulation and voicing features are selected at random. Since manner of articulation information is retained, the random selection of place and voicing features will result in within-category (manner of articulation) substitution errors --the obtained pattern.

The final issue we wish to address concerns the absence of substitution errors in IGR's production of sentences (both in spontaneous speech and in sentence repetition--see Language Evaluation section). This result is, on the face of it, inconsistent with the hypothesis we have proposed for IGR's pattern of impairment. We have argued that single-word production in reading and repetition does not involve the phonological buffer because of the possibility of direct access of lexical-articulatory representations. However, we have also argued that the phonological buffer is necessarily involved in sentence production and therefore, if damaged (as we have hypothesised), sentence production should be impaired even though single-word production would be spared. The results we have reported for IGR's spontaneous production of sentences and sentence repetition would appear to be inconsistent with the predicted dissociation between sentence and word production processing performance. Fortunately, there is a construal of the interaction among the phonological buffer, the phonological output lexicon, and the lexical-articulatory system in sentence production which, in fact, allows us to predict that damage (of the sort we have hypothesised) to the phonological buffer need not result in impaired sentence production.

The modified functional architecture for reading and repetition postulates a lexical-articulatory system that can be addressed either directly from the phonological output lexicon or from the phonological buffer. In the case of sentence production, the lexical-articulatory system must be addressed from the phonological buffer where lexical-phonological representations are temporarily stored for assembly into sentence patterns. Thus, suppose that the patient is trying to produce the sentence "The man bought the book." The information in the phonological buffer should correspond to the phonological representation for that sentence which we could represent as "ðə mæn bɔt ðə bʊk" (considering only segmental information). However, by our hypothesis of the nature of damage to the phonological buffer, some of the lexical-phonological representations will be underspecified; for example, for "mæn" we might only have that the initial segment is an obstruent followed by "æn." This information is not sufficient to access "man" in the lexical-articulatory system; it is "equally"[3] likely to access "man" as "ban," "can," and so on. Thus, if the only information used to select lexical-articulatory representations is that stored in the phonological buffer, we would expect IGR to make errors in sentence production. We could assume, however, that other information may be involved in the selection of lexical-articulatory representations. Specifically, we could assume that lexical-phonological representations activate the corresponding lexical-articulatory representations directly and that the primary role of the phonological representations held in the phonological buffer is to specify the order in which the activated lexical-articulatory representations should be produced. In this case, the underspecified representation "obstruent + æn" would pick out "man" as the lexical articulatory representation to be produced, resulting in intact production of sentences.

The fact that it has been possible to elaborate the functional architecture of the cognitive systems that underlie reading, writing, and repetition so as to serve as the basis for explaining IGR's pattern of performance is not trivial--not just any functional architecture could serve as the basis for explicating the complex pattern of performance reported here. However, the model must not only account for IGR's pattern of performance; it must also serve as the basis for explaining other patterns of performance such as that in other forms of dyslexia and dysgraphia, as well as being compatible with other cognitive systems (e.g., sentence production). Ultimately, our confidence in the explanatory value of a functional architecture depends on its generality as an explanatory framework. It is encouraging, therefore, that functional architectures of this type have been successful in accounting for various patterns of dysgraphia (e.g., Ellis, 1982; Patterson, in press) and dyslexia (e.g. Caramazza & McCloskey, in press; Coltheart, in press).

CONCLUSION

We take it that the goal of cognitive neuropsychology is to articulate the functional architecture of cognitive systems consistent with observed patterns of impairment in brain-damaged patients. By "consistent with," we mean that the relationship between functional architectures and impaired patterns of performance is specified in terms of conditions which must obtain for a proposed functional architecture to generate an observed pattern of impairment. These conditions consist of hypotheses about the locus of damage to a functional architecture. Thus, the explication of a given pattern of impairment consists of articulating a functional architecture which, when "lesioned" appropriately, results in the observed pattern of impairment. Success in this task constitutes empirical support for the proposed functional architecture.

In this paper, we have described in some detail the performance of a patient in reading, writing, and repetition tasks. The patient's performance in these tasks had a remarkably consistent structure--errors were made in repeating, writing, and reading nonwords, and, in each case, the errors were explicable in terms of phonological principles. We have argued that this pattern of impaired performance can be explained as resulting from the proposed functional architecture (see Figure 3) in which the phonological buffer is damaged. However, to provide a successful account of IGR's patten of impairment, we had to make specific assumptions about the role of the phonological buffer. Specifically, we had to assume that the phonological buffer is operational only in those cases where a phonological representation is to be operated upon by a mechanism in which its units of analysis are smaller than the representation over which it is to operate. Furthermore, in order to distinguish between the processing of nonwords and words, we had to assume that lexical-phonological representations can address lexical-articulatory representations directly, obviating the need to assume that processing single words implicates the phonological buffer. By contrast, processing nonwords necessarily implicates the phonological buffer, which, if damaged, would result in a pattern of impairment in reading, writing, and repetition of nonwords, but not words.

The postulation of an independent lexical-articulatory system in the proposed functional architecture is not without cost--it increases the system's power substantially. However, neither is the proposed modification without its benefits. Thus, in addition to providing a principled account for the pattern of impairment found in IGR, the modified functional architecture may provide the basis for explaining an often-noted pattern of performance in cognitively impaired patients that has not received satisfactory explanation. We are referring to that curious situation in which a patient may show considerable difficulty in producing a word in some context but not in another. We can illustrate this point by considering the number-reading performance of a patient (RR) we have studied recently (Caramazza & McCloskey, in press; McCloskey, Caramazza, & Basili, 1985).

This patient shows severe difficulties in reading arabic numbers (e.g., 348 → "two hundred and forty-one"). His pattern of performance is such that it has been possible to locate the locus of impairment within the number reading system, at the level of retrieval of number words from the phonological lexicon. And, yet, the patient can count without major difficulty. This dissociation undermines the hypothesis that the locus of damage in this patient is in retrieving lexical-phonological representations, since he appears not to have difficulties in retrieving these representations in counting. Thus, we are forced to conclude either that our hypothesis of damage to the lexical-phonological system is false, or that counting involves number-production mechanisms different from those implicated in number reading. But the hypothesis of damage to the retrieval process of lexical-phonological representation is too elegant an explanation of RR's complex pattern of number reading impairment for us to want to reject this hypothesis. It is important, then, to entertain seriously the possibility that counting could be accomplished through a process that does not implicate the lexical-phonological retrieval system used in number reading. One possibility is that counting involves the retrieval of a preassembled articulatory routine instead of word-by-word retrieval of number words in the counting sequence. A consequence of this proposal is that it is possible to damage the number reading process without affecting counting. For our purposes, however, the point is that there appears to be good reason to postulate the existence of preassembled articulatory representations for well-learned speech sequences and words. In short, then, although the postulation of preassembled articulatory representations increases considerably the power of functional architectures, it may be necessary to include this level of representation in a complete model of language performance.

ACKNOWLEDGEMENTS

The research reported here was supported by a grant from the Centro Nazionale Delle Ricerche (Italy), by NIH Grant No. 14099 to The Johns Hopkins University, and by Biomedical Research Support Grant S07-RR07041, Division of Research Resources, National Institutes of Health. We would like to thnak Michael McCloskey, Bill Badecker, Howard Egeth, and Roberta Goodman for their comments on an earlier version of this paper. We thank Karalyn Patterson and two anonymous reviewers whose criticisms forced us to consider important factors we had overlooked. We also thank Kathy Sporney for her help in various stages of the preparation of this manuscript.

REFERENCES

Beauvois, M. F. & Dérouesné, J. (1981).	Lexical or orthographic agraphia. Brain, 104, 21-49.

Caramazza, A. (1986).	On drawing inferences about the structure of normal cognitive systems from the analysis of patterns of impaired performance: The case for single-patient studies. Brain and Cognition, 5, 41-66.

Caramazza, A., Berndt, R. S. & Basili, A. (1983).	The selective impairment of phonological processing:	A case study. Brain and Language, 18, 128-174.

Caramazza, A. & McCloskey, M. (in press). Number system processing: Evidence from dyscalculia. In Cohen, Schwartz & Moscovitch (Eds.), Advances in cognitive neuropsychology. New York, NY:	Guilford Press.

Caramazza, A., Miceli, G., Silveri, M. C. & Laudanna, A. (1985). Reading mechanisms and the organization of the lexicon:	Evidence from acquired dyslexia. Cognitive Neuropsychology, 2, 81-114.

Coltheart, M. (in press). Cognitive neuropsychology and the study of reading. Attention and Performance XI. Hillsdale, NJ:	Lawrence Erlbaum Associates, Inc.

DeRenzi, E. & Faglioni, P. (1978). Normative data and screening power of a shortened version of the Token Test. Cortex, 14, 41-49.

Ellis, A. W. (1982). Spelling and writing (and reading and speaking). In A. W. Ellis (Ed.), Normality and pathology in cognitive functions. London:	Academic Press.

Ellis, A. W. (in press). Modelling the writing process. In G. Denes, C. Semenza, P. Bisiacchi & E. Andreewsky (Eds.), Perspectives in cognitive neuropsychology. London: Lawrence Erlbaum Associates Ltd.

Ellis, A. W., Miller, D. & Sin, G. (1983). Wernicke's aphasia and normal language processing: A case study in cognitive neuropsychology. Cognition, 15, 111-144.

Garrett, M. F. (1980). Levels of processing in sentence production. In B. Butterworth (Ed.), Language production. New York, NY: Academic Press.

Goodman, R. & Caramazza, A. (1986). Dissociation of spelling errors in writing and oral spelling: The role of allographic conversion in writing. Cognitive Neuropsychology, 3, 179-206.

Hatfield, F. M. & Patterson, K. E. (1983). Phonological spelling. Quarterly Journal of Experimental Psychology, 35A, 451-468.

Marcel, T. (1980). Surface dyslexia and beginning reading: A revised hypothesis of the pronunciation of print and its impairments. In M. Coltheart, K. E. Patterson & J. C. Marshall (Eds.), Deep dyslexia. London: Routledge & Kegan Paul.

McCarthy, R. & Warrington, E. K. (1984). A two-route model of speech production: Evidence from aphasia. Brain, 107, 463-485.

McCloskey, M., Caramazza, A. & Basili, A. (1985). Cognitive mechanisms in number processing and calculation: Evidence from dyscalculia. Brain and Cognition, 4, 171-196.

Miceli, G., Silveri, M. C. & Caramazza, A. (1985). Cognitive analysis of a case of pure dysgraphia. Brain and Language, 25, 187-212.

Miller, D. & Ellis, A. W. (in press). Speech and writing errors in "neologistic jargon aphasia": A lexical activation hypothesis. In M. Coltheart, R. Job & G. Sartori (Eds.), Cognitive neuropsychology of language.

Morton, J. (1980). The logogen model and orthographic structure. In U. Frith (Ed.), Cognitive processes in spelling. London: Academic Press.

Nolan, K. A. & Caramazza, A. (1983). An analysis of writing in a case of deep dyslexia. Brain and Language, 20, 305-328.

Patterson, K. (in press). Acquired disorders of spelling. In G. Denes, C. Semenza, P. Bisiacchi & E. Andreewsky (Eds.), Perspectives in cognitive neuropsychology. London: Lawrence Erlbaum Associates Ltd.

Shallice, T. (1981). Phonological agraphia and the lexical route in writing. Brain, 104, 413-429.

Wing, A. M. & Baddeley, A. D. (1980). Spelling errors in handwriting: A corpus and a distributional analysis. In U. Frith (Ed), Cognitive processes in spelling. London: Academic Press.

APPENDIX 1 ERRORS MADE BY IGR IN READING
Abbreviation key: m=masculine; f=feminine; sg=singular; p=plural)

A) Words

ossia	(that is)	ossia	
notati	(noticed, m.pl.)	nottati	
tirano	(they pull)	tirano	
saluti	(cheers)	salute	(health)
stavolta	(this time)	talvolta	(sometimes)
macchina	(car)	macchine	(cars)
contento	(happy, m.sg.)	contenta	(happy, f.sg.)
toglievo	(I was taking away)	coglievo	(I was picking)
dimostro	(I show)	timosto	
rimarrai	(you will remain)	rimarrei	(I should remain)

B) Nonwords

sote	sode (firm, f.pl.)	cevini	chevini
drugga	grugga	isco	isto
viveta	vivete (you live)	novve	noffe
cotova	cotove	ghita	chita
raporto	rapporto (relationship)	vicro	vistro
tieno	dieno	zicri	zieri
ucchido	ugghido	vuldo	fundo
giodere	gioghere	dagno	bagno (bath)
fispico	fispito	fomigna	fomiglia
mirpe	mirne	ferdire	verdire
diffa	biffa	ebbiomo	ebbiono
caroi	cardi	bammine	babbine
tulma	tulpa	dregupo	gregulopo
brelve	prelve	resteto	certeto
padone	patone	arrasti	arasti (you sowed)
pascri	pastri	ripano	rippano
dochio	doglio	refleto	repleto
frusca	frusta (whip)	getruva	cetruva
mansote	sansote	uttico	uttito
libongi	lipongi	scurpe	urpe
ulebbia	uleppia	sfuppa	sfulpa
salcoti	santoti	slomba	splomba
sghioto	schioto	mucrile	mutrile
fistrelo	fisprelo	pamugno	pamuglio
lerucedo	lerugedo	bilotro	pilotro
antruspa	altruspo	ghennia	chiennia

fiutirei	fiuterei (I would sniff)	cabonti	capunti
garnace	carnace	trefova	trevova
teleffono	telefono (telephone)	saziuto	sazionto
spalute	spallute	pulzova	sulzova
fotopravi	fototravi	destevi	destivi
sinistaro	sinistraro	turbeto	turbito
sfergande	sfercande	albergio	alberghio
cisbustri	cispustri	ghiurare	chiurare
occulesti	oddulisti	pecrolio	petrolio (oil)
compensei	ponsensei	scoltondo	scoltoldo
elvitare	elvidare	priginondo	priginundo
asodunte	osodunte	fributeggia	friputelgia
chiagico	chiasico		

APPENDIX 2 ERRORS MADE BY IGR IN WRITING TO DICTATION

A) Words

anzi	(to the contrary)	alzi	(you lift)
dello	(of the, m.sg.)	tello	
rango	(rank)	zango	
padre	(father)	badre	
pacco	(package)	Bacco	(Bacchus)
invaso	(invaded, m.sg.)	indaso	
talora	(sometimes)	dallora	
alzare	(to life)	anzare	
ritiene	(he thinks)	ridiene	
ventura	(venture)	fentura	
discorso	(discourse)	discordo	(I disagree)
soltanto	(only)	soltando	
eseguite	(executed, f. sg.)	eseguire	(to execute)
altronde	(on the other hand)	altromte	
tendenza	(tendency)	tentenza	
scrissero	(they wrote)	scrissono	

B) Nonwords

zibo	zito	giorovi	giovovi
deie	beie	fentota	ventota
izzi	izi	ebbiomo	ebiomo
voda	foda	ebbiomo	ediomo

A. Caramazza

laci	lasi	ebbiomo	ebieno
pefi	befi	omunqua	nomqua
nafo'	naffo'	cimpito	incito
egne	egnie		(I incite)
delto	telto	cimpito	cimbito
vicro	vidro	pidogno	pidognio
vicro	vigro	pidogno	biodogno
tieno	dieno	bammine	bamine
derso	terso (terse)	bammine	babamba
cecchio	ciechio	besmi	besni
cecchio	cechio	efile	evile
stedere	stetere	astirova	aspirova
birdi	birti	dirando	tiramdo
ospao	ostao	intarno	indarno
mopie	motie	battivi	battavi
pinco'	pinco	sarciti	serciti
chebo	chepo	fermiva	ferviva
oldine	oltine	sentuti	sentute
dochio	docchio	abitire	apitire
prelmo	prelpo	salvite	alvite
pascri	pasri	baltovi	bantovi
siglio	silio	cardune	cartutine
siglio	sillio	nortedi	nordeti
vosato	fosado	effista	efista'
ledria	letria	chiedva	chietiva
everti	eferti	grendine	grentine
imieto	inieto	cancetto	cancietto
pascri	pastri	cerriera	ceriera
guirta	ciurta	cerriera	cieriera
tolori	taloli	eristoti	eristovi
cudore	codore	somprovi	sonprovi
dettro	detto (said, m.sg.)	scastovi	stastovi
somitovi	somitoi	cemigiana	ciemigiana
ripano	repano	sposendo	spovendo
uttico	uttito	dormerei	dormenei
pedovi	pebovi	deleguto	teleguto
veveta	fefeti	scartivi	startivi
letimi	lepini	dettimmo	detimmo
fomignia	fomiglia	scampotte	stampotte
fomignia	foninia	cirbatoio	cirbattoio
santando	sandando	sfergande	sfergante
patremmo	papremmo	guanciasi	guanciavi

sontommo	sontonmo	sinistaro	sinistraro
gambiano	ganbbiano	aerocrano	aerotrano
crodezza	crobezza	cavalieno	cavallieno
crodezza	grodezza	coragghio	coraghio
opprenso	oppremso	atmorpera	ar.....
altiande	altiante	ciomunque	ciononque
tondinza	contimza	fumpelcri	funchelgri
strivule	strivune	occulesti	occhulesti
aiupotte	aupotte	crastulpa	grastulpa
cirenghi	cirenchi	cisbustri	cisburti
vallunde	valunde	orenghino	orengino
paruntri	parundrie	nurzioche	unzioche
gotadepo'	catadepo	cruzialpo	truzialpo
sfanciova	svangiova	blapistro	blatrispo
bindrista	binti...	posciggio	posiggio
bindrista	bintrista	diventufe	diventuse
nedasbori	nebasbori	taccormia	tattormia
tasciolfo	tasciolvo	canquirpa	cancui...
tasciolfo	casciolvo	tatografo	dato...
landrasto'	landrasto	scrissovo	sgri...
landrasto'	lantraspo	ghinderte	ghinterte
madessipi	mate....	doccarbia	docarbia
madessipi	madespiti	zobralgio	zobrancio
colaziofi	colazionfi	corbattovi	corbatovi
forettore	forrettore	fributeggia	frimuteggia

APPENDIX 3 ERRORS MADE BY IGR IN REPETITION

Nonwords

codo	goto	tacro	tagro
pepo	peco	frice	frige
bade	pade	pascri	pastri
piga	biga	refona	revona
tobo	pogo	pedita	petita
daca	cada (that he falls, subjunctive present)	goduto	do...
pagodo	pagoto	cadata	gadata
Tapico	capico	cubaco	cupaco
sgatro	scatrio	atmorpera	atmopera
brasna	crasna	fumpelcri	fumpeltri
maveca	maveva,	orisivati	orusivati
		blapistro	blatrispo

	mavesa	siocciono	schioccono
zobuti	sobuti	boltistia	boltischia
pazoli	padzorli	gramidota	draminota
telpito	telpido	garzucali	gra....
gamorda	damorta	tadrupari	tal....
asemugo	asemuco	rafubrasa	raudrasa
psilone	stilone	sacrivagi	sacrivasi
sganutta	sganuta	ganaltiza	nada...
laffusco	lass...	lapriveco	lat....
moccalno	moccarno	gacrupite	gacopite
zirreplo	zinreplo	vazaltine	zav....
crodezza	crotezza	castizuvo	castezugo
santando	santanto	zavarsufi	zavarstufi
fronista	frondista	fularsade	fularzate
marmosca	marmoscia	darolcigo	dalorcigo
canfegna	canvegna	pavrutiga	pavu...
riadruse	riacruse	saduborli	sadi...
viarbafe	riar...	poltriglia	boltriglia
sdarablo	stara..	sgacrastia	sgatrastia
draspico	traspico	riadrascio	riagrasico
brisnavo	brismago	viarbusilo	viasbusilo
valosafo	valosavo	brasnupora	brammu...
secuvego	ve....	flumangera	flumangela
buferipe	b.....	spamorbico	spamorpilo
dizegiva	zid...	carpestice	cas....
metinace	metinacce	prunirceva	prumircela
sodubeli	sonubeli	mastablica	mastag...
zapafise	zafa...	taldaprico	talpaprico
madiraco	madirago	gartosmini	gartosbini
cosazuva	cozu...	mircolnita	mircolmita
sadabulo	sagabulo	pradistosa	pratistosa
petudino	petiu...	frumponesal	fruntonesa
vazelena	vaze....	ragruntire	ran...tran...
radisaga	raddisago	sganormile	sganormire
cemigiana	genegiana	mircalpave	mircanpave
orenghino	ortenghino	sfabindile	sfabindire
venocchio	fenocchio	tarmancona	tarbangona
madessipi	madespidi	gratmovica	gratmoviga
bindrista	bindirista	larfascuni	larfantuni
poltrilia	poltriglia	drampizone	tranpizone
aerocrano	aerotrano		

NOTES

[1] Alternative functional architectures of the reading and writing systems have been proposed which do not implicate grapheme/phoneme and phoneme/grapheme conversion processing components (e.g., Marcel, 1980). However, given the relatively underspecified nature of the two types of functional architectures--the lexically-based and non-lexically-based models--we have little basis for choosing between the two at this time (see Caramazza, 1986).

[2] We are unsure whether we ought to distinguish between an output and an input phonological buffer, or whether we need only assume a single phonological buffer that is used both in input and output processing--hence the parentheses around output.

[3] We have placed equally in quotation marks to indicate that the probability of choosing any one of the representations compatible with the input may not, in fact, be equal but may be determined by other factors, for example frequency of usage.

CHAPTER FOUR

THE ANALYSIS OF
MORPHOLOGICAL ERRORS IN A CASE
OF ACQUIRED DYSLEXIA

INTRODUCTION

The linguistic analysis of words provides a rich array of formal and functional characteristics that would appear to be at least potentially relevant to an understanding of language processing.[1] However, while the description and explanation of numerous phenomena from the domain of grammatical competence rely importantly on these concepts, there has been little progress in demonstrating their relevance to the explanation of linguistic performance. The crux of the problem is that, if we wish to construct a psychologically valid model of lexical processing, theoretically minimal, linguistic solutions cannot be given precedence over the actual mechanisms that subjects employ. The question of whether a morphologically complex word will be generated by a rule-like mechanism or will simply be listed in the lexicon, for example, must be given the same answer by the linguist and the psychologist at some level of description.[2] In this paper we will consider some of the issues that are special to the study of processing mechanisms, and we will examine how they bear on demonstrations of the effects of word structure on lexical processing. In particular, we will focus on the analysis of lexical mechanisms as revealed by neurolinguistic data.

Studies of lexical processing by subjects with selective language deficits have tended to deal primarily with the processing of visually presented stimuli. With regard to the effect of lexical structure on lexical processing, the question that has received the most attention is whether morphologically complex words are decomposed and, if so, whether decomposition occurs prior to or after lexical access. Many researchers have argued from the occurrence of dyslexic errors such as reading *initiate* as *initiative*, or *slavery* as *slaving* that complex words are indeed decomposed by one means or another (see, for example, Patterson, 1980, 1982; and Job and Sartori, 1984); and have referred to such paralexias as derivational errors. In order to avoid confusion with linguistic terminology regarding the types of affixation (inflectional vs. derivational), we will adopt the more apt term "morphological error" when referring to paralexias of this kind. Commonly, morphological errors are distinguished in neurolinguistic reports from visual errors (e.g., reading *threat* as *thread*) and semantic errors (e.g., reading *spout* as *nozzle*, or *contents* as *index*). Ideally, though, the classification of errors should reflect the nature of the functional impairment that results in their production: visual errors following from deficits in the (visual) input processing stages of reading, semantic errors resulting from some less peripheral impairment in the lexical system (e.g., a lexical-semantic system), and morphological errors engendered by damage to some morphological processing component. Nevertheless, the fact that subjects who produce morphological reading errors in many cases also produce one or both of these other error types makes it quite difficult to establish that the functional locus of the effect leading to the morphological errors is indeed a processing component that is organized according to the morphemic structure of words. A visual error often cannot be construed as being semantically related to the target (as with *threat* and *thread*), just as many semantic errors are visually dissimilar from the stimulus (e.g., when *harder* was read as *strong*, or *common* as *freight*). When the same subject reads a word like *disconnect* as *connection*, though, we have an error response that is both visually and semantically related to the stimulus.[3] How can we establish (one way or the other) whether these so-called morphological errors are actually visual, semantic or (true) morphological errors? (That is, errors resulting from damage to visual and/or semantic and/or morphological processing mechanisms?) More generally, do these errors in any way reflect morphological principles of organization in the lexicon?

In order to answer these questions in a particular case, one must begin by selecting some sort of theoretical framework within which these errors could be explained. The model of lexical processing that appears most tenable to us is one which distinguishes mechanisms according to level (positing distinct lexical input and output mechanisms in addition to central, semantic processing mechanisms) as well as discriminating input- and output-component modalities. That is, the model posits separate lexical input mechanisms for visual and for auditory stimuli (and similarly for lexical output mechanisms). Figure 1 indicates the relational characteristics of such a model.

One consequence of this functional architecture is that it should be possible for the components of this system to be selectively compromised by brain damage, and this selective disruption should be reflected in the patterns of performance on various tasks. For example, a deficit in the Orthographic Input System should not affect a subject's performance on repetition tasks, although it would be expected to impair performance on reading and auditory/visual stimulus matching tasks. In particular, damage to a visual processing component of this input system may be expected to result in the production of visual error responses, since this component is, by hypothesis, organized along dimensions corresponding to the visual properties of words. Similarly, errors resulting from a disruption in the lexical semantic system (which should be evident in performance on tasks involving either input modality) should reflect those lexical properties according to which that system is organized (e.g., semantic associations). If a morphological processing mechanism has been disrupted, then it is also reasonable to expect that, for example, reading errors resulting from this disruption will reflect the lexical characteristics which organize the impaired component (including the morphological properties of words).

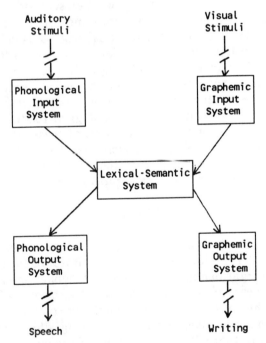

Figure 1.

In addition to the lexical properties that we have identified in terms of this broadly specified architecture of lexical mechanisms, there are certain other factors which are known to affect lexical processing, among which are included letter length, concreteness (e.g., Kroll and Merves, 1986), frequency (e.g., Gordon, 1983), and grammatical category (e.g., Miceli, Silveri, Villa and Caramazza, 1984). However, an appeal to these or other lexical factors to account for a subject's performance on lexical tasks can only make sense in the context of a tenable theory of how and when these lexical characteristics induce their effects under various conditions of dysfunction. For example, in the models of lexical processing we accept, it is not the characteristics of an item in isolation, but only the characteristics of an item in the context of the set of items related along particular dimensions that may affect reading performance. Furthermore, there are instances where a deficit in one lexical component can induce a pattern of performance that reflects the organizing principles of another, intact mechanism which interacts with the disrupted processing component--a point which we will elaborate on below. We would contend that a major flaw in most studies of patients whose lexical paraphasias include morphological errors is that they have not formulated their analysis in the context of any theory of when such performance patterns can occur. In this paper we will present some hypotheses concerning the influence of these factors in cases of lexical processing deficits, presenting our suggestions primarily in a discussion of our own attempts to analyze the reading performance of one subject, FM, whose errors include those of the type operationally defined as morphological. After presenting this subject, we will return to a discussion of the standard arguments concerning the interpretation of morphological reading errors of brain damaged subjects. We will argue that most of these attempts to establish the existence of a morphological deficit have been unsuccessful, largely because they have failed to pursue their analyses in the context of a sufficiently explicit model of lexical processing.

CASE HISTORY

FM is a 43 year old, right-handed, male high-school graduate who suffered a large left middle cerebral artery infarct in 1981, which left him with moderate right hemiparesis and with language impairments. A CT scan done two years after his CVA showed a large area of lucency on the left involving the posterior inferior frontal lobe, the inferior parietal lobe, the anterior temporal lobe, and the underlying white matter and lateral basal ganglia, together with some atrophy of the cortex of the remainder of the left frontal convexity.

At the time of this study (four years post onset), FM's speech is considered nonfluent with reduced phrase length, and his performance on sentence processing tasks such as sentence-picture matching reveals "asyntactic" comprehension (i.e., he was significantly worse on matching thematically "reversible" sentences like *the boy kissed the girl* than on "nonreversible" sentences like *the boy threw the rock*). His speech is labored, and he produces literal paraphasias and some morphological errors. FM's reading performance includes errors of visual, semantic, inflectional (*sew → sewing*; *decayed → decays*; or *walks → walk*), derivational (*achieve → achievement*; *disconnect → connection* or *worker → work*), and other (unclassified) types, as well as correct responses. Morphological errors (especially affix deletions and substitutions) were the most common error type for morphologically complex stimuli, although FM's reading errors also include a substantial number of affix insertions for monomorphemic stimuli.

Summary of Reading Performance

FM's reading was evaluated extensively (Gordon, Goodman and Caramazza, reference note 1; Caramazza, 1985), with emphasis on analysis of his visual and semantic errors. The resulting corpus of reading responses serves here as the basis for a preliminary description of his performance. The pattern of his analyzable responses is indicated in Table 1.

Table 1. Summary of reading responses and breakdown of number and overall percentage of error types (reported in Caramazza, 1985).

Analyzable Responses	Number	Percent
Correct	1778	43%
Incorrect	2393	57%
Derivational errors	202	5%
Inflectional errors	478	12%
Visual errors	556	13%
Semantic errors	461	11%
Other classifiable errors	709	17%

As Gordon, Goodman and Caramazza (reference note 1) report, words that were read incorrectly were consistently longer (by letter length) and less concrete than those that were read correctly, although the over-all frequency comparison between stimuli and responses was equivocal. However, for both the visual and semantic errors, FM's responses tended to be more frequent than the stimuli (as determined from the Kucera and Francis, 1967, norms), in addition to being shorter and less abstract.

A. Caramazza

In reading and lexical comprehension tasks, visual and semantic errors were shown to be distinguishable in terms of the lexical processing stage that is compromised. For example, because he tended on retesting to produce visual errors on words that he had **previously** responded to with a visual error (and because he was similarly consistent for items which induced semantic errors), it was possible to determine whether these stimuli were understood correctly. FM showed "good" comprehension of words which he had consistently read correctly and for which he had produced semantic errors (86% and 80% correct respectively), while he demonstrated correct comprehension of words which had induced visual errors on previous presentations substantially less often (36% correct response rate). Similarly, preliminary results from a single-subject lexical decision experiment with FM indicate that there is semantic priming when the prime is a word that had been read correctly or had induced a semantic error, but not when the priming stimulus is a word which he had produced a visual error for on earlier occasions (Raymer and Caramazza, reference note 2). These results provide strong evidence concerning where the lexical processing system breaks down for particular words. A word that is read correctly activates an entry in both the graphemic input lexicon and the phonological output lexicon, while a word which induces a semantic error activates the proper entry in the graphemic input lexicon, but not the correct entry in the phonological output lexicon. This could be because the lexical-semantic system has been compromised, or because of damage to the phonemic output lexicon. Finally, a word which induces a visual error fails to activate the correct entry in the orthographic input lexicon.[4] These aspects of FM's reading performance provide an important starting point for an interpretation of the morphological errors he produces.

An analysis of the inflectional and derivational errors referred to in Table 1 revealed two interesting contrasts: FM performed better on words with the agentive -er suffix than with the comparative -er suffix (54% vs. 2% correct responses), and was more likely to mistakenly insert or substitute the agentive suffix (21 insertions, 5 substitutions) than the comparative suffix (zero insertions and substitutions).[5] Similarly, the plural morpheme -s was read correctly more often than the third person singular suffix -s (75/240 correct vs. 2/28 correct), and the plural morpheme was also inserted more often than the verbal inflection (103 vs. 2 insertions).[6] While it was entirely possible that some of these contrasts merely reflect a disparity in the number of nouns, verbs and adjectives that occurred in the corpus[7] (especially in the case of morphological insertion and substitution errors), this could not be the entire story (as, for example, with the correct responses and deletions).

Furthermore, there were some interesting contrasts with the visual and semantic errors that FM produced. Recall, for example, that when he produced a visual or semantic error, the response was consistently more frequent than the stimulus. This was also the case when FM produced a morphological deletion error on the agentive and comparative stimuli (e.g., *dancer → dance* and *smaller → small*). However, when the agentive *-er* was either inserted or substituted for another suffix, the response was less frequent than the stimulus in 21 of the 26 cases. Given that the comparative *-er* was never inserted or substituted for another suffix, we have a strong candidate for a dissociation defined along a morphological dimension. For these reasons, it might appear that some of the errors FM produced were the result of a deficit to a morphological processing component. To test this hypothesis, FM was given a series of reading tests with new controlled lists.

Controlled Morphological Processing Tasks

The first reading tasks to be described here were administered to determine whether the factor most affecting the likelihood of FM producing a morphological error is the visual similarity between the stimulus and morphologically related response. Three separate lists of test items were composed, each matching items that contain pseudo-stems (like *earn* in *earnest*) with affixed and unaffixed controls. If morphological errors result from a visual processing deficit simply because the stem of an affixed stimulus competes with the whole stimulus item for activation, then lexical items with embedded words (the pseudo-stems) should induce analogous, pseudo-morphological errors (i.e., where the pseudo-stem is preserved in the response, but the "affix" has either been deleted or replaced with an actual prefix or suffix).

(1) *Pseudosuffix list.* There were 43 monomorphemic, pseudo-suffixed words (e.g., *wicked, corner,* etc.) matched in surface frequency[8] and letter length with 43 regularly suffixed and 43 unaffixed controls. Frequencies ranged from 200.4 to 0.1 on the Carroll et al. U distribution, (mean frequencies for the three sublists were 44.8, 31.2 and 43.6 for pseudosuffixed, suffixed and unaffixed words respectively); and letter length ranged from 5 to 9 (with mean length of 5.9, 6.5 and 6.1 for the pseudosuffixed, suffixed and unaffixed lists).

(2) *Embedded words list 1 ("suffixed").* There were 85 monomorphemic words[9] containing initial letter sequences which are also words (e.g., *yearn, dogma, pierce,* etc.) matched in surface frequency and letter length with 85 regularly suffixed and 85 unaffixed controls. The "suffixes" attached to the embedded words in the test items (*-n, -ma,* and *-ce* in the

examples) ranged from one to two letters in length. Frequency values ranged from 173.6 to 0.1 on the Carroll et al. U distribution, with means of 17.4, 17.4, and 17.3 for the embedded words, affixed controls and unaffixed controls respectively. Letter length ranged from 5 to 7, with a mean value of 5.5 on each list.

(3) *Embedded words list 2 ("prefixed").* There were 52 monomorphemic words containing final letter sequences which are also words (e.g., *bland*, *borough*, *frock*, etc.) matched in letter length and surface frequency with 52 prefixed and 52 unaffixed controls. The "prefixes" attached to the embedded words in the test list ranged in length from one to three letters. Frequency values ranged from 179.7 to 0.1 on the U distribution (with means of 14.3, 13,9 and 13.1 on the embedded, prefixed and unaffixed lists respectively); and letter length ranged from 4 to 9 (with means of 5.5, 6.4 and 5.9 on embedded words, prefixed controls and unaffixed controls respectively).

Stimuli from these three sets of items were typed on 3x5 unlined index cards and were presented in pseudo-random, unblocked order. Responses were transcribed at the time of testing, and were recorded on a cassette tape recorder for comparison when needed. Errors were scored as morphological, visual, semantic or other; and morphological errors were further categorized as deletions, substitutions or insertions. The results for the three tasks are presented in Tables 2-4.

At first blush, the results for these lists appear to support the hypothesis that visual similarity between stimuli and responses cannot account for FM's morphological errors: while differences between correct and incorrect reading of the test words and unaffixed controls were not significant in any of the three tasks, this was not true for comparisons between test words and suffixed controls (X^2 = 41.27, p < 0.001, two-tailed) from the first embedded words list, nor between test words and prefixed controls (X^2 = 13.05, p < 0.001, two-tailed) from the second embedded words list. (The comparison between pseudosuffixed words like *corner* and suffixed words, however, failed to reach significance: X^2 = 3.46, p < 0.10, two-tailed.) Pseudomorphological errors like *fleece → fled* or *device → vice* occurred much less often than morphological errors like *bowled → bowling* or *deport → import, outport.* If FM's "true" morphological errors (in the operational sense) arise because of the visual similarity between a stimulus and his morphologically related response, one would not expect to find differences between the test items from the embedded words lists and their affixed controls. The fact that FM produces more pseudomorphological errors (e.g., deletions like *corner → corn*, and substitutions like *earnest → earning*) on the pseudosuffix list might, in fact, serve as evidence for an input deficit affecting whole word recognition, but not morphological parsing, as in the model of lexical processing proposed by Caramazza, Miceli, Silveri and Laudanna (1985).

Table 2. Numbers (and proportions) of reading response types for the pseudoaffixed word list.

	Pseudoaffixed Words	Affixed Controls	Unaffixed Controls
Correct	23 (.53)	14 (.33)	29 (.67)
Errors			
Morphological	7 (.16)	19 (.44)	2 (.05)
Deletions	4*	16	--
Substitutions	2*	3	--
Insertion	1	--	2
Semantic	4 (.09)	2 (.05)	4 (.09)
Visual	5 (.12)	3 (.07)	5 (.12)
Other	4 (.09)	5 (.12)	3 (.07)
Total	43	43	43

* These numbers represent pseudomorphological errors like <u>earnest</u> → <u>earning</u>.

Table 3. Number (and proportion) of reading response types for the embedded words list #1 ("suffixes").

	Embedded Words	Suffixed Controls	Unaffixed Controls
Correct	52 (.6)	11 (.13)	55 (.65)
Errors			
Morphological	15 (.18)	57 (.67)	3 (.04)
Deletions	10*	49	--
Substitutions	1*	8	--
Insertions	3	--	3
Semantic	5 (.06)	7 (.08)	4 (.05)
Visual	10 (.12)	4 (.05)	14 (.16)
Other	2 (.02)	6 (.07)	9 (.11)
Total	84	85	85

* These numbers represent pseudomorphological errors: e.g., <u>castle</u> → <u>cast</u>.

However, a rival account of FM's performance on these tasks attributes the differences between the error patterns on the embedded words lists and the affixed controls to differences in surface frequency and stem frequency[10] patterns. Given that it is generally true that the stem of an arbitrary affixed word is more frequent than its surface form, apparent

Table 4. Number (and proportion) of reading response types for embedded words list #2 ("prefixes").

	Embedded Words	Prefixed Controls	Unaffixed Controls
Correct	25 (.48)	7 (.13)	27 (.52)
Errors			
Morphological	10 (.19)	25 (.48)	5 (.10)
Deletions	8*	20	--
Substitutions	--	1	--
Insertions	2	4	5
Semantic	2 (.04)	8 (.15)	1 (.02)
Visual	15 (.29)	7 (.13)	15 (.29)
Other	--	5 (.10)	4 (.08)
Total	52	52	52

* This number represents pseudomorphological errors like crevice → vice.

morphological deletion errors might arise from a visual processing deficit that favors the access of the more frequent form. So, on this account, if the (pseudosuffixed) stimulus *wicked* activates both *wick* and *wicked* in the orthographic input system, one factor that can reasonably be expected to affect the outcome of the competition between the two items is their frequency relative to one another. Thus, one might predict that, given the frequency sensitivity evidenced in the pattern of visual error responses in FM's corpus of errors, FM would be more likely to produce a morphological deletion or substitution error if the stem or pseudostem of an item is more frequent than the stimulus. On this account we need only posit a visual processing deficit to explain the pattern of responses indicated in Tables 2-4. An analysis of FM's errors on the pseudosuffix words list and the embedded words list #1 (suffixed), broken down according to the relative frequency of the surface form and pseudostem, was carried out to determine the proportion of errors that were scored as pseudomorphological in the different frequency categories. FM's errors were more likely to be pseudomorphological errors on forms whose pseudostem frequency exceeded their surface frequency than on forms whose surface frequency was greater than their pseudostem frequency. 46% (17/37) of FM's errors were scored as pseudomorphological for items whose pseudostems were more frequent than their surface form, while only 17% (2/15) of the errors on items whose surface form was more frequent than the corresponding pseudostem were pseudomorphological errors. (Chi-square comparisons fall just shy of significant levels: $X^2 = 3.59$, $df = 1$, $p < 0.10$, two-tailed.) Since stem frequency is known to have an effect on the access of morphologically complex words (Taft, 1979; Bradley, 1980; Burani, Salmaso and Caramazza, 1984), and since most of FM's morphological and pseudomorphological errors are deletion errors, one must entertain the possibility that the better performance on the pseudosuffix and embedded words lists is the product of a number of converging factors (including visual similarity and lexical frequency) that simply favored the production of more "functionally" visual errors on the morphologically complex control items. That is, the fact that FM read the stimulus *center* correctly, but read *faster* as *fast*, may simply be due to the fact that <u>enter</u> is more frequent than its pseudostem *cent*, while *faster* is much less frequent than its stem *fast*, and the lexical representation corresponding to the more frequent item--whether it be the actual stimulus or its (pseudo-) stem--is significantly easier to access. As we already mentioned, this proposal is especially relevant given that the visual errors in the reading corpus were generally more frequent than their corresponding stimuli.

One way to circumvent the frequency-effect counter-argument is to look at cases where the morphemes involved are known not to be governed by the relative frequency of the stem morpheme. Recall that in the corpus of errors, the agentive suffix *-er* was not only preserved more often than the comparative *-er* suffix, but it was also produced more often in morpheme insertion errors. Since the form produced in the case of insertion errors was virtually always (21/26 instances) less frequent than the stimulus item, stem frequency would not appear to be the controlling factor in the production of the agentive ending. Furthermore, the fact that the distribution of the two *-er* morphemes differed in the corpus is also important, as it appears to provide a good candidate for a pattern of reading performance that is definable in morphological terms. In order to test whether this contrast would stand up under controlled conditions another reading task was administered comparing the two types of *-er* words. While we could not expect to induce specific morpheme insertion errors on the controlled tasks, we can expect to see if a similar pattern of correct responses vs. morphological deletions and substitutions will obtain.

(4) *Agentive vs. Comparative -er List.* There were 34 deverbal nouns formed with the agentive *-er* suffix matched in surface frequency and letter length to 34 comparative adjectives formed with the regular *-er* suffix. Frequency values range from 183.0 to 3.7; with mean frequency of 38.6 (s.d. = 43.9) and letter length of 6.2 for the comparative adjectives, and frequency and letter length of 19.5 (s.d. = 26.6) and 6.3 respectively for the agentive nominals.[11]

Of course, one stimulus feature that could not be controlled for in this comparison is the grammatical category of the stimulus item. This is particularly relevant because of a grammatical category asymmetry found in FM's reading corpus: he read nouns correctly more often than adjectives and verbs (63%, 42% and 30% correct respectively). Thus, even if FM does perform better on the agentive forms in list (4), this might only be because these words are deverbal nouns. If the verbs that constitute the stems of these words are more difficult to access than the agentive nominal they are embedded in, then superior performance on these words could result even if the underlying deficit were a visual (i.e., orthographic) processing impairment. So, in order to test the effects of grammatical category on FM's reading performance, two additional sets of stimuli were presented: list (5) was presented to test the effect of surface grammatical category on FM's performance; and list (6), the effect of stem category.

(5) *Part of Speech List.* High frequency, monomorphemic nouns, verbs and adjectives (7 monosyllabic, 7 bisyllabic each) were matched in letter and syllable length with low frequency, monomorphemic nouns, verbs and adjectives (7 monosyllabic, 7 bisyllabic each). The mean frequency for nouns, verbs and adjectives in the high frequency lists was 142, 141 and 139 respectively, and 7, 6, and 7 respectively for the low frequency lists.

(6) *Derived Noun and Verb List.* There were 50 morphologically derived verbs (25 denominal verbs like *scandalize* and *hospitalize*, and 25 deadjectival verbs like *intensify* and *equalize*) matched in letter length and surface frequency with 50 morphologically derived nouns (25 deverbal nouns like *betrayal* and *spillage*, 25 deadjectival nouns like *intensity* and *blindness*). Frequency norms for this list were derived from Francis and Kucera (1982): mean frequency for deverbal and deadjectival nouns was 8.7 and 9.0 respectively; and for denominal and deadjectival verbs, 8.7 and 8.4 respectively.

The materials for the three lists were prepared in typed form on 3x5 unlined index cards and were presented pseudo-randomly in unblocked order along with a large set of monomorphemic fillers of varying frequency and letter length. Results for the agentive vs. comparative -*er* list and the derived noun vs. derived verb lists are presented in Tables 5 and 6.

As expected from the data from the corpus we discussed earlier, FM's reading performance showed an effect for surface grammatical category on the part of speech list (correct vs. incorrect: $X^2 = 8.99$, $df = 1$, $p < 0.02$, two-tailed) and on the derived noun vs. derived verb list (correct vs. morphological error vs. other error type X verbs vs. nouns: $X^2 = 11.00$, $df = 2$, $p < 0.01$, two-tailed). Nouns were read reliably more often than adjectives, which were read correctly more often than verbs. However, when comparisons were made within derivational types (deverbal nouns vs. deadjectival nouns vs. denominal verbs vs. deadjectival verbs), the results were not significant (X^2 = 10.93, df = 6, p > 0.05, two-tailed). We should note, though, that this may be a floor effect: FM's overall performance level was quite low for this task (perhaps due to the relatively low frequency of the items), so it should not be taken as showing that stem category has no effect.

Table 5. Response types for agentive and comparative -er forms.

	Agentive Nominals	Comparative Adjectives
Correct	23 (.68)	--
Errors		
Morphological	9 (.26)	29 (.85)
Deletions	7	28
Substitutions	2	1
Semantic	--	3 (.09)
Visual	1 (.03)	1 (.03)
Other	1 (.03)	1 (.03)
Total	34	34

Results for the agentive vs. comparative -er list replicated the pattern found in the corpus: scores for agentive and comparative -er forms differed significantly on correct vs. morphological errors vs. other errors: X^2 = 34.86, df = 2, p < 0.001, two-tailed). Furthermore, when we compare the surface-to-stem frequency ratios for the agentive words read correctly and those which induced morphological deletions or substitutions, there is no reliable difference (t = 1.15, df = 29, p > 0.05, two-tailed). Thus, the convergence of frequency and visual similarity effects cannot be used to argue from these data that FM's morphological errors are functionally attributable to a "visual" input processing impairment in entirety. Nevertheless, there are additional factors which could in fact contribute to the production of visual errors in the case of the comparative adjectives: grammatical category and concreteness. Given that FM's visual errors analyzed in the corpus of responses showed effects for both of these factors, it might be objected that the difference in FM's performance arises in this case as in others because of the convergence of these four factors: visual similarity of stimulus to response, the grammatical category of the stimulus items, and the asymmetries of frequency and concreteness between stimuli and responses.

Table 6. Numbers (and proportions) of reading response types for morphologically derived nouns and verbs.

| | Derived Nouns | | Derived Verbs | |
	Deverbal	Deadjectival	Denominal	Deadjectival
Correct	7 (.28)	2 (.08)	--	1 (.04)
Errors				
Morphological	7 (.28)	14 (.56)	18 (.72)	17 (.68)
Deletions	4	11	14	14
Substitutions	3	3	4	1
Insertions	--	--	--	2
Semantic	1 (.04)	5 (.20)	2 (.08)	4 (.16)
Visual	5 (.20)	4 (.16)	4 (.16)	--
Other	5 (.20)	--	1 (.04)	3 (.12)
Total	25	25	25	25

Unfortunately, there does not appear to be any way to construct a list of morphologically complex stimuli that controls for all of these factors. One way around this problem, though, is to try a bootstrap approach to the comparisons we need in order to rule out an input processing explanation of FM's morphological errors. We extracted a sublist from the embedded words (suffix) list and the pseudosuffix list of test items by taking all stimuli which met the following criteria: (i) the item's surface frequency is lower than that of the corresponding pseudostem; (ii) the embedded word is a noun, and the surface form is either a verb or an adjective; (iii) the pseudostem is more concrete than the item it is embedded in. (Of course, all of these words would meet the requirement of having a pseudostem that is visually similar to the entire test item.) Of the 21 items obtained in this manner, 10 were from the pseudosuffix list and 11 from the embedded words list #1 ("suffixed"). FM's reading performance on these and the agentive and comparative words is summarized in Table 7.

Chi-square comparisons between the embedded words (e.g., *rustle*) and the comparative -*er* items (e.g., *taller*) were significant both when correct responses, morphological errors and other errors are analyzed separately ($X^2 = 22.4$, $df = 2$, $p < 0.001$, two-tailed), and when error types were collapsed ($X^2 = 14.03$, df = 1, p < 0.001, two-tailed). The comparison of the agentive -*er* list (containing items like *reader*) with the embedded words also revealed a statistically reliable difference when morphological errors and other errors are separated ($X^2 = 8.02$, $df = 2$, $p < 0.02$, two-tailed), but not when the error types are collapsed ($X^2 = 2.79$, $df = 1$, $p > 0.05$, two-tailed).[12] It would appear, then, that the differences between the agentive and comparative -er lists cannot be attributed to the effect of these various factors at the input (visual) level of lexical processing. This, of course, does not mean that none of the morphological errors that FM produces are actually visual in nature, but it does entail that *some* of these errors are not visual errors.

Table 7. Numbers (and proportions) of reading response types for agentive and comparative -er forms and embedded words with pseudo-stems that are more concrete and more frequent than the complete word.

	Agentive -er	Comparative -er	Embedded Words
Correct	23 (.70)	--	9 (.43)
Errors*			
Morphological	9 (.27)	29 (.89)	6**(.29)
Semantic	--	3 (.09)	3 (.14)
Visual	1 (.03)	1 (.03)	3 (.14)
Total	33	33	21

*   There were two "other" errors, one each in the two -er categories.
** There were five pseudomorphological errors (e.g., pierce → pier) and one morphological error (carve → carves) in this category.

An additional bit of evidence to this effect derives from FM's performance on delayed repetition tasks. The reader will recall that in the model of lexical processing we proposed in the introduction to this paper we posited two modality specific lexical input systems: an orthographic input system and a phonological input system. The predictions made by this division are clear. If FM's morphological reading errors were actually all visual input errors, then he shouldn't produce any such errors in a lexical processing task that doesn't involve the orthographic processing components of the input system. If, on the other hand, these errors are (at times) the product of a lexical semantic and/or morphological output deficit, then any task which involves these components (such as repetition) should also induce error responses comparable to the morphological errors found in FM's reading. So, in order to compare his performance in reading and repetition, FM was asked to read items which contrasted regularly and irregularly inflected words with uninflected controls:

(7) *Inflectional Regularity List.* There were 50 irregularly inflected words (e.g., *fought, broke, swam*, etc.) matched in letter length and surface frequency with 50 regularly inflected words (e.g., *waited, standing*, etc.) and 50 uninflected words. Frequencies ranged from 390.8 to 17.8 from the Carroll et al. U distribution: mean frequency was 102.4 for the irregularly inflected words, 101.0 for the regularly inflected words, and 102.5 for the uninflected controls. Mean word length in letters was 4.6,

5.3, and 5.1 for irregularly inflected, regularly inflected, and uninflected words respectively.

The materials were presented typed on 3x5 unlined index cards in unblocked, pseudo-random order, with monomorphemic fillers of varying letter length and frequency. FM's reading performance is indicated in Table 8.

Table 8. Numbers (and proportions) of reading response types for regularly inflected, irregularly inflected and uninflected controls.

	Irregularly Inflected	Regularly Inflected	Uninflected Controls
Correct	17 (.34)	5 (.10)	26 (.52)
Errors			
Morphological	19 (.38)	35 (.70)	7 (.14)
Deletions	14	28	--
Substitutions	5	7	--
Insertions	--	--	7
Semantic	2 (.04)	2 (.04)	6 (.12)
Visual	7 (.14)	5 (.10)	7 (.14)
Other	5 (.10)	3 (.06)	4 (.08)
Total	50	50	50

Comparisons of scores for the three test conditions (with morphological errors analyzed separately from other error types) were significant (X^2 = 35.03, $df = 4$, $p < 0.001$, two-tailed), and pairwise comparisons between regularly and irregularly inflected words, and between irregularly inflected and uninflected words were also significant (respectively, X^2 = 11.95, $df = 2$, $p < 0.01$, two-tailed; and $X^2 = 7.71$, $df = 2$, $p < 0.02$, two-tailed). FM performed best on the uninflected items, and better on the irregular words than the regular ones.

This same list of items was employed as stimuli for the following repetition task: FM was read items one word per trial and was asked to repeat the word after he had counted to five.[13] FM's repetition performance in indicated in Table 9.

While FM produced fewer errors in the repetition task (and X^2 comparisons were not significant), we cannot compare these aspects of performance on the different tasks directly. For example, the fact that FM's performance was better on the repetition task may be due to the availability of a phonological record of the stimulus that is not present in the case of reading tasks. Nevertheless, the remarkable thing about his responses on these two tasks is that he produces the same types of errors (with the obvious exception of the occurrence of visual errors in the reading task and phonological errors on the repetition task). The memory task does introduce an additional source of potential impairment (memory), but there is no motivated reason for suggesting that the morphological errors produced in the two tasks are caused by different sorts of impairment. Since we have been operating under the assumption that there are separate input systems for visual and auditory lexical processing, we conclude parsimoniously that the morphological errors that FM produces in these and other reading tasks are not all visual input processing errors. That is, some of these morphological errors are the result of a lexical semantic and/or morphological output deficit. Otherwise one would have to hypothesize two independent input deficits (orthographic and phonological) that have exactly the same consequences for production.

Table 9. Numbers (and proportions) of repetition response types for matched irregularly inflected, regularly inflected and uninflected words.

	Irregularly Inflected	Regularly Inflected	Uninflected Controls
Correct	37 (.74)	28 (.36)	31 (.62)
Errors			
Morphological	10 (.20)	13 (.26)	8 (.16)
Deletions	4	12	--
Substitutions	6	1	1
Insertions	--	--	7
Semantic	--	1 (.02)	3 (.06)
Phonological	2 (.04)	2 (.04)	3 (.06)
Other	1 (.02)	6*(.12)	5*(.10)
Total	50	50	50

*Includes two perseverative responses.

The question remains, however, as to whether we can unambiguously determine if, in addition to the deficit which induces FM's semantic errors, FM has an impairment to an output processing component that is organized along morphological lines. That is, can we establish whether or not the morphological errors he produces are actually semantic errors (in the functional sense)? One possibility for doing so would be to establish an intact morphological ability in another output modality (writing), which would thereby rule out a lexical-semantic deficit as an account of these errors. Unfortunately, FM's writing performance is impaired to the point that we could not attempt to establish a reliable dissociation of this sort (between speech and writing).[14] In fact, since it is plausible that the phonological and orthographic output systems might share a common morphological processing component, indeed it may not be possible to find a morphologically specified dissociation as defined by output modality even in a true instance of a post-semantic, output morphological deficit. If the orthographic and phonological output systems share such a morphological processing component, an impairment in this component should have the effect of inducing morphological errors in both output modalities. Furthermore, it is an obvious consequence of the phenomena that we are concerned with here that the items that tend to induce morphological errors (i.e., morphologically complex words) will tend to be linked semantically to all of their morphologically related cohorts. Given the fact that FM produces both semantic and morphological errors on reading and repetition tasks, then, it is unlikely that one could design a task that could unambiguously tease these two types of errors apart in this case.

GENERAL DISCUSSION

It has not been the goal of the preceding discussion to place into doubt the role of morphological decomposition in normal language processing. Evidence that the surface forms of words are parsed into morphological components during lexical access, and that morphologically complex words are generated from more basic stems and inflections during production has been derived from psycholinguistic experimentation with normal subjects (e.g., Taft, 1979, 1981, 1984; Stanners, Neiser, Hernon and Hall, 1979, Burani et al., 1985), from research with brain damaged subjects (e.g., Caramazza, Miceli, Silveri and Laudanna, 1985), and from studies of normal speech errors (e.g., Garrett, 1980a, b, 1982; MacKay, 1979). What has been at issue, beyond the characterization of a particular instance of reading impairment, is whether the type of error operationally defined as morphological in acquired dyslexia can be attributed to impairments to these hypothesized morphological processing components. FM, whose pattern of reading responses is commonly associated with such a deficit (e.g., Morton and Patterson, 1980; Coltheart, 1985), provides an excellent opportunity for exploring just what is involved in making such an assessment. However, before we summarize our characterization of FM's lexical processing abilities, especially with regard to the processing of morphologically complex words, it would be useful to consider in more detail the architecture of the normal lexical processing system that we have been assuming.

The psychological lexicon is not, in the models that we consider tenable, a unitary functional structure. What corresponds to a single "lexical entry" in linguistic grammars is considered here to be a distributed representation relating parts of several input, output, and central processors that comprise a modular lexical system. Furthermore, it is hypothesized that at least some of the processing components of the psychological lexicon are modality specific. On the basis of studies such as those mentioned above, we have also assumed, for example, that the graphemic input system can be further analyzed into a set of morphological parsing and whole-word address procedures, and an orthographic input lexicon (see Caramazza et al., 1985, for details). With these uncontroversial assumptions, though, we must still confront the issue of what constraints they impose on the interpretation of impaired lexical processing. When FM's lexical processing is examined closely, a number of additional properties of the lexical system emerge for consideration in this regard.

Besides the errors that are operationally defined as morphological, FM's reading responses include those which can be clearly attributed to separate visual and non-input lexical processing deficits. In the former case, the stimulus activates visually similar items in the input processing components, but due to an impairment at this processing stage, a cohort of the stimulus representation in the input system erroneously succeeds in activating its own corresponding representation in the semantic system. For our concerns, the characteristic of FM's visual errors that is important to bear in mind is that, in addition to being more frequent than the stimulus, visual error responses tended to be more concrete than the stimulus word as well. Despite the fact that a concreteness effect has been found for errors that we suggest originate in a visual processing component, we do not mean to imply that this "semantic" parameter functions to organize the visual input lexicon (the hypothesized locus of impairment). Instead, we consider this feature of FM's visual errors to constitute a convincing demonstration of how errors induced by impairment to one component can reflect organizing characteristics of another, interfacing component. For example, suppose, as in this case, that there is a disruption in the graphemic input system which impedes the mechanisms of these components in terms of their ability to access representations in the lexical-semantic system. If concrete words are more easily activated in the semantic system than abstract words, then the composition of the set of visually related response candidates may indeed be influenced by this asymmetry. (For expository purposes, we will refer to this phenomenon as interface influence.) It is because of this very phenomenon that it has proved difficult to unambiguously account for FM's morphological errors in terms of the functional impairments which give rise to them. In a controlled study of his performance on morphologically complex words, we have demonstrated that at least some of these errors are not visual errors reflecting interface influences (or other, nonmorphological properties which organize the input mechanisms themselves); yet we have not been able to demonstrate that these remaining cases do not follow from the independently motivated processing deficit that induces semantic errors (i.e., a deficit for which evidence is available that is independent of the occurrence of morphological errors).

It is important to keep in mind at this point that a deficit in a semantic processing or representational system is not the only type of impairment that could be expected to induce "semantic" errors. Reading *priest* for *pastor*, for example, could also plausibly result from a disruption in the phonological output lexicon. That is, if an entry in the lexical semantic system cannot activate a representation in an impaired phonological output lexicon, it may still be possible for spreading activation in the semantic system to result in the activation of a corresponding entry in the output lexicon--the net effect of which is a semantic error.[15] (There are, in fact, reasons why this account of FM's semantic errors is preferable to positing a semantic deficit. See Gordon et al., reference note 1.) However, even if we want to maintain that the phonological output lexicon is organized along morphological dimensions, one need not appeal to that aspect of the output lexicon in order to account for the production of morphological errors. As long as the deficit in question results in the production of semantic errors, and given the semantic relatedness of morphologically related words, only those features of the system that allow for the production of the semantic errors need be invoked. Thus, regardless of the origin of FM's semantic errors, we cannot demonstrate that the source of these errors differs from that of FM's morphological errors.

Nor has it been ruled out, however, that these errors are indeed induced by an impairment directly affecting the functioning of one or more morphological processing components. If one examines FM's scores on the various reading lists, for example, a strikingly suggestive feature of his performance can be seen: The proportion of responses corresponding to correct plus morphological errors combined is approximately equal across conditions for each list! The problem is that this could be because FM's morphological errors are the product of a separate morphological processing deficit; or because these errors reflect the effects of deficits which otherwise result in visual and semantic errors, when various lexical and nonlexical factors converge in a particular category of stimuli (i.e., morphologically complex words).

While these findings may remain incorrigible with respect to the goal of formulating a concise account of the functional nature of FM's lexical impairment, they have at least succeeded in making one thing apparent: The standards that should be demanded of evidence for a morphological impairment are underrepresented in studies of subjects whose dyslexic errors include deletions, substitutions, and/or insertions of affixes. In what follows we provide a brief survey of such studies and the arguments raised for interpreting these errors as reflecting the operation of morphological processing mechanisms. Included are reports of subjects whose overall pattern of reading responses is very similar to FM's (i.e., including visual, semantic and morphological errors when operational standards are applied), as well as subjects who produce only a subset of these error types.

In his discussion of the multiple-lexicon account of the clinical category of deep dyslexia, Coltheart (1980) cites the following explanation (provided by Patterson, 1978) for why affix errors should not be considered as special cases of visual or semantic errors:

> Patterson (1978) has argued that derivational errors cannot be semantic errors because they differ with respect to the confidence ratings assigned to them by patients, and also because the two types of errors yielded different results in her forced-choice task. She has also argued that derivational errors are not visual errors either, since the two error types also yield somewhat different patterns of results (p. 371).

However, since subjects' confidence ratings for their reading responses may be affected by how "close" the stimulus and response are semantically, as well as how visually similar they are, the fact that these different ratings were obtained for different operational error types cannot be construed as evidence for different loci of associated deficit. Similarly, interface influences could be responsible for "the somewhat different patterns of results" for visual and "derivational" errors. Patterson (1980) concedes nearly as much in her discussion of these results:

> Though suffix deletions and substitutions in reading seem compatible with the notion of morphological decomposition, these phenomena cannot be localized to a prelexical stage of word recognition, or even to word recognition (as opposed to production) at all (p. 290).

The results of Patterson's (1980) lexical decision studies of these subjects, while potentially capable of identifying the presence of a lexical input deficit, were not designed to distinguish morphological from other (i.e., more purely visual) input impairments.

Job and Sartori (1984) argue, in their discussion of the reading performance of patient Leonardo, that the morphological errors he produces are the result of an impairment to a morphological decomposition mechanism (i.e., that the errors are functionally morphological). Leonardo's overall pattern of reading performance is as follows: he produces affix errors (with the same stem), stem errors (with the same affixes), and visual errors for words, and his nonword reading was poor (with mostly visually similar word and nonword responses). Job and Sartori also report that in the early stages of his dyslexia, Leonardo's errors included gross semantic paraphasias. This last observation is worth mentioning simply because one could argue from it that Leonardo's improved performance was not devoid of semantic paraphasias, but only now they involve less dramatic shifts in meaning--i.e., they are limited to morphologically related cohorts. Even if we disregard this possibility, though, the explicit arguments that are advanced in support of a morphological deficit can be seen as inadequate.

Job and Sartori (1984) present two main arguments for their analysis. First, they argue that, if there were an impairment affecting a morphological parsing component, then only regularly inflected words should be affected, since (they hypothesize) only regular words are subject to morphological parsing. In fact, Leonardo did perform better on irregular than regular inflected forms (15/33 vs. 6/33 correct respectively). Second, he produced only one pseudomorphological error on pseudoprefixed words (substituting a stem for the stimulus's pseudostem: *ricordo → ritardo*), though he performed much worse on words with true prefixes. This too, they argue, is to be expected if a morphological parsing device has been compromised by brain damage, since only words that are composed of actual stems and prefixes should be affected by such an impairment. As we argued from similar patterns in FM's performance, however, this is not the only reasonable account of these results. For example, we have suggested, in our discussion of interface influences, that the likelihood of producing a visual error that can be operationally defined as morphological can depend on some factors which organize the lexical-semantic system. (Concreteness vs. abstractness is one such factor.) Whether or not the activation of visually similar words at the visual stage of processing results in the activation of a set of words that are related in the lexical-semantic system could also affect the probability of whether a visual deficit will result in a morphological error. To use an English example, we are suggesting that, while a pseudoprefixed stimulus like *religion* may have a potential cohort of visually related items (such as *legion*, *lion*, etc.), these representations will not be related in the lexical-semantic system. An affixed word like *repayment*, on the other hand, will have a cohort of visually related words that are also semantically related (*payment*, *repay*, *pay*, *repaying*, *paying*, etc.); and this may contribute to the probability of producing a morphologically related form even if the deficit which induces such errors is visual in nature. Thus, in the case of the pseudo-prefixed words, one could expect fewer visual errors than for true prefixed forms because there are fewer (or no) lexical representations that are visually confused with the pseudostem in the input system (and that will converge on the same stem in the lexical-semantic system).[16] Similarly, since regularly inflected words will, almost by definition, be more visually similar to inflectional paradigm cohorts than irregular forms will be, the fact that Leonardo makes fewer reading errors on irregular verbs fails to differentiate the visual and morphological deficit hypotheses. In fact, if only regular words are parsed by the morphological processing mechanisms, then by the very logic of Job and Sartori's (1984) argument, there should not have been instances of reading errors involving substitutions of regular forms for irregular forms, contrary to what they report.[17]

Patterson (1982) describes a dyslexic subject, AM, who presents with the following pattern of reading performance: he (i) has difficulty in assembling phonology from print (i.e., reading nonwords); (ii) makes errors reading function words (mostly function word substitutions); (iii) produces morphological paralexias (i.e., deletes, inserts, and substitutes affixes as in *initiate → initiative*); and (iv) "makes some visual errors." The argument she presents for treating AM's morphological errors as functionally morphological is constructed out of observations about the different error types and her explanation of the clustering of AM's performance characteristics:

> (1) so few of his errors are visual but clearly not derivational; (2) on a **purely** visual basis, <u>initiate</u> for example is probably more similar to <u>imitate</u> than to <u>initiative</u>; (3) AM's reading performance constitutes a more coherent and more theoretically interesting pattern if we can conclude that only one type of paralexic error, derivational, occurred often enough to require an account (p. 87).

The lynch pin of her argument is her explanation of co-occurring impairments, so we will address this part of her argument first.

Patterson (1982) attempts to account for the co-occurrence of (i)-(iii) with the following dual-route model of normal lexical processing. The lexical route is best suited to stem processing, while affix and function-word processing relies heavily on sound-based (i.e., grapheme-to-phoneme mapping) mechanisms. An impairment to the latter mechanisms can thus account for the first three aspects of AM's performance. The embarrassment for Patterson's explanation is that there have been reported instances of subjects who exhibit a pervasive nonword reading deficit (and who produce affix errors), but whose performance shows no grammatical category effects (e.g., Funnell's, 1983, subject WB), as well as instances of nonword reading deficits without morphological impairment (Caramazza et al.'s, 1985, subject AG). Yet Patterson's theory would suggest that the

A. Caramazza

function-word and "morphological" deficits should not be dissociable from the impairment affecting nonwords. Thus, even if AM's "morphological paraphasias" and nonword processing deficits are functionally linked in AM's case, it would appear that hypothesizing an independent impairment affecting function-word reading would be required. Since the theories of lexical processing such as the one Patterson invokes are not sufficiently explicit to differentiate the deficits of AM, WB and AG, the explanatory force of the account is much diminished.

The removal of this theoretical support for treating AM's "morphological paralexias" as functionally morphological topples the remaining legs of Patterson's argument much as one would expect. In order to reason to her conclusion from the facts that fewer "pure" visual errors than "affix errors" are produced, and that (by some unspecified criteria) there may be less visual similarity between the stimulus and a morphologically related response than between the stimulus than some other visually related word, one must assume that only purely visual properties of a stimulus word will have any bearing on the composition of the set of response candidates for visual errors. As we argued in our discussion of interface influences, this assumption is unlikely to be true.

The foregoing discussion may well have created the impression that, with the complexity of the language processing models that we consider plausible, it might not ever be possible to identify true instances of morphological processing deficits. This is not a conclusion that should be drawn, however; and so we describe a recent case study of an Italian-speaking subject, FS (Miceli and Caramazza, reference note 3), in order to make this clear.

In addition to producing function word errors, FS makes morphological errors in spontaneous speech, as well as in reading and repetition tasks. Notably, nearly all of the morphological errors he produces are inflectional substitutions. Given the constancy of this feature across the different tasks, a parsimonious approach to this pattern of performance requires a common account. That is, while it is logically possible, we would argue that it is highly unlikely that FS has two or more distinct deficits that result independently in the same restricted type of morphological errors in reading, repetition and spontaneous speech. Miceli and Caramazza (reference note 3) reason from his spontaneous speech and repetition performance that the deficit is in fact a morphological output processing impairment, as opposed to a lexical-semantic or phonological output impairment. For example, in controlled repetition tasks involving inflected adjectives, FS's responses showed a strong tendency to favor the masculine singular form, regardless of whether this form of the item took the -o or -e suffix, or whether masculine singular was the most frequent inflected form for the stem. Thus, lexical frequency cannot explain this pattern of errors: FS's errors tend to be the "basic" form of the inflectional paradigm (see Bybee, 1985). Similarly, one feature of FS's linguistic output which argues against a lexical-semantic deficit account is the performance asymmetry between inflectional and derivational morphology. Furthermore, his performance on auditory/visual stimulus matching tasks is quite good, in contrast to performance on the production tasks--a fact that would be left largely unexplained if the morphological errors FS produces were not attributed to an output processing deficit. In the absence of phonological or form-class effects, and given the fact that FS does not produce any semantic errors (either in reading or repetition tasks), we must appeal to those factors, specified by our theory of lexical processing, which **are** known to affect FS's performance on production tasks. Since the primary determinant of the probability of producing a particular inflected adjectival form, for example, appears to be a morphological principle; the evidence for a true morphological processing impairment is quite compelling.

In summary, we have argued that despite the possibility that many instances of reported reading errors which involve affix deletions, substitutions and insertions are indeed the product of deficits to morphological processing mechanisms, there have been few convincing arguments to this effect. Most putative examples of morphological deficit can be subsumed under the consequences of independently motivated visual and/or semantic processing deficits. What sets the convincing example that we have discussed apart from the rest is that the examples of true morphological error have had to satisfy both linguistic and psychological criteria for their classification as such. The linguistic criteria, dissociation along a purely morphological dimension, is significant; but our discussion of FM's performance on agentive vs. comparative -*er* words demonstrated the importance of processing considerations as well. The difference, in the case of FS, is that the effect corresponding to the linguistic contrast cannot be derived from independent linguistic or psychological properties of the processing mechanisms or representations (e.g., frequency, phonological complexity, concreteness, etc.).

In the case we have reported here, though, we have not been quite as successful in demonstrating a morphological deficit. We cannot exclude the possibility that a significant proportion of FM's morphological errors are induced by such a deficit, nor can we exclude the possibility that these errors result from the influence of converging factors governing the effects of independently motivated processing impairments that induce visual and semantic errors. The linguistic contrasts which emerged in

A. Caramazza

various reading tasks could not, on their own, suffice to settle this issue. Nevertheless, FM's pattern of performance is instructive because it reveals the complexity of the process whereby one may reason validly from observable patterns of performance to the nature of the impairments responsible for them.

ACKNOWLEDGEMENTS

The research reported here was funded by NIH grant NS23836 to The Johns Hopkins University. We would like to thank Roberta Goodman and Barry Gordon for allowing us access to their data and research reports, and to Gabriele Miceli, Kathy Straub, and an anonymous reviewer for helpful comments on an earlier draft of this paper.

REFERENCES

Anderson, S. (1985a). Typological distinctions in word formation. In T. Shopin (ed.), Language Typology and Syntactic Description, Vol III: Grammatical Categories and the Lexicon. Cambridge: Cambridge University Press.

Anderson, S. (1985b). Inflectional morphology. In T. Shopin (ed.), Language Typology and Syntactic Description, Vol III: Grammatical Categories and the Lexicon. Cambridge: Cambridge University Press.

Aronoff, M. (1976). Word Formation in Generative Grammar. Cambridge, MA: MIT Press.

Bradley, D. (1980). Lexical representation of derivational relation. In M. Aronoff & M.-L. Kean (Eds.), Juncture. Saratoga, CA: AnmaLibri.

Burani, C., Salmaso, D. & Caramazza, A. (1984). Morphological structure and lexical access. Visible Language, 18, 342–352.

Bybee, J. (1985). Morphology: A Study of the Relation Between Meaning and Form. Amsterdam: John Benjamins Publishing Co.

Caramazza, A. (1985). Reading and lexical processing mechanisms. Reports of the Cognitive Neuropsychology Laboratory, Number 12, The Johns Hopkins University.

Caramazza, A., Miceli, G., Silveri, M. & Laudanna, A. (1985). Reading mechanisms and the organization of the lexicon: Evidence from acquired dyslexia. Cognitive Neuropsychology, 2, 81–114.

Carroll, J., Davies, P. & Richman, B. (1971). Word Frequency Book. New York, NY: American Heritage Publishing Co.

Coltheart, M. (1980). Deep dyslexia: A right hemisphere hypothesis. In M. Coltheart, K. Patterson & J. Marshall (Eds.), Deep Dyslexia. London: Routledge & Kegan Paul.

Francis, W. & Kucera, H. (1982). Frequency Analysis of English Usage. Boston, MA: Houghton Mifflin Co.

Garrett, M. (1980a). Levels of processing in sentence production. In B. Butterworth (Ed.), Language Production, Vol 1. New York, NY: Academic Press.

Garrett, M. (1980b). The limits of accommodation. In V. Fromkin (Ed.), Errors in Linguistic Performance. New York, NY: Academic Press.

Garrett, M. (1982). Production of speech: Observations from normal and pathological language use. In A. Ellis (Ed.), Normality and Pathology in Cognitive Functions. New York, NY: Academic Press.

Gordon, B. (1983). Lexical access and lexical decision: Mechanisms of frequency sensitivity. Journal of Verbal Learning and Verbal Behavior, 22, 24-44.

Job, R. & Sartori, G. (1984). Morphological decomposition: Evidence from crossed phonological dyslexia. The quarterly Journal of Experimental Psychology, 36, 435-458.

Kroll, J. & Merves, J. (1986). Lexical access for concrete and abstract words. Journal of Experimental Psychology: Learning, Memory and Cognition, 12, 92-107.

MacKay, D. (1979). Lexical insertion, inflection, and derivation. Journal of Psycholinguistic Research, 8, 477-498.

Matthews, P. (1984). Morphology: An Introduction to the Theory of Word-Structure. Cambridge: Cambridge University Press.

Miceli, G., Silveri, M., Villa, G. & Caramazza, A. (1984). On the basis for the agrammatic's difficulty in producing main verbs. Cortex, 20, 207-220.

Morton, J. & Patterson, K. (1980). A new attempt at an interpretation, or, an attempt at a new interpretation. In M. Coltheart, K. Patterson & J. Marshall (Eds.), Deep Dyslexia. London: Routledge & Kegan Paul.

Patterson, K. (1978). Phonemic dyslexia: Errors of meaning and the meaning of errors. Quarterly Journal of Experimental Psychology, 30, 587-601.

Patterson, K. (1980). Derivational errors. In M. Coltheart, K. Patterson & J. Marshall (Eds.), Deep Dyslexia. London: Routledge & Kegan Paul.

Patterson, K. (1982). The relation between reading and phonological coding: Further neuropsychological observations. In A. Ellis (Ed.), Normality and Pathology in Cognitive Functions. New York, NY: Academic Press.

Stanners, R., Neiser, J., Hernon, W. & Hall, R. (1979). Memory representation for morphologically related words. Journal of Verbal Learning and Verbal Behavior, 18, 399-412.

Taft, M. (1979). Recognition of affixed words and the word frequency effect. Memory and Cognition, 7, 263-272.

Taft, M. (1981). Prefix stripping revisited. Journal of Verbal Learning and Verbal Behavior, 20, 638-647.

Taft, M. (1984). Evidence for an abstract representation of word structure. Memory and Cognition, 12, 264-269.

REFERENCE NOTES

1. Gordon, B., Goodman, R., and Caramazza, A. 1986. Separating the stages of reading errors. Unpublished Manuscript, The Johns Hopkins University.

2. Stacie Raymer and Alfonso Caramazza. In preparation. Semantic priming in a patient with acquired dyslexia. The Johns Hopkins University.

3. Miceli, G., and Caramazza, A. 1986. Dissociation of inflectional and derivational morphology. Unpublished manuscript, The Johns Hopkins University.

NOTES

[1] For example, lexical items may be unanalyzable units of meaning (i.e. monomorphemic), or they may be composed of two or more meaningful parts (morphemes). Formally, we may distinguish between stem and affixal morphemes, between prefixes, infixes and suffixes, and between affixation and compounding to name just a few of the defining contrasts in the typology of word formation. The contrasts between inflectional and derivational morphological processes, and between regular and suppletive inflection straddle the formal/functional opposition; and there are other concepts of lexical typology which lie more squarely in the camp of functional properties of word formation--grammatical function and productivity being the two most obvious of these. For detailed discussions of these formal and functional aspects of morphology, the reader should consult Matthews (1974), Aronoff (1976), Anderson (1985a,b) and Bybee (1985).

[2] Note that this requirement would not rule out a (motivated) psychological analysis that posited both decomposed and non-decomposed representations for (certain) morphologically complex words when linguistic criteria by themselves require morphological decomposition alone. Whereas this sort of disparity can be tolerated, though, contradictory analyses cannot.

[3] These errors were, in fact, produced by the same subject (FM), whose lexical processing we describe in greater detail below.

[4] Another sort of evidence that visual and semantic errors arise from different functional loci is the fact that FM produces visual-to-semantic errors like minstrel → (minister) → gospel and trifles → (rifle) → hunter, where hypothesized intermediate representations appear in parentheses.

[5] These figures are of course based on the assumption that when the -*er* suffix is added to a verb, it is the agentive ending and not the comparative (which only attaches to adjectives). Since there are very few (three) instances in which FM produced a morphologically illegal nonword response, in comparison to the hundreds of morphologically legal complex words he has produced as a morpheme insertion or substitution error, this would appear to be a rather safe assumption.

[6] Another suffix, -y, was also mistakenly inserted often in comparison with the other affixes in the corpus: 13 insertions, 18 deletions, and 10 correct responses.

[7] There were 2987 nouns, 936 verbs and 783 adjectives in the corpus.

[8] By "surface frequency" we mean the frequency measure of a particular word (e.g., untying), as opposed to the combined frequency of inflected variants (which would include untie, untied, etc.) or the cumulative frequency of the root (tie). Except where otherwise noted, surface frequency matching and frequency comparisons for this and the other controlled lists discussed here were based on the U distribution of frequency norms from Carroll, Davies and Richman (1971).

[9] One item, fatal, was miscategorized as monomorphemic, and was discarded in the analysis of FM's performance.

[10] By stem frequency we refer to the surface frequency of the morphological stem or pseudostem of the stimulus: happy in the case of happier, and earn in the case of (the morphologically unrelated) earnest. Clearly, this frequency rating will underestimate the cumulative frequency of stems.

[11] These lists could not be controlled for abstractness and concreteness. See our comments below concerning the problems this raises.

[12] If the morphological errors (operationally defined) are actually visual, then it is the latter comparison, with error types collapsed, that is most relevant to the discussion: i.e., if morphological errors are in fact visual errors, then they should be grouped as such in the comparisons.

[13] The delay component of the task was introduced to bring FM's performance down from ceiling levels. Ideally, the stimuli in the repetition task should have been controlled for syllable length and stress pattern, but this is not possible when comparing regular and irregular verbs without introducing other confounds such as consonant cluster complexity. However, these problems do not affect our argument since it does not rely on quantitative differences in repetition performance on the

sublists, but rather on qualitative similarities in performance on the reading and repetition tasks.

[14] FM produces some semantic errors in writing words (e.g., cattle → cow), and cannot write nonwords. However, so many of his responses to words are either entirely unrelated to the target (e.g., cheer → tully) or only partially related to the target (e.g., trout → tucat) that it is not possible to assert one way or the other whether FM's writing responses include morphological errors.

[15] Similarly, it could be that activation of a semantic representation normally results in the activation of a whole cohort of (semantically related) items in the phonological output lexicon, and it is this many-to-one nature of the mapping that enables a deficit in the phonological output lexicon to result in the production of a semantic error.

[16] In order for pseudoprefixed words to be comparable to affixed words in this regard, we have assumed that, minimally, they must have lexical pseudostems. On this point, see Caramazza et al., 1985.

[17] We would also contend that their argument from inflectional regularity for a morphological deficit underrepresents the complexity of the situation. There are two sorts of inflectional irregularity in Italian (although from Job and Sartori's discussion, they appear to have been conflated in their experiments): suppletive forms (e.g., and-are "to go" has the suppletive forms vado "I go" and va "he goes") and irregular verbs with small inflectional sub-paradigms (e.g., fing-ere "to pretend" has irregular stems in participial and indicative past tense forms: fint-o, fint-a, fint-i, fint-e are the third person m.sg, f.sg., m.pl., and f.pl. past participle forms respectively; and fins-i, fins-e, fins-ero are the 1st.sg., 3rd.sg., and 3rd.pl. forms of the irregular root used in the past tense). While Job and Sartori's claim that irregular verbs are not morphologically parsed is reasonable for the suppletive forms, this is not clearly so for the irregular verbs with irregular sub-paradigms. It is reasonable to suppose that, pressed on this point, Job and Sartori would make differing predictions regarding Leonardo's performance on these two kinds of verbs, although no such judgments appear in their paper (nor is Leonardo's performance described in terms of this difference). In any event, our arguments concerning the visual similarity between regular and irregular forms of verbs hold for both varieties of irregular verb.

CHAPTER FIVE

GENERAL TO SPECIFIC ACCESS TO WORD MEANING:
A CLAIM REEXAMINED

INTRODUCTION

Considerable research in cognitive psychology has been dedicated to determining the structure of the lexical semantic system. Recently, research with neurologically impaired subjects has provided data relevant to issues concerning the processing of word meaning. Warrington (1975), Warrington and Shallice (1979) and Warrington and McCarthy (1983), using data from neurologically impaired subjects, have proposed a view of access to word meaning according to which "The precise meaning of a word may well be accessed only as the end result of a process which involves the attaining of increasingly specific semantic representations" (Warrington and Shallice, 1979 p.61). We will refer to this view of semantic access as the 'general to specific' hypothesis of access to word meaning and, for the sake of convenience, we will refer to Warrington, Shallice, and McCarthy as WSM. In this paper we examine the data and arguments that WSM present in support of the general to specific hypothesis. We also present analyses of a patient's performance that have implications for the hypothesis proposed by WSM.

WSM base their claim of general to specific semantic access on their observation of the performance of a number of patients who apparently fail to comprehend the meaning of words for which they indirectly demonstrate knowledge of their superordinates when asked to make forced-choice decisions about their category membership. Warrington (1975) reported data obtained from three patients: A.B., E.M., and C.R. who, adequately fluent in oral expression, were described as both agnosic for pictorial representations of objects and impaired in their comprehension of auditorily presented words. In spite of an impairment in their ability to name or describe the function of items presented auditorily or pictorially, further testing indicated that these patients had the ability to correctly make certain yes/no judgements about the meaning of words and pictures. Furthermore, their decisions were more often correct when the questions referred to superordinate information than when the questions required knowledge of subordinate characteristics. For each item the patients were presented with a series of yes/no questions ordered from general to specific (e.g., for animal words and pictures: is it an animal? is it a bird? is it foreign? is it bigger than a cat?; for objects:

Reproduced, with permission, from Cognitive Neuropsychology, Vol. 6. Copyright 1989 by Lawrence Erlbaum Associates Ltd.

is it an animal? is it used indoors? is it heavier than a telephone directory? is it made of metal?). Subjects performed significantly above chance on both pictorial and auditory presentations with the most general question: is it an animal? However, their performance was at chance in answering most of the other questions.

Warrington and Shallice (1979) have reported further evidence in support of their hypothesis. They have interpreted the performance of their patient A.R. as suggesting that he had a deficit which prevented him from gaining *full* access to stored semantic information from written stimuli. This conclusion was based on the patient's significantly above chance performance on a number of categorization tasks with words that he could neither read nor identify. A.R. had been asked to read various sets of words and for each word that he could *not* read or identify he was asked to make a forced-choice, superordinate-level decision (e.g., Is this word a surname/forename; boys'/girls' name; author/politician; subject/measurement) as well as a decision concerning subordinate traits (e.g., for 'cabbage': is it green, brown or grey?). He performed above chance level in categorizing those words he had failed to read or to describe accurately.[1]

WSM interpreted these data as indicating: 1) that there is a distinction between the representation of superordinate and subordinate information, generally supporting the hypothesis that the semantic system is organized hierarchically (Collins & Quillian, 1969; Quillian, 1969), and 2) that, in terms of the time course of access to semantic knowledge, superordinate information becomes available prior to subordinate information. However, the fact that the patients presumably had access primarily or exclusively to superordinate information was considered by WSM to be incompatible with one of the basic assumptions of a hierarchically structured semantic network--that the activation of a concept proceeds from the node where item specific knowledge is stored, upwards through the hierarchy, to progressively more general superordinate nodes. That is, the apparent finding of selective sparing of superordinate information in the face of damage to subordinate information cannot be accommodated within a spreading activation theory of semantic memory which both assumes that 1) semantic knowledge is organized in a hierarchical structure and 2) the access point to this knowledge is at the level where item-specific information is represented--one (or both) of these assumptions must be rejected. WSM chose to reject the assumption that access to the semantic network takes place at the level of item-specific information and proposed, instead, that the access procedure must be initiated at the superordinate node with progressive activation downward resulting, over the time course of access, in an increasingly specific semantic representation. Thus, we might imagine that, according to the hypothesis of general to specific semantic access, when one hears the word 'collie' one first accesses the fact that it is living then that it is an animal, a dog, and finally that it is large, has pointed ears and muzzle, long hair, etc.

Before addressing the empirical status of WSM's hypothesis we must discuss a theoretical difficulty that becomes apparent when we attempt to make explicit the (implicit) processing claims in WSM's hypothesis of general to specific semantic access in a hierarchical network. If, as argued by WSM, entry to the hierarchy is via the superordinate it is not clear how the downward paths of items sharing a common entry point are individuated: Both fern and collie share the common entry point living, yet, their downward paths soon diverge. The activation associated with fern must proceed to the next lower hierarchical level that corresponds to it--presumably the plant node, whereas collie requires the activation of the animal node. WSM do not indicate how these decision points are to be negotiated nor can we come up with an acceptable solution that retains a hierarchical organization. It would appear that the hypothesis of semantic access proposed by WSM may not be theoretically coherent--it may not be possible to articulate a spreading activation model of semantic processing which assumes both that semantic knowledge is organized hierarchically and that access to this knowledge is at the level of superordinate information.

Although apparently not interpretable within a hierarchical network framework, the general to specific view of access to word meaning, nonetheless, consists of two interesting proposals: 1) superordinate and subordinate semantic information are represented autonomously (i.e., access to superordinate information can occur without access to subordinate information) and 2) in the course of accessing a semantic representation, superordinate knowledge becomes available prior to subordinate information. These proposals, if correct, would place important constraints on a theory of semantic processing. It is important, therefore, to determine whether, as WSM argue, there is empirical support for these proposals.

It must be emphasized that the proposals under consideration are based on the observation that a number of patients can correctly categorize words which they cannot identify. These proposals, however, do not automatically follow from this observation--they depend on a strong assumption that may be false. WSM assume that performance on the categorization tasks provides a "direct" measure of the type and amount of semantic information available to patients when they are presented with a stimulus (word or picture as the case may be). On this assumption, patients' ability to classify items which they cannot identify may be taken as evidence that they have accessed superordinate level information for these items without having access to their subordinate or item-specific features. However, this assumption may be unwarranted.

In this paper we address the following question: Can we, in fact, assume that the ability to categorize items that are not identified is best understood as the result of gaining access to only superordinate information? We address this question first by presenting data from patient J.E. which establishes that he exhibits a performance pattern comparable to the other patients described by WSM. Then, in order to determine if the WSM interpretation of their data is a necessary one, we will, through further testing with J.E., examine some of the implications of the general to specific hypothesis of semantic access.

CASE STUDY

J.E., a right handed, fifty year old male, participated in this study from 2/86-6/87. He had a resection of the left parietal-occipital lobe in 1979 as a result of intervention for treatment of an arterio-venous malformation. He was a college graduate in Wildlife Management and employment prior to 1979 included high school science teaching and working as an upper level administrator in a government agency. Upon evaluation in our laboratory he exhibited severe dyslexia and dysgraphia, though oral spelling abilities were relatively less impaired. His spontaneous speech was fluent with some anomic difficulties which were accentuated in confrontation naming. His language comprehension performance was adequate though impaired (see Caramazza & Berndt, 1985, for a description of his sentence comprehension performance and McCloskey, Sokol, Goodman-Schulman and Caramazza, in press, for a report on his number processing abilities).

TEST RESULTS
Oral Reading

Partial administration of the Johns Hopkins University Reading Battery (designed to assess dimensions of reading performance such as: frequency, word length, concreteness/abstractness, and nonword reading abilities) indicated severe reading difficulties: He read a total of 6% (13/231) of the items correctly (11/186 words; 2/45 nonwords). Errors consisted largely of don't know responses. The low rate of correct responding makes it difficult to draw conclusions about the parameters affecting J.E.'s reading performance. We may note, however, that of the eleven words read correctly nine were high frequency words. The two nonwords read correctly were pseudohomophones. (e.g., 'windoe' and 'cherch').

Naming and Oral Production

Results of a picture naming task which included pictures of both common objects and actions indicated a moderate impairment in naming with performance at 75% (15/20) accuracy.

In a sentence completion task J.E.'s performance was at 100% (10/10) accuracy (e.g., he was asked to complete the following auditorily presented sentence: The teacher expected the student....)

J.E.'s expressive ability to convey the meaning of words was evaluated through a task in which he was required to define 70 aurally presented words. He was able to provide satisfactory definitions for all items tested (e.g., a note: "a piece of paper with writing"; home: "where your abode is").

Reading Comprehension

In order to assess reading comprehension and compare it to auditory comprehension abilities the Peabody Picture Vocabulary Test (PPVT) Form L (Dunn & Dunn, 1981) was administered presenting even items 2-100 auditorily and odd items 1-99 in written form. He scored 98% correct (49/50) for the auditory presentation and 38% correct (19/50) with presentation of written words; with chance set at 25% in this task, JE's performance with written words was just above chance ($X^2 = 3.84$, $p < .05$). He clearly demonstrated a selective impairment in comprehension of written materials.

Categorization of Written Words (Blocked Trials)

J.E. was presented with a list of 164 words to read. If he could either read or define a word correctly it was set aside; likewise, if a word was read incorrectly it was discarded. If he produced a "don't know" response even after being provided with ample time and encouragement to define the word, he was asked to choose from among three aurally presented category names the one he thought the word might belong to. The words were divided into three lists. The lists were presented in a blocked manner such that each list contained only three categories of words (matched for frequency, letter, and syllable length) and the same three category names were presented for each categorization judgement. For example, List I consisted of professions, clothing, and names of people; he was presented with a word such as 'pilot,' if unable to read or describe it he was asked

A. Caramazza

if it was a profession, clothing, or a person's name. Each list consisted of 50-60 items and was presented twice on separate occasions separated by two weeks.

The results, summarized in Table 1, indicate that 26% (85/327) of the words were either read or identified correctly; 6% (19/327) of the words were read incorrectly and 68% (223/327) elicited a "don't know" response. Categorization performance with the 223 "don't know" responses indicate a 70% accuracy level (157/223) which is significantly above chance (X^2 = 136.24, p < .001).

Table 1. Results of the categorization task (blocked presentation).

		Read/ identified correctly	Read incorrectly	Don't know responses correctly categorized
List 1				
NAMES	time 1	10% (2/20)	0% (0/20)	67% (12/18)*
	time 2	20% (4/20)	0% (0/20)	63% (10/16)*
PROF	time 1	7% (1/14)	0% (0/14)	31% (4/13) ns
	time 2	13% (2/15)	13% (2/15)	64% (7/11)*
CLOTH	time 1	0% (0/15)	0% (0/15)	60% (9/15)*
	time 2	7% (1/15)	13% (2/15)	75% (9/12)*
List 2				
ANIM	time 1	50% (10/20)	0% (0/20)	70% (7/10)*
	time 2	80% (16/20)	0% (0/20)	50% (2/4) ns
FOODS	time 1	35% (7/20)	25% (1/20)	100% (12/12)*
	time 2	60% (12/20)	25% (5/20)	100% (3/3)*
BODY	time 1	0%	5% (1/20)	63% (12/19)*
	time 2	10% (2/20)	10% (2/20)	50% (8/16)ns
List 3				
PLACES	time 1	21% (4/19)	0% (0/19)	87% (13/15)*
	time 2	47% (9/19)	5% (1/19)	89% (8/9)*
TRANSP	time 1	33% (5/15)	7% (1/15)	56% (5/9)ns
	time 2	33% (5/15)	7% (1/15)	77% (7/9)ns
HOUSE	time 1	10% (2/20)	20% (1/20)	94% (16/17)*
	time 2	15% (3/20)	10% (2/20)	87% (13/15)*
TOTALS		26% (85/327)	6% (19/327)	70% (157/223)**

* binomial P < 0.05
** X^2 = 136.24, P < 0.001

(NAMES=people's names; PROF=professions; CLOTH=clothing; ANIM=animals; FOODS=foods; BODY=body parts; PLACES=place names; TRANSP=transportation; HOUSE=household items)

Categorization of Written Words (Mixed Trials)

Because of the blocked nature of the previous task, J.E. always knew prior to being administered an item which of three categories it could belong to; thus, for example, for List 1 he knew that all items were either clothing, professions or the name of a person. This information might have allowed him to generate exemplars of the categories in a block which he could then match with the item presented, thus facilitating his performance. In an attempt to reduce the efficient use of this strategy the task was readministered. The second administration differed from the first in that the words were not presented in blocked lists according to category membership, instead words were administered in random order. Furthermore, for each category decision the patient was asked to choose among the target category and two others randomly selected from the remaining eight categories. This task was administered 10 weeks after the blocked presentation.

Table 2. Results of the categorization task (mixed presentation).

	Read/ identified correctly		Read incorrectly		Don't know responses correctly categorized	
List 1						
NAMES	20%	(4/20)	15%	(3/20)	69%	(9/13)*
PROF	13%	(2/15)	0%	(0/15)	61%	(8/13)*
CLOTH	0%	(0/15)	7%	(1/15)	53%	(8/15)*
List 2						
ANIM	85%	(17/20)	0%	(0/20)	100%	(3/3)*
FOODS	45%	(9/20)	5%	(1/20)	90%	(9/10)*
BODY	5%	(1/20)	0%	(0/20)	58%	(11/19)*
List 3						
PLACES	58%	(11/19)	0%	(0/19)	100%	(8/8)*
TRANSP	53%	(8/15)	0%	(0/15)	43%	(3/7)ns
HOUSE	5%	(1/20)	5%	(1/20)	67%	(12/18)*
TOTALS	32%	(53/164)	4%	(6/164)	68%	(71/105)**

* binomial $p < 0.05$
** $x^2 = 54.82$, $p < 0.001$

(NAMES=people's names; PROF=professions; CLOTH=clothing; ANIM=animals; FOODS=foods; BODY=body parts; PLACES=place names; TRANSP=transportation; HOUSE=household items)

The results obtained in this task (Table 2) were virtually identical to those obtained with the blocked presentation: 32% (53/164) of the words were read or identified correctly; 4% (6/164) were read incorrectly; and 64% (105/164) elicited a "don't know" response. Of the items that were not identified 68% (71/105) were categorized correctly--significantly above chance level performance (X^2 = 54.82, p < .001). (Although the items were not administered in a blocked manner according to list type, Table 2 is organized according to list number for ease of comparison with Table 1).

These results establish the fact that J.E. displayed the performance pattern described for all the patients WSM cite in support of the general to specific semantic access hypothesis: J.E. demonstrated a discrepancy between his ability to read or describe the meaning of words and his ability to make forced-choice category judgements for these same words. Consequently, J.E.'s performance may be used to explore WSM's account of the discrepancy between categorization and reading performance.

Word/Picture Verification Task

If for this patient, in fact, presentation of a written word resulted in access only to information concerning an item's superordinate then items sharing a superordinate should be indistinguishable in terms of meaning. At the very least we would predict that items belonging to the same superordinate category should be confused more often than items belonging to different superordinate categories. Thus, for example, if upon presentation of the word 'dog' J.E. had access only to the information that it is an animal and if subsequently upon presentation of 'cat' he also had access only to the fact that it is an animal, he should not be able to distinguish the two words in terms of their meaning--they both would mean 'animal.' By contrast, if a pair of words do not share a superordinate then knowledge of their category membership should be sufficient to allow the two items to be distinguished in terms of meaning. To continue with our example, 'dog' would access the superordinate animal and 'hat' would be associated with the category clothing and the two words could be differentiated.

A word/picture verification task was designed to evaluate this prediction. J.E. was presented with a word which he was asked to read or define. If the word was identified either correctly or incorrectly it was discarded. If he could not identify a word it was removed from sight and a picture was presented. J.E. was asked to decide if picture and word matched.

This task allowed us to evaluate the hypothesis that accuracy on the categorization tasks reported previously was due to access to category level information from the printed word. This hypothesis predicts that in situations where word and picture name differ in superordinate membership J.E. should be able to correctly determine that the word/picture pair differ in meaning; for example, when shown the word 'domino' followed by a picture of a donkey he should be able to recognize that they do not match since, presumably, he has "normal" access to the superordinate information for both the printed word and the picture.

The variables manipulated in this task were the degree of semantic and orthographic similarity between each word and the name of the picture presented for verification. Word and picture name were either semantically similar (SS) (e.g., the word 'sock' and a picture of a glove) in that they shared a common superordinate (in this example the category clothing) or semantically dissimilar (SD) (e.g., 'domino'/donkey) indicating membership in different superordinate classes. Word/picture name pairs were either visually similar (VS) (e.g., 'cone'/cane) or visually dissimilar (VD) (e.g., 'pilot'/dentist). Furthermore, there were two levels of visual similarity: A and B. Level A of visual similarity required that the pair at least share a common initial letter and approximately equal letter and syllable length (e.g., 'pear'/plum). Level B required a higher degree of visual similarity in that the word and picture name pairs shared common initial letter, approximately equal letter and syllable length, and necessarily 50% or more of letters in common (e.g., 'toe'/tie). A VD relationship was established by the absence of initial letter identity and fewer than 50% letters in common (e.g., 'mouth'/suit). Based on these criteria, six different word-picture name relationship types were established:

(1) MATCHES: word and picture name were identical (e.g., 'toe'/toe);
(2) VSA,SD: word and picture name were visually similar at level A but did not share a superordinate (e.g., 'domino'/donkey);
(3) VSA,SS: word and picture name were visually similar at level A and shared a common superordinate (e.g., 'pear'/plum);
(4) VSB,SD: word and picture name were visually similar at level B but did not share a superordinate (e.g., 'toe'/tie);
(5) VD,SS: word and picture pairs were visually dissimilar but semantically similar (e.g.,'sock'/glove);
(6) VD,SD: word and picture pairs were visually and semantically dissimilar (e.g., 'pie'/bow).

Word lists for each of the six conditions were approximately matched for average frequency, word length, and syllable length (see Table 3). The ratio of trials with matches to those with non-matches was 1:2. Test items were presented in four blocks such that no word was presented more than once in each block. Blocks were presented with one non-testing day between each block.

If J.E. had access only to superordinate information for written words specific predictions can be made about his performance on the word/picture verification task described above. The critical expectation is that when two word/picture pairs have the same level of visual similarity (e.g., 'hut'/ham and 'chin'/cheek) the pair whose members belong to different semantic categories ('hut'/ham) should have the benefit of this additional discriminating semantic information. The prediction in this case is that there would be a greater probability of correct rejection of pairs such as 'hut'/ham than pairs such as 'chin'/cheek. Based on this reasoning we can make the following predictions: 1) we expect a superior correct rejection rate for list VSA,SD ('hut'/ham) compared to list VSA,SS ('chin'/cheek); and, 2) we expect greater accuracy of rejection for list VD,SD ('pie'/bow) than for the VD,SS list ('spoon'/fork).

The overall results obtained on this task are presented in Table 4. A comparison of the specific predictions and the results obtained are presented in Table 5.

The results indicate no significant difference in correct rejection rates between lists VSA,SD and VSA,SS ($X_2 = 1.16$, ns) nor between lists VD,SD and VD,SS ($X_2 = .99$, ns) Thus, when word/picture pairs are matched for level of visual similarity there is no significant advantage for those pairs belonging to different superordinate categories. This result is clearly inconsistent with WSM's assumption that the ability to categorize words not identified implies access to superordinate knowledge of those words.

Table 3. Characteristics of word lists for word picture verification task.

Type	n	Mean cumulative frequency	Mean letter length	Mean syllable length
MATCHES	144	31.5	4.9	1.4
VSA,SD	56	43.7	4.9	1.5
VSA,SS	69	32.0	4.9	1.7
VSB,SD	72	35.9	4.6	1.3
VD,SS	73	29.3	5.5	1.4
VD,SD	27	42.8	4.4	1.1

Table 4. Word/picture verification results.

Pair type	% Categorized correctly	% Read correctly	% Read incorrectly
Matches (toe-toe)	79% (95/120)	13% (18/144)	4% (6/144)
VSA,SD (net-neck)	69% (34/49)	7% (4/56)	5% (3/56)
VSA,SS (toe-tooth)	59% (30/51)	19% (13/69)	7% (5/69)
VSB,SD (toe-tie)	45% (29/65)	7% (5/72)	3% (2/72)
VD,SS (toe-ear)	65% (35/54)	26% (19/73)	0% (0/73)
VD,SD (pie-bow)	83% (19/23)	4% (1/27)	11% (3/27)

(The discrepancy between the n categorized and total n is the result of the fact that items correctly or incorrectly identified were discarded before the patient was asked to make a yes/no decision.)

We can also make an overall comparison of the effect of semantic similarity/dissimilarity by collapsing lists across the various levels of visual similarity to compare performance on SD vs. SS lists. A chi-square analysis of the results (Table 5) indicates a non-significant difference between SD and SS lists in the direction contrary to the one predicted (x^2 = .04, ns).

Table 5. Predictions and results of the word/picture verification task.

	Predictions	Results
(1) % correct rejections:	VSA,SD > VSA,SS	69% / 59% (x^2 = 1.16 ns)
(2) % correct rejections:	VD,SD > VD,SS	83% / 65% (x^2 = 0.99 ns)
(3) total across lists*:	SD > SS	60% / 62% (x^2 = 0.04 ns)

* SS includes VSA,SS and VD,SS. SD includes VSA,SD; VD,SD and VSB,SD)

A further set of expectations for J.E.'s performance on this task can be derived from the view that this patient had access only (or primarily) to superordinate information. When two word/picture pairs consist of items belonging to different semantic categories (e.g., 'skin'/skunk and 'soup'/clown) in both instances there is sufficient information to allow the patient to correctly reject the match independently of the degree of orthographic similarity between word and picture name. For example, if the patient knows that 'skin' is a body part and also recognizes the picture of the skunk he would know that they do not match; likewise, if the word 'soup' is identified as a food, the patient should not confuse it with a picture of a clown. This reasoning is reflected in predictions 3-5 in Table 6. We can expect equivalent accuracy in correct rejection rates on each of these lists since the words are matched for frequency and letter and syllable length--a correct rejection can be made for all pairs on the basis of superordinate information alone. However, these predictions, unlike predictions 1 and 2, are not critical to the position taken by WSM. One might imagine an interaction between visual and semantic similarity such that visually similarity makes the discrimination between word and picture pairs more difficult. Nonetheless, this task, which requires matching across different surface forms of stimuli (picture-word), is a semantic task and it is not easy to imagine that this patient would not avail himself of the necessary semantic information if it were available to him.

As indicated in Table 6 for comparisons 3-5, where equivalent results were expected on the list pairs, a chi-square analysis reveals significantly superior performance in comparisons 3 and 4 for those lists containing visually dissimilar items. For comparison 3 the correct rejection rate was superior on list VSA,SD as compared to list VSB,SD ($X^2 = 5.97$, $p < .02$). For comparison 4 performance was significantly more accurate on list VD,SD than on VSB,SD ($X^2 = 8.42$, $p < .01$). Only comparison 5: VSA,SD/VD,SD did not reveal a significant difference ($X^2 = .81$, ns) in rejection accuracy.

Table 6. Further predictions and results of the word/picture verification task.

	Predictions	Results
(3) % correct rejections:	VSB,SD = VSA,SD	45% / 69% ($X^2 = 5.97$, $p<.02$)
(4) % correct rejections:	VSB,SD = VD,SD	45% / 83% ($X^2 = 8.42$, $p<.01$)
(5) % correct rejections:	VSA,SD = VD,SD	69% / 83% ($X^2 = .81$ ns)
(6) total across lists*:	VS = VD	56% / 70% ($X^2 = 3.62$, $p<.05$, one-tailed)

* VS includes VSA,SD; VSA,SS and VSB,SD. VD includes VD,SD and VD,SS

To examine the overall significance of orthographic factors we can collapse across lists and compare similar (VS) vs. visually dissimilar (VD) lists. A chi-square analysis of the frequencies of correct matches indicate a statistically significant difference ($X^2 = 3.62$, $p < .05$; one-tailed) between VS and VD conditions. These results indicate that the patient is sensitive to orthographic information since discrimination between visually dissimilar word and picture names is superior to discrimination between visually similar pairs.

Auditory Presentation of the Word/Picture Verification Task

The entire task was readministered auditorily in order to ensure that the subject's deficits did not involve either a central semantic impairment or an impairment in picture identification. It was necessary to determine that this patient had no difficulty, for example, in making the comparison required in the verification task. J.E.'s accuracy with auditory presentation was 95% correct (420/442). The 22 errors occurred principally on word/picture pairs that were semantically similar regardless of the degree of orthographic similarity between word and picture name. The distribution of the 22 errors was as follows: Matches: 6/144 (4%); VSA,SD: 1/56 (2%); VSA,SS: 7/69 (10%); VSB,SD: 1/72 (1%); VD,SD: 0/27 (0%); VD,SS: 7/73 (10%). The discrepancy in performance between the written and aural versions of the task demonstrates that neither a central semantic impairment nor an impairment in picture identification can account for the pattern of results obtained by J.E. in the written word/picture verification task.

DISCUSSION

We have documented the case of a patient (J.E.) whose performance shows above chance accuracy in forced-choice categorization tasks in spite of an apparent inability to identify more precisely the very items he is able to categorize correctly--a pattern of performance that WSM have interpreted as support for their view of general to specific access to semantic information. This patient's performance in a word/picture verification task was used to test WSM's proposal according to the following reasoning: If this patient has access only to the superordinate class of written words then he should have greater difficulties in distinguishing between words that share a superordinate than between those that do not. The results obtained with J.E. do not support this prediction. Consequently, the general to specific access view of WSM is weakened. The question now becomes: If correct categorization of items that cannot be specifically identified does not necessarily imply support for the hypothesis of general to specific semantic access, how can we explain the categorization results?

We briefly describe two classes of accounts that are consistent with the data reported thus far. We shall call the two classes of accounts the 'partial semantic activation explanation' and the 'restricted search explanation.' We present these accounts, without discounting the possibility that other explanations are also plausible, simply to indicate that there are indeed other ways of thinking about the performance patterns under review besides that proposed by WSM.

The general form of the 'restricted search explanation' can be found in Riddoch and Humphreys' (1985) criticism of the interpretation that Warrington and Shallice (1979) provide for A.R.'s categorization abilities. Riddoch and Humphrey suggest that the discrepancy between this patient's impaired performance in item identification and his ability to correctly categorize these items resides in differences in task demands: In the identification task there is a large number of possible response choices whereas in the yes/no, forced-choice, categorization task there is a limited set of possible responses.

The restricted search explanation suggests that the information available when a written word is presented to J.E. is insufficient for the successful identification of that word amongst all possible words in the English language. However, when he is able to reduce the set of possible responses to those that are members of the category choices presented him, he is often able to make a correct forced-choice judgement. It is important to realize that when a subject is provided with a category choice for items he cannot identify, the task structure has been changed in substantive ways. First of all, a fuller description of the item is provided to the subject--the subject now knows that the word is spelled p-e-a-r and that it is either a fruit or a profession. This fact not only enriches the search process but allows for another starting point to the search, that is, the subject can begin with the category and attempt to retrieve orthographic representations of its exemplars. Second, a slightly different question is being asked of the subject, the question is now: to which is the letter string p-e-a-r more related? to fruit or profession?

The restricted search explanation is actually a class of explanations. There are a number of different architectures and processes that would be consistent with and subsumed under the rubric of restricted search hypotheses. In this discussion, and without independent motivation to prefer one particular instantiation over another, we will limit ourselves to examining the relevance of this sort of explanation to the categorization abilities of this patient.

We can reexamine the results of the word/picture verification task with respect to the restricted search hypothesis. On this hypothesis, we do not expect any advantage for word/picture pairs that do not share a superordinate over those that do; that is, given the word "pilot" a picture of a policeman should be as helpful (or unhelpful) as a picture of a pillow in reducing the search space. J.E.'s performance on the word/picture verification task is consistent with this expectation derived from the restricted search hypothesis. Thus, both the categorization and the picture/word verification results are consistent with a restricted search explanation of J.E.'s performance.

Also consistent with the restricted search explanation are categorization results obtained with J.E. that demonstrate the strong influence of: 1) the degree to which the word is typical of its category and 2) the number of choices in the category decision. J.E. was tested with a categorization task in which the variables of typicality and number of choices were manipulated. Word stimuli were presented in written and auditory forms on separate occasions. Stimuli were either highly typical or less typical exemplars of their categories. The Battig and Montague norms (1969) were used to select highly typical items--items from positions 1-10 in a given category--and less typical items--items below position 24 in a given category. These norms were constructed on the basis of the order and frequency with which subjects provided examples of a particular category; that is, the order in which category exemplars 'came to mind' (e.g., according to these norms dentist and carpenter are highly typical professions, whereas priest, butcher, and chef are less typical professions). As a further manipulation of the decision structure, J.E. was asked either to choose between two or among four categories.

J.E. performed the categorization task with 100% accuracy when the word stimuli were presented auditorily. The results of his performance with the written stimuli are presented in Table VII. Statistical analyses reveal a significant difference in overall categorization accuracy between high and low typicality items ($X^2 = 6.33$, $p < .02$). Highly typical items were categorized at above chance levels in the two-choice condition ($X^2 = 6.33$, $p < .02$) and at a level that approached significance in the four-choice condition ($X^2 = 3.44$, $p < .1$). Accuracy with items of low typicality was not significantly above chance levels in either the four-choice or the two-choice conditions ($X^2 = 1.38$, $p < .05$ and binomial $p < .05$ respectively). Typicality appears to be a variable that distinguishes between those items correctly categorized and those which were not. In order to directly compare accuracy of high typicality items in the two versus the four-choice condition a correction for guessing was calculated[4]. The correction for guessing yields: two-choice: 46% accuracy; four-choice: 20% accuracy. A chi-square analysis indicates that accuracy in the two-choice condition was superior to that in the four-choice condition ($X^2 = 6.6$, $p < .01$). Thus, J.E. was more successful in categorizing items when he was asked to decide between two rather than among four categories.

Within the restricted search framework the typicality effects reported above could be the result of an advantage in the search process for those items that subjects encounter first in their search for category exemplars. Words such as carpenter and barber, which normal subjects retrieve first

Table 7. Two/four choice categorization with low and high typicality items (items read or identified correctly or incorrectly are excluded).

	Hi Freq.	Mid Freq.	Lo Freq.	TOTALS
Two Choices				
HI TYP	86% (12/14)	67% (6/9)	64% (9/14)	73% (27/37)*
LO TYP	44% (4/9)	38% (3/8)	32% (6/19)	36% (13/36)**
Four Choices				
HI TYP	50% (5/10)	50% (5/10)	27% (4/15)	40% (14/35)***
LO TYP	36% (4/11)	30% (3/10)	35% (7/20)	34% (14/41)****

*   binomial $\underline{P}$ <.01)
**   binomial $\underline{p}$ > .05
*** $\underline{\chi}^2$ = 3.44, $\underline{P}$ < .1
**** $\underline{\chi}^2$ = 1.38, $\underline{P}$ > .05

when asked to give exemplars of professions, may be the words that J.E. examines when searching the category of professions. Finally, a two-choice decision situation provides a greater reduction of the search space than does a four-choice decision.

Consistent with this view, Patterson and Kay (1982) reported what they believed to be an example of this type of "artifact." Working with a "letter-by-letter" reader they presented words tachistoscopically and the patient was asked to make category judgements for words she was unable to read with such a brief exposure. The patient typically reported seeing only the first one or two letters of most words she could not read. Nonetheless, her performance on a categorization task was above chance on certain lists. Concerned that the patient was using partial orthographic information to make correct category decisions without actually accessing the words' meanings, several weeks later the authors aurally presented the subject with only those letters she herself had reported seeing during the task and asked her to make the same category decisions as in the previous task. She was correct in 9/10 cases. The authors concluded that this patient's categorization abilities did not constitute evidence for comprehension but rather for a limited-choice, decision-making process.

The other explanation of the pattern of performance under consideration in this paper, the 'partial semantic activation explanation,' assumes that J.E. is able to access the semantic representation corresponding to a written word but that this representation is only *partially* available or activated. By partially activated we mean that a subset of the possible semantic information available for a given concept is accessed. The critical difference between this view and that proposed by WSM is that according to the 'partial semantic access hypothesis' the information accessed is not strictly about the superordinate category of a word. Nonetheless, access to this partial information may allow for accurate category judgements. For example, if upon presentation of the word "ostrich" any part of its semantic representation (e.g., flies, eats, runs, has feathers, or has a particular type of neck) becomes available one could, without knowing that it is an ostrich, choose between the categories animal/transportation. However, the word/picture verification task used in the reported experiments was not specifically designed to test the partial semantic activation explanation. That is, although we would expect items from different superordinate classes to generally share fewer features and therefore be more discriminable, strong predictions cannot be generated.

J.E.'s performance in the categorization experiment in which the typicality of words and the number of category choices were manipulated is also consistent with the 'partial semantic access hypothesis.' If we were to assume that items of low typicality differ from those of high typicality in that the first share fewer characteristic features with their superordinates (Smith et al.,1974), we can account for J.E.'s superior categorization performance for high-typicality words compared to low-typicality words: the incompletely activated semantic representations of high-typicality words are more likely to contain features that can support a correct categorization of these words than would be the case for low-typicality words. Furthermore, on the assumption that the patient may only have available partial semantic information for a word, a two-choice categorization task not only allows for less complex decision making but provides fewer opportunities for categories to overlap in terms of their features and, therefore, offers a more discriminable contrast than a four-choice categorization task. This account may be the basis for J.E.'s better performance for the two-choice than the four-choice categorization task.

From the above it is clear that there are alternative accounts that may be offered for the apparently paradoxical dissociation between item identification and categorization. Furthermore, it would appear that the general to specific hypothesis is undermined by the results we have reported for J.E. in the word/picture verification task. One may wish to attempt to save the general to specific hypothesis by arguing that J.E. differs in principled ways from the patients whose performance led to the proposal of the hypothesis in the first place. We note, however, that J.E. was selected for this study because he presented with the critical dissociation between item identification and categorization. Still, had the other patients described by WSM been tested on the tasks used with J.E.-- the word/picture verification and the two- and four-choice discrimination tasks--they might have differed in significant ways in their performance on these tasks. However, unless and until these other patients are tested on the relevant tasks such an objection cannot be given serious consideration. Before concluding we briefly return to the performance of the patients described by WSM and consider their performance in the light of the data and arguments presented above.

In her study, Warrington (1975) reported data obtained from the presentation of pictures as well as from words presented auditorily. There are some difficulties in the interpretation of the results obtained with picture stimuli. These results, rather than providing information regarding the structure of the semantic system, may instead reflect the ability of agnostic patients to extract a reduced amount of information from the visual array. One can assume that in order to precisely identify an object the object recognition system must extract all of the visual features needed to distinguish that object from all other objects known to the subject. These patients, although unable to perform a complete visual analysis of pictures, may have been able to extract sufficient information from the pictorial stimuli to make certain forced-choice decisions. To distinguish between an animal and an object the identification of only one of a large number of features would suffice: leg, wing, eye, mouth, ear, fur, feather, etc. The determination that a picture represents a bird can be made from a more reduced subset of features: wing, feather, beak, etc. and consequently would be more difficult. Finally, knowledge of whether an object is English/non-English, larger than a cat, heavier than a telephone directory and so forth is only available after a subject has uniquely identified the object. Within this framework, it is not surprising that animal/object decisions were the most accurate, bird/non-bird were less accurate but still above chance, and that the patients were essentially at chance in recognizing the name, size, or country of origin of an object or animal. In other words, subjects' performance is consistent with the hypothesis that they base their classification decisions on a limited number of visual features.

The results of the auditory task are more interesting as they do not allow for the type of explanation given above. One cannot identify aspects of a word's meaning from its phonetic or phonological features. Nonetheless, two of three patients described by Warrington (1975) exhibit significant differences in accuracy between superordinate and subordinate judgements. These results can, however, be equally well explained by the partial semantic activation explanation. The superior performance for superordinate judgements may merely reflect the fact that these latter judgements can be made on the basis of any one of a large number of semantic properties. As noted above, access to any one of the following properties: fur, legs, living, moves, and so forth, would be sufficient for a correct animal/non-animal decision. By contrast, for an English/foreign discrimination precisely that piece of information must be retrieved.

The restricted search account can also explain the reported results if we assume that certain cues such as English, heavier than a telephone directory, metallic, larger than a cat, and so forth are not as effective as others. It is reasonable to suppose that the facility with which exemplars can be retrieved is dependent on the system of cross referencing and indexing a subject has developed and that all cues do not equally facilitate the retrieval of exemplars. That is, although it may be fairly easy to retrieve exemplars from the categories animal, bird, and indoor objects it may be less straightforward to retrieve exemplars of items heavier than a telephone directory or larger than a cat (and, in any case, the set of items in these latter categories is indeterminately large).

The performance of the other well-studied patient, A.R. (Warrington & Shallice, 1979), that has been used to support the general to specific hypothesis can also be explained by the alternative hypotheses considered above. What is puzzling about Warrington & Shallice's discussion of case A.R. is that, although the authors conclude that access to word meaning involves addressing increasingly specific semantic representations this patient, in fact, performs similarly with superordinate and subordinate choices: 54/72 and 53/72 respectively. This finding is inconsistent with the view that general information is accessed prior to item specific information. The general to specific view predicts that for a patient who cannot fully activate semantic representations, the information required to make superordinate choices should be available more often than the information required to make decisions regarding item specific characteristics. The finding of equal accuracy on superordinate and subordinate decisions for items that cannot be identified suggests that superordinate and subordinate information may not be independent but rather, as would be consistent with the partial semantics explanation, that the limited semantic information available to this patient was sufficient to support both category and subordinate judgements. Alternatively, within the restricted search framework, the subordinate cues offered were as effective as the superordinate cues in reducing the search space.

In conclusion, the general to specific hypothesis of access to word meaning presented by WSM has been shown to have a number of weaknesses. First, the instantiation of a general to specific access procedure in a hierarchical semantic system structure is problematic--it is not obvious how movement downward through the hierarchy is to be negotiated, and WSM do not offer any concrete proposals in this regard. Second, a number of alternative explanations can be formulated which account equally well for the relevant data reported by WSM. The general to specific explanation is, consequently, not obligatory. Finally, and most importantly, we have reported results that directly undermine predictions derived from the general to specific view.

ACKNOWLEDGEMENTS

The research reported in this paper was supported by a grant from the Seaver Institute. We would like to express our appreciation to JE for his participation in this study. We also would like to thank Caroline Carrithers, Neal Cohen, Roberta Ann Goodman-Schulman, and Scott Sokol for their helpful comments.

REFERENCES

Albert, M. L., Yamadori, A., Gardner, H. & Howes, D. (1973). Comprehension in alexia. Brain, 96, 317-328.

Battig, W. F. & Montague, W. E. (1969). Category norms for verbal items in 56 categories: A replication and extension of the Connecticut category norms. Journal of Experimental Psychology, 80, 3, 1-46.

Caramazza. A. & Berndt, R. S. (1985). A multicomponent deficit view of agrammatic Broca's aphasia. In M. L. Kean (Ed.), Agrammatism. London: Academic Press.

Collins, A. M. & Quillian, M. R. (1969). Retrieval time from semantic memory. Journal of Verbal Learning and Verbal Behavior, 8, 240-248.

Dunn, J. M. & Dunn, L. M. (1981). The Peabody Picture Vocabulary Test. Circle Pines, MN: American Guidance Service.

McCloskey, M, Sokol, S., Goodman-Schulman, R. & Caramazza, A. (in press). Cognitive representations and processes in number production: Evidence from cases of dyscalculia. In A. Caramazza (Ed.), Advances in Cognitive Neuropsychology and Neurolinguistics. Hillsdale, NJ: Lawrence Erlbaum Associates, Inc.

Patterson, K. & Kay, J. (1982). Letter-by-letter reading: Psychological descriptions of a neurological syndrome. Quarterly Journal of Experimental Psychology, 34A, 411-441.

Quillian, M. R. (1969). The teachable language comprehender: A simulation program and theory of language. Communications of the ACM, 12, 8, 459-475.

Riddoch, M. & Humphreys, G. (1985). Semantic Systems or System? Neuropsychological Evidence Re-examined. Cognitive Neuropsychology Conference, Venice, Italy.

Schwartz, M. F., Marin, O. S. M. & Saffran, E. M. (1979). Dissociations of language function in dementia: A case study. Brain and Language, 7, 277-306.

Smith, E., Shoben, E. & Rips, L. (1974). Structure and process in semantic memory: A featural model for semantic decisions. Psychological Review, 81, 214-241.

Warrington, E. K. (1975). The selective impairment of semantic memory. Quarterly Journal of Experimental Psychology, 27, 635-657.

Warrington, E. K. & McCarthy, R. (1983). Category-specific access dysphasia. Brain, 106, 859-878.

Warrington, E. K. & Shallice, T. (1979). Semantic access dyslexia. Brain, 102, 43-63.

NOTES

[1] See the Discussion section for problems with the interpretation WSM give for their results.

[2] Warrington and Shallice (1979) also refer to a case reported by Schwartz, Marin and Saffran (1979) and another by Albert, Yamadori, Gardner and Howes (1973) in support of their view of general to specific access to word meaning. However, the data reported in these papers are not easily applicable to the current discussion: These latter researchers were not explicitly addressing the issues of semantic system structure raised here and, consequently, the tasks used in their studies are not readily interpretable in the current context. Furthermore, the tests used by these authors often included an inadequate number of stimuli, making interpretation of results problematic.

[3] In the two choice condition it is assumed that the number of errors produced (10/37) reflects the number of incorrect guesses. Furthermore, given that chance level is 50%, we assume that an equal number of correct responses were also obtained by chance. By subtracting 10 from the total number of correct responses we can get an approximate measure of performance having eliminated the possible effects of guessing. The same logic applies to the four-choice condition if we assume that the number of incorrect responses reflects 3/4 of the total responses made by guessing.

C. Writing

Introduction to Section on Writing

The study of writing (spelling) has not received nearly the same degree of attention enjoyed by reading and reading disorders. Despite this relative neglect, in recent years there has been a considerable amount of work directed at understanding the nature of the spelling process and its disorders (excellent reviews may be found in Ellis, 1982; 1987; Ellis & Young, 1988; Roeltgen & Heilman, 1985; Shallice, 1988; for reviews). A brief overview of this work was presented in the General Introduction, and will not be repeated here. I will, instead, proceed directly to a brief presentation of the papers included in this collection.

Chapter 6, written with Roberta Goodman, presents a detailed analysis of a patient, JG, who was unable to access lexical-orthographic information and consequently had to rely on knowledge of phonology-to-orthography mapping rules in order to spell words and nonwords: JG made many phonologically plausible errors in oral and written spelling of words (e.g., known → none) but spelled nonwords virtually flawlessly. This pattern of performance allowed ut to investigate two issues. One issue concerned whether there is a direct link between the phonological input and the orthographic output lexicon. This issue was investigated through the analysis of JG's performance in spelling homophones. JG's spelling errors for these words consisted primarily in the production of the spelling of the high frequency member of a pair (e.g., hare → hair). This performance was interpreted as support for the hypothesis that there is a direct link between phonological input and orthographic output lexicon. However, I now think that that conclusion is probably incorrect--or, at least, that the results are equally compatible with a model that does not assume any such direct link, but assumes instead that the production of lexical-orthographic forms is the result of the summation of activation of lexical representations from the semantic component and the phonology-to-orthography conversion mechanism (see Hillis & Caramazza, in press).

The principal focus of the paper, however, concerned questions about the nature of the phonology-to-orthography conversion procedure. Beauvois and Dérouesné (1981) had already documented quite clearly that the choice of a grapheme option for a given phoneme was not consistent. An analysis of the distribution of spelling errors produced by JG showed that the particular choice of a grapheme for a given phoneme was a function of the frequency of that phoneme-grapheme option in the language. Thus, given the sound /s/, JG was more likely to produce the grapheme <s> than the grapheme <c>, consistent with the relative frequency of those two option in English orthography. More importantly,

189

the probability of a particular grapheme option was <u>context dependent</u>. That is, the choice of a grapheme option was determined by the within-syllable position of a phoneme (e.g., syllable-initial versus syllable-final) and the immediately surrounding graphemes (e.g., /s/ was rendered as <s> or <c> when preceding <e, i, and y> but only as <s> when preceding <a, u, and o>. The implication of these results is that the unit of phonology-to-orthography conversion is not the phoneme but a larger unit, most likely the syllable. The latter conclusion is consistent with other results which show that graphemic representations are not simply linear sequences of graphemes but, instead, consist of multidimensional structures specifying the consonant/vowel (CV) status of graphemes and graphosyllabic structure (see Caramazza & Miceli, 1989; in press).

The claim that the selection of a grapheme option reflects the distribution of phoneme-grapheme mapping options in the language has not gone unchallenged, however. Baxter & Warrington (1987) reported the performance of a dysgraphic patient which they interpreted as showing that when spelling is accomplished by the application of sub-lexical phonology-to-orthography conversion procedures the selection of a grapheme option for a phoneme is not, as proposed in Goodman and Caramazza, a direct function of the <u>relative</u> frequency of phoneme-grapheme mappings in the language but is simply based on which phoneme-grapheme mapping is the most frequent one (but see Goodman, 1988; Baxter & Warrington, 1988). However, the analysis of the performance of another dysgraphic patient (see Sanders & Caramazza, 1990) and reconsideration of the analyses reported by Baxter and Warrington, suggest that the conclusion reached in Goodman and Caramazza is probably correct. Independently of which account ultimately turns out to be correct, it is clear that analyses such as those first reported by Beauvois and Dérouesné (1981) and subsequently by Hatfield and Patterson (1983), Goodman & Caramazza (1986), Baxter and Warrington (1987), and Sanders and Caramazza (1990) will help us understand the structure of the sub-lexical phonology-to-orthography conversion procedure.

It has been known for some time from research reported by Kinsbourne and his colleagues (Kinsbourne & Warrington, 1963; Kinsbourne & Rosenfield, 1974) that oral and written spelling may be affected differentially by brain damage. These investigators have reported both cases of relative sparing of oral spelling in the face of impaired written spelling, and the reverse pattern. In Chapter 7, written with Roberta Goodman, we report the spelling performance of a complex case, MW, who had a deficit in activating lexical-orthographic representations and, consequently spelled words through the application of sub-lexical phonology-to-orthography conversion procedures: many of his spelling errors for words consisted of phonologically plausible misspellings (e.g., immense → immence). These errors were observed both in oral and written spelling. However, MW also made many errors in written spelling of words and nonwords that were not phonologically plausible (e.g., starve → starze). The presence of the latter type of errors only in written spelling was interpreted as suggesting an additional deficit at the level of allographic conversion--the mechanism that converts graphemes into specific letter shapes for subsequent motor processes. This case illustrates that it is possible to distinguish the contribution of multiple deficits on performance.

Although computational considerations led to the postulation of a graphemic buffer in the spelling process (e.g., Ellis, 1982), it was not until the report by Caramazza, Miceli, Villa, and Romani (1987) (Chapter 8) that clear empirical evidence for this component was obtained. This case was summarized in the general discussion, and will not be considered again here.

Chapter 9, written with Gabriele Miceli, briefly summarizes the results of a detailed investigation of the spelling errors produced by patient LB. A more detailed report may be found in Caramazza and Miceli (in press). The interest in this case stems from the fact that it represents the first report to consider seriously the possibility of articulating specific claims about the structure of graphemic representations (as already alluded to in the general introduction). LB's spelling errors respected a highly specific set of constraints. Thus, for example, he virtually always substituted consonants for consonants and vowels for vowels, and he virtually only omitted consonants when these were flanked by at least another consonant and vowels when these were flanked by at least another vowel. The presence of these constraints on spelling errors is difficult to explain if only assume that graphemic representations consist of linearly ordered sets of graphemes. On this latter assumption it is not obvious why consonants are only substituted for consonants or why singleton consonants are never omitted but they are when they occur in clusters. Furthermore, the assumption of a linear sequence of graphemes would fail to explain LB's performance with geminate consonants (e.g., sorella). Geminates behaved as a single entity so that substitutions and transpositions involved both members of a geminate cluster (e.g., troppo → trocco; soffre → fossre). To account for these and other constraints on LB's spelling errors, we had to assume that graphemic representations are multidimensional structures representing not only the identity and order of the graphemes that comprise the spelling of a word, but also their CV status and graphosyllabic structure. It is quite possible that the specific assumptions we have made about graphemic structure are wrong. However, it is unlikely that we are mistaken about the need to assume a multidimensional structure for graphemic representations.

References

Baxter, D. M. & Warrington, E. K. (1987). Transcoding sound to spelling: Single or multiple sound unit correspondence? Cortex, 23, 11-28.

Baxter, D. M. & Warrington, E. K. (1988). The case for biphoneme processing: A rejoinder to Goodman-Schulman. Cortex, 24, 137-142.

Beauvois, M.-F. & Dérouesné, J. (1981). Lexical or orthographic agraphia. Brain, 104, 21-49.

Caramazza, A., Miceli, G., Villa, G. & Romani, C. (1987). The role of the Graphemic Buffer in Spelling: Evidence of a case from acquired dysgraphia. Cognition, 26, 59-85.

Caramazza, A. & Miceli, G. (1989). Orthographic structure, the graphemic buffer and the spelling process. In C. von Euler, I. Lundberg & G. Lennerstrant (Eds.), Brain and Reading. MacMillan/Wenner-Gren International Symposium Series.

Caramazza, A. & Miceli, G. (in press). The structure of graphemic representations. Cognition.

Ellis, A. W. (1982). Spelling and writing (and reading and speaking). In A. W. Ellis (Ed.), Normality and pathology in cognitive functions. London: Academic Press.

Ellis, W. W. (1987). Intimations of modularity, or, the modularity of mind: Doing cognitive neuropsychology without syndromes. In M. Coltheart, G. Sartori & R. Job (Eds.), The cognitive neuropsychology of language. London: Erlbaum.

Ellis, A. W. & Young, A. W. (Eds.). (1988). Human cognitive neuropsychology. Hillsdale, NJ: Lawrence Erlbaum Associates.

Goodman-Schulman, R. (1988). Orthographic ambiguity: Comments on Baxter and Warrington. Cognitive Neuropsychology Laboratory. The Johns Hopkins University, Baltimore, MD.

Goodman, R. A. & Caramazza, A. (1986). Dissociation of spelling errors in written and oral spelling: The role of allographic conversion in writing. Cognitive Neuropsychology, 3, 179-206.

Hatfield, M. & Patterson, K. E. (1983). Phonological spelling. Quarterly Journal of Experimental Psychology, 35, 451-468.

Hillis, A. & Caramazza, A. (in press). The reading process and its disorders. In D. Margolin (Ed.), <u>Cognitive Neuropsychology In Clinical Practice</u>. New York, NY: Oxford University Press.

Kinsbourne, M. & Rosenfield, D. B. (1974). Agraphia selective for written spelling: An experimental case study. <u>Brain and Language</u>, <u>1</u>, 215-225.

Kinsbourne, M. & Warrington, E. K. (1963). Jargon aphasia. <u>Neuropsychologia</u>, <u>1</u>, 27-37.

Roeltgen, D. P. & Heilman, K. M. (1985). Review of agraphia and a proposal for an anatomically based neuropsychological model of writing. <u>Applied Psycholinguistics</u>, <u>6</u>, 205-230.

Sanders, R. & Caramazza, A. (1990). Operation of the phoneme-to-grapheme conversion mechanism in a brain-injured patient. <u>Reading and Writing</u>, <u>2</u>, 61-82.

Shallice, T. (1988). <u>From Neuropsychology to Mental Structure</u>. Cambridge: Cambridge University Press.

CHAPTER SIX

ASPECTS OF THE SPELLING PROCESS:
EVIDENCE FROM A CASE OF ACQUIRED DYSGRAPHIA

INTRODUCTION

Within the last decade, we have witnessed a radical change in the approach to the study of acquired spelling disorders (dysgraphias). Researchers have shifted their attention from classification schemes that describe global characteristics (e.g., agraphia without alexia) to more detailed and explicit accounts of how the spelling system is organized and the possible forms its dissolution may take (see Newcombe & Marshall, 1980; Shallice, 1981; Beauvois & Dérouesné, 1981; Bub & Kertesz, 1982; Hatfield & Patterson, 1983, 1984; Caramazza, Miceli, & Villa, 1986; Goodman & Caramazza, 1986; Patterson, in press; Ellis, 1982, in press).

Two patterns of impaired performance in particular have provided support for a distinction between two sets of processes used in spelling--one for accessing whole-word orthographic information (i.e., addressed orthography) and one for applying sound-to-spelling rules to a phonological sequence (i.e., assembled orthography). One pattern of performance, first described by Shallice (1981), is characterized by inability to accurately spell dictated nonwords in the presence of relatively intact word spelling skills. The other, first described by Beauvois & Dérouesné (1981), is characterized by impairment in accurately spelling orthographically 'regular' and 'irregular' words in the presence of relatively intact nonword spelling skills. The spelling errors produced by Beauvois & Dérouesné's patient primarily took the form of phonologically plausible responses--responses that are explicable in terms of the use of phoneme-grapheme conversion rules in generating a candidate spelling (e.g., 'serfiss' for SURFACE) (see also Hatfield & Patterson, 1983).

The double dissociation between word and nonword spelling performance and the production of phonologically plausible errors by patients with intact nonword spelling skills has been interpreted as support for the view that functionally distinct sets of processes are used in spelling familiar and novel words. Spelling of familiar words involves processes that allow access to lexical-graphemic representations. The component in which these representations are accessed is referred to here as the Graphemic Output Lexicon. Spelling of nonwords (functioning here as

A. Caramazza

novel words) involves nonlexical processes that convert the phonological sequence into a graphemic representation (see Beauvois & Dérouesné, 1981; Caramazza, Miceli, & Villa, 1986; Goodman & Caramazza, 1986). The system in which sound-to-spelling correspondence mappings are selected is referred to here as the Phoneme-Grapheme Conversion Mechanism.[1]

Other case reports in the literature provide evidence for the important role of three other processing mechanisms involved in spelling: A working memory component that temporarily stores addressed or assembled graphemic representations prior to the implementation of more peripheral processes for oral or written spelling--the Output Graphemic Buffer (see Caramazza, Miceli, Villa, & Romani, in press; Miceli, Silveri, & Caramazza, 1985); a mechanism by which each graphemic unit of an addressed or assembled graphemic representation is transcoded into the appropriate case (upper versus lower), type (script versus print), and visual shape associated with each case-type format for written spelling--the Allographic Conversion Mechanism (see Kinsbourne & Rosenfield, 1974; Rothi & Heilman, 1981; Goodman & Caramazza, 1986); and a component by which each graphemic unit of an addressed or assembled graphemic representation is converted into the associated letter-name for oral spelling--the Letter-Name Conversion Mechanism (see Kinsbourne & Warrington, 1965; Hier & Mohr, 1977). These processes are referred to here as "post-graphemic" in order to capture the fact that a graphemic representation for spelling has already been computed. (For a discussion of the more peripheral processes involved in writing such as the organization of handwriting or typewriting, the reader is referred to the work of van Galen, 1980; Viviani & Terzuolo, 1983; Margolin & Wing, 1983; Roeltgen & Heilman, 1983; Margolin, 1984; Baxter & Warrington, in press.)

The general architecture of the spelling system that emerges from a consideration of the nonlexical, lexical, and post-graphemic processing mechanisms required for oral or written spelling of familiar and novel words is schematized in Figure 1. In this paper, we attempt to further elucidate the general structure of the spelling system and to articulate hypotheses about the organization of two of the processing mechanisms critical for accurate spelling performance. More specifically, we addressed the issue of whether or not graphemic representations in the Graphemic Output Lexicon can be directly accessed in response to input from a Phonological Lexicon by considering a dysgraphic patient's pattern of errors in spelling homophonic (nonhomographic) words. We further discuss aspects of the internal structure of the Phoneme-Grapheme Conversion Mechanism by considering the factors that determine whether or not the patient spells a word correctly and the pattern of phonologically plausible responses produced as errors.

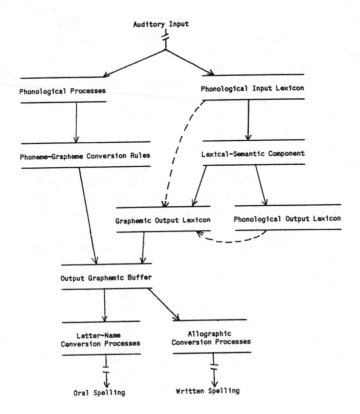

Figure 1. Model of the nonlexical, lexical, and post-graphemic processing mechanisms used for spelling.

CASE HISTORY

JG, a 24 year old right-handed female, sustained a closed-head injury in September, 1983. The patient was found lying unconscious within a half hour of having sustained a fall. At the time of admission to the hospital, JG was described as being somewhat confused and agitated. Her spontaneous speech and language production skills were intact, and she responded appropriately to multiple order commands and answered complex questions accurately. However, JG had some difficulty in confrontation naming, perseverating on some responses and exhibiting mild word finding problems on others.

Neurological examination, performed within 24 hours of admission, revealed that JG had sustained lambdoid suture and basal skull fractures. She suffered a *grand mal* post-traumatic seizure during evaluation. CT-scan revealed a small intercerebral hematoma in the left temporoposterior region. Surgery was not indicated. Motor functioning and cranial nerve examination were intact. At the time of discharge from the hospital one week after admission, JG's naming abilities had greatly improved. A second CT-scan, performed in November, 1983 revealed an area of edema compatible with porencephaly in the left temporoparietal area adjacent to the occipital and temporal horns.

JG was referred to the Cognitive Neuropsychology Laboratory of the Johns Hopkins University in September, 1984 from the University of Maryland Speech and Language Clinic for an assessment of her spelling skills. Her major complaint was that she now produced spelling errors that either sounded like the word but that were not "real" words or that were word substitutions that sounded like the words she intended to write but which had the "other meaning." Examples of errors provided by JG and family members indicated that the patient was referring to phonologically plausible errors (e.g., writing 'kach' for 'catch') and homophone confusion errors (e.g., writing 'pear' instead of 'pair').

JG participated as a subject for the present study over a seven month period. During this time, her spelling performance remained highly stable. JG and the other members of her immediate family report that her reading and spelling skills were normal prior to her accident. JG is a high school graduate. She has been employed as a hair stylist for six years.

SPEECH AND LANGUAGE ASSESSMENT

JG was administered some formal and clinician-devised tests to evaluate her overall language functioning.

Boston Diagnostic Aphasia Examination (Goodglass & Kaplan, 1972)
JG's spontaneous speech was fluent with normal intonation contours, articulation, and word usage. Grammatical complexity and vocabulary were judged to be within normal limits for her age and education level. Repetition of single words and phrases was performed perfectly. Responsive naming and visual confrontation were performed perfectly and JG scored 15 on the 'animal naming/fluency in controlled association' subtest. Auditory comprehension, in terms of word discrimination, body-part identification, commands, and complex ideational material were all performed quickly and accurately. Reading comprehension of sentences was intact and oral reading of single words was perfect;

however, JG produced a few errors in performing oral sentence reading
(i.e., a visually similar nonword response and a function word
substitution). The most difficult section of the battery for JG was the
written language expression section. Copy transcoding ability was intact,
however oral and written spelling of single words and sentences was
impaired. JG uses her preferred right hand for all writing tasks.

Boston Naming Test (Goodglass & Kaplan, 1983)
JG scored 36 of 60 correct on this test. On the BNT norms, normal adults
in JG's age range average 55.86 (SD=2.86). She responded well to
phonemic cuing (16 of 24 correct) but not to stimulus (semantic) cuing (1
of 25 correct). JG did not respond well to phonemic or stimulus cuing for
six of the last eight items on the test, possibly a reflection of her lack of
knowledge of these words premorbidly.

Peabody Picture Vocabulary Test-Revised (Dunn & Dunn, 1981)
For auditory presentation of all items that comprise this test, JG scored
144 of 175 correct. On the PPVT norms, this score falls into the 28th
percentile rank for normal adults within her age range. The majority of
errors (22 of 31) were produced for stimuli in the most difficult section of
the test (items 146-175). As was the case for results of the Boston Naming
Test, this finding may simply reflect the fact that JG never had these
particular words in her vocabulary prior to her accident.

*The Johns Hopkins University Dyslexia Battery (Goodman & Caramazza,
1984)* JG was administered subtests from the Johns Hopkins University
Dyslexia Battery in order to further assess the possibility of her having a
reading deficit at the single word level. She was administered 216 words
and 68 nonwords (e.g., wessal) as an oral reading task. JG was 82%
(177/216) and 44% (30/68) correct for reading of words and nonwords,
respectively ($X^2 = 39.55$, $p < .001$). Analyses performed on preselected
subsets of word stimuli revealed that grammatical word class, concreteness,
orthographic regularity, and word length (i.e., how many letters were in
each word, holding constant the number of phonemes across words of
different letter lengths) did not significantly influence JG's oral reading
performance. However, she was 89% (81/91) and 71% (65/91) correct for
high and low frequency open-class words, respectively ($X^2 = 8.88$, $p < .01$)
indicating that word frequency did significantly affect oral reading
performance. Errors produced for word and nonword reading included
visually similar word (e.g., CURTAIN for 'certain'; CIRCLE for 'sarcle')
and nonword (e.g., /strʌv/ (STRUV) for 'starve'; /gralb/ (GRIBE) for
'ghurb') responses. For words, morphologically related errors (e.g.,

CATCH for 'caught,' SPEECH for 'speak') were also observed. The general pattern of reading performance suggests that JG may have a disruption to the nonlexical Grapheme-Phoneme Conversion Mechanism and a deficit to a lexical reading mechanism, the loci of which cannot be specified from the data presented. This pattern of deficit is in contrast to what was observed in JG's spelling, as will be extensively described in the remainder of the paper.

EXPERIMENTAL SPELLING TASKS

JG was administered a number of spelling and associated tasks. The tasks and results are presented in four sections. Section I describes results obtained from administration of the Johns Hopkins University Dysgraphia Battery (Goodman & Caramazza, 1985), a battery designed to discriminate among functional deficits to various components of the writing system in patients with acquired spelling disorders. In this section, we use results of the battery to hypothesize the locus/loci of deficit(s) to one or more of the three major processing components of the spelling system (i.e., lexical, nonlexical, and post-graphemic processes) responsible for the observed pattern of spelling impairment.[2] We introduce results from specially designed tasks in conjunction with the analysis of spelling errors to more precisely localize the deficit implicated in our patient's impaired pattern of spelling performance. The remaining sections are devoted to a finer-grained analysis of the patient's performance in an effort to further develop and refine hypotheses about the general structure of the lexical spelling system (Section II) and of the internal structure of the Phoneme-Grapheme Conversion Mechanism (Section III).

Results obtained for the battery and associated tasks (accuracy levels)
Writing to Dictation. JG was administered 326 words and 34 nonwords to be written to dictation. Accuracy levels were obtained for preselected subsets of stimuli that systematically differ along dimensions (e.g., grammatical word class) assumed to reflect differential involvement of the hypothesized processing components of the spelling system. We discuss results obtained for subsets of stimuli associated with lexical, nonlexical, and post-graphemic processing skills required for accurate spelling.

1. Lexical Spelling Processes. JG exhibited no significant grammatical word class or concreteness effects (see Table 1). The only lexical factor influencing performance was word frequency. JG was 85% (124/146) and 46% (67/146) correct for high and low frequency open-class words, respectively ($X^2 = 49.18$, $p < .001$). This finding suggests that she has a

deficit to a lexical mechanism in contrast to an impairment to nonlexical or post-graphemic processes.[3]

2. Nonlexical and Post-Graphemic Spelling Processes. JG was 100% (34/34) correct for writing nonwords indicating that phoneme-grapheme conversion processes are intact (see Table 1). She was more accurate for writing nonwords (100% (34/34)) than words (65% (212/326)) ($X^2 = 17.97$, $p < .001$). JG's impairment for word spelling relative to her intact nonword spelling performance provides additional support for the view that she has a deficit at some level of a lexical component. JG's excellent performance for nonword spelling rules out the possibility of a post-graphemic processing deficit as an explanation of her deficit for word spelling since both words and nonwords require an intact Output Graphemic Buffer and Allographic Conversion Mechanism for accurate performance. Further, word length (i.e., varying the number of letters that form a word but keeping the number of phonemes constant across words of different letter lengths), a factor that has been related to an impairment to a post-graphemic spelling mechanism (i.e., Output Graphemic Buffer), did not significantly affect JG's spelling performance.

In sum, results of the writing to dictation task indicate that JG has a deficit to a lexical component in the face of intact nonlexical and post-graphemic processing abilities. In the next section, we explore the level of the lexical impairment implicated in JG's spelling performance.

A lexical deficit implicated in impaired ability to accurately spell words may be the result of a deficit at the level of the Phonological Input Lexicon, the Lexical-Semantic Component, or the Graphemic Output Lexicon (or any combination thereof). In order to try to specify the level of the lexical deficit implicated in JG's pattern of impaired spelling of words, we administered oral spelling, meaning/writing to dictation, written naming, and written picture description tasks, each of which is described in turn.

Oral Spelling. According to our model of spelling, a deficit in any of the lexical or nonlexical spelling mechanisms should affect performance for written and oral spelling of words and nonwords. Therefore, we explored JG's performance for oral spelling with the expectation that the same lexical (i.e., word frequency) and nonlexical (i.e., ability to implement phoneme-grapheme correspondence mappings) factors that influenced spelling under the written spelling condition would also affect spelling under the oral spelling condition. JG was administered the same set of stimuli used for the writing to dictation task as an oral spelling to dictation task (i.e., given an auditory presentation of a word or nonword, JG was to spell the word aloud). These stimuli were administered within a two month period following the completion of the writing to dictation tasks.

At least one month lapsed between written and oral spelling of any particular stimulus.

Table 1. JG's performance for written spelling of dictated words and nonwords.

			Percent Correct
1. Word frequency[a]			
	High	(N=146)	85%
	Low	(N=146)	46%
2. Grammatical word class[b]			
	Nouns	(N=28)	61%
	Verbs	(N=28)	68%
	Adjectives	(N=28)	43%
	Functors	(N=20)	75%
3. Concreteness[c]			
	Concrete	(N=21)	57%
	Abstract	(N=21)	52%
4. Word/nonword status[d]			
	Words	(N=326)	65%
	Nonwords	(N=34)	100%
5. Word Length[e]			
	4-letters	(N=14)	57%
	5-letters	(N=14)	71%
	6-letters	(N=14)	79%
	7-letters	(N=14)	57%
	8-letters	(N=14)	43%

[a] High versus low frequency: $x^2=49.18$, $p<.001$
[b] Grammatical word class:
　Nns versus vbs+adjs　$x^2=0.21$, NS
[c] Concreteness:　$x^2=0.10$, NS
[d] Words versus nonwords:　$x^2=17.96$, $p<.001$
[e] Word Length:
　4-5 versus 7-8 letters　$x^2=1.16$, NS

As was expected, JG performed similarly in written and oral spelling of dictated words and nonwords (see Table 2; JG's performance on the written spelling task is reproduced from Table 1 for ease of comparison). She correctly spelled 97% (33/34) of nonwords, a result consistent with intact phoneme-grapheme conversion and post-graphemic processing skills. Grammatical word class and concreteness did not significantly affect spelling performance. The only lexical factor influencing oral spelling performance was word frequency. JG correctly spelled 89%

(130/146) and 60% (88/146) of high and low frequency open-class words, respectively ($X^2 = 31.94$, $p < .001$).

Table 2. JG's performance for oral (and written) spelling of dictated words and nonwords.

Spelling to Auditory Dictation:		Percent Correct	
		Oral Spelling	Written Spelling
1. Word frequency[a]			
High	(N=146)	89%	(85%)
Low	(N=146)	60%	(46%)
2. Grammatical word class[b]			
Nouns	(N=28)	71%	(61%)
Verbs	(N=28)	68%	(68%)
Adjectives	(N=28)	57%	(43%)
Functors	(N=20)	75%	(75%)
3. Concreteness[c]			
Concrete	(N=21)	76%	(57%)
Abstract	(N=21)	76%	(52%)
4. Word/nonword status[d]			
Words	(N=326)	74%	(65%)
Nonwords	(N=34)	97%	(100%)
5. Word Length[e]			
4-letters	(N=14)	64%	(57%)
5-letters	(N=14)	64%	(71%)
6-letters	(N=14)	79%	(79%)
7-letters	(N=14)	79%	(57%)
8-letters	(N=14)	43%	(43%

[a] High versus low frequency: $X^2=31.94$, p<.001
[b] Grammatical word class:
  Nns versus vbs+adjs $X^2=0.66$, NS
[c] Concreteness: $X^2=0.00$, NS
[d] Words versus nonwords: $X^2=11.98$, p<.001
[e] Word Length:
  4-5 versus 7-8 letters $X^2=0.06$, NS

The results reported thus far indicate that JG has a deficit at some level of a lexical mechanism. There are two possible loci of impairment that could account for JG's impaired pattern of spelling performance. One possibility is that JG has a deficit at the level of the Phonological Input Lexicon not allowing for access to the corresponding entries in the Lexical-Semantic Component. Another possibility is that JG can in fact obtain the meaning of the auditorily presented stimulus (i.e., has an intact ability to gain access to the Lexical-Semantic Component from the Phonological Input Lexicon) but has a disruption in accessing whole-word spelling representations in the Graphemic Output Lexicon. If the former hypothesis is correct, then when JG is asked to provide the meaning of an auditorily presented word prior to spelling the word, she should not be able to do so for words in which she subsequently produces spelling errors. However, if the latter hypothesis is correct, then JG should be able to provide the meaning for all auditorily presented words whether they are subsequently spelled correctly or incorrectly. In order to discriminate between these two alternatives, we administered the following task.

Meaning/Writing to Dictation Task. JG was administered a list of 188 words auditorily, one word at a time, and asked to first write a short definition of each stimulus and upon completion of this to then write the word that had been presented by the examiner. She supplied an adequate definition for 98% (185/188) of the words. However, she misspelled 42% (77/185) of the words for which an adequate definition had been provided as seen in the following examples taken from the error corpus:

STIMULUS	RESPONSE-DEFINITION/TARGET
CUSHION	something that goes on a couch - *coushin*
PITY	feel sorry for someone - *pitty*
NUISANCE	pain in the butt - *newcence*
URGE	feel for you - *erge*, urge
ODOR	smell - *odar*
ANCIENT	old, history - *anchant*
CHORUS	singers - *couras*
RATION	limited - *rasson*

JG also produced errors in spelling of words that were part of the definitions (23% (43/185)) whether the target word was subsequently spelled correctly (56% (24/43)) or incorrectly (44% (19/43)) as seen in the following examples taken from the error corpus (words misspelled in the definitions have been underlined with the intended target placed in brackets to the right of the misspelled word):

STIMULUS	RESPONSE-DEFINITION/TARGET
ANNOY	*earatate* (irritate), bother - *anoye*
FRAGILE	*easly* (easily) *brocken* (broken)/broken - *fragel*
MERCY	*spear* (spare) them no *merse* (mercy) if tampered with! - *mersy*

LAUGH   *silley* (silly) - laugh
ARGUE   difference in *apinon* (opinion)- argue
MOOSE   hair *jell* (gel) or *fome* (foam); animal - moose
               (Note: 'mousse' is the name of a hair gel.)

These results indicate that JG correctly addresses the semantic representation of words that she misspells. Hence, the locus of the deficit responsible for her impaired performance for oral and written spelling of auditorily presented words is *not* in addressing lexical-semantic representations but, most likely, in gaining access to whole-word spelling representations in the Graphemic Output Lexicon. According to this hypothesis, any written spelling task requiring access to the Graphemic Output Lexicon, regardless of the modality of input to this mechanism (e.g., phonological, visual) will produce the same pattern of impaired performance. The following written spelling tasks were administered in order to further examine this possibility.

Additional Written Spelling Tasks
1. *Written Naming.* JG was shown 51 pictures of single objects and asked to write the name most often associated with that picture. One-third of these pictures are associated with a low frequency name, one-third with a mid frequency name, one-third with a high frequency name; the names associated with the pictures were counterbalanced for word frequency, syllabicity, and word length (i.e., the number of letters forming each word).

JG produced seven errors in spelling these words, all to words associated with low-to-mid frequency names. Thus, she was 100% (17/17), 76% (13/17), and 82% (14/17) accurate for high, mid, and low frequency words, respectively (X^2 = 4.05, p < .05 for high versus low-to-mid frequency words).

2. *Written Picture Description.* JG was asked to provide a written description to the Cookie Theft scene of the Boston Diagnostic Aphasia Examination (Goodglass & Kaplan, 1972). Of the 84 words she produced, five (4%) were misspelled. JG's low error rate for this task is most probably a reflection of the fact that almost all of the words she selected to use in her description were high frequency words.

The results of these additional tasks are consistent with the hypothesis that JG has a selective deficit in gaining access to whole-word spelling representations in the Graphemic Output Lexicon.

Assessment of Pre- and Post-morbid Spelling Ability. The overall pattern of converging results for written and oral spelling indicates that JG has a selective deficit to the Graphemic Output Lexicon. A major source of evidence in favor of this hypothesis is the patient's marked difficulty in spelling low frequency words. It could be maintained, however, that this difficulty is not an acquired impairment but reflects instead JG's premorbid inability to spell low frequency words. In order to explore this possibility, a premorbid (reportedly uncorrected) sample of JG's written spelling was obtained; a poem that had been written one and a half years prior to the accident. In the sample (containing approximately 200 words), two phonologically *im*plausible nonword errors, taking the form of letter transpositions, were observed. Thus, no phonologically plausible errors or homophone confusion errors had been produced. From the correctly spelled words, 40 stimuli, varying in word frequency, were selected and administered, one at a time, as a writing to dictation task (see Table 3). JG produced 12 errors, 11 of which took the form of phonologically plausible errors, one a substitution error (i.e., 'surrow' for SORROW). These results indicate that JG's spelling impairment is an acquired disorder.

Error Analysis
Up to this point, we have used only the overall pattern of *accuracy* of performance to help identify the level of impairment responsible for JG's spelling deficit. We have ruled out the possibility of explaining JG's performance in terms of disruption to either nonlexical or post-graphemic processing components and have postulated that she has a selective deficit in gaining access to whole-word spelling representations in the Graphemic Output Lexicon.   Given these general hypotheses regarding which components of the spelling system (i.e., lexical, nonlexical, or post-graphemic) are impaired or spared, we can make predictions about the pattern of *errors* we expect our patient to produce. If JG has a deficit to one of the lexical processes, thus making a representation inaccessible for output, but has intact nonlexical and post-graphemic processing mechanisms, we expect her to use the alternative nonlexical mechanism in order to attempt to provide a candidate spelling for the word. Hence, we should observe phonologically plausible errors (PPEs), errors that are explicable in terms of the implementation of phoneme-grapheme correspondence mappings in generating that spelling option.[4] Table 4 shows a breakdown of errors produced to the set of 326 words that were dictated under both oral and written spelling conditions.

The great majority of spelling errors produced took the form of PPEs. PINs represent phonologically *im*plausible nonword responses (e.g., 'ploot' for PLOT). "Other" errors represent responses that do not fall into the error categories of PPEs or PINs--including visually similar word responses. JG did not produce morphologically related responses (e.g.,

'running' for RUNS), semantically related responses (e.g., 'deep' for
SURFACE), or function word substitutions (e.g., 'you' for ME). These
results are consistent with our account of the spelling processes implicated
in JG's pattern of spared and impaired performance.

Table 3. JG's performance for written spelling of words obtained from a
pre-morbid writing sample.[a]

Wd Freq	Stimulus	Response	Wd Freq	Stimulus	Response
2426	EACH	+	90	FIGHT	+
1105	JUST	+	87	HAPPENS	+
821	PLACE	+	82	WONDER	+
468	KEEP	+	74	TOUCH	+
445	ENOUGH	+	60	WORTH	+
389	SOON	+	50	CLIMB	+
313	LEARN	+	48	LOSE	+
292	TURN	+	36	SILENCE	sylence
258	KNOWN	none	35	FROZEN	+
227	FEEL	+	26	BIRTH	berth
173	CARRY	+	19	WAKE	+
155	BOTTOM	+	11	BEATEN	beton
155	MUSIC	+	7	SORROW	surrow
155	FRIEND	+	7	GOALS	goles
155	FIGURE	+	6	DEALS	deales
128	HUMAN	+	3	STRIDE	+
120	REACH	+	2	UNISON	+
108	GUESS	+	2	BETRAYED	betrade
100	MEANT	ment	2	SPEECHLESS	speachless
96	DECIDE	deside	0.4	SURVIVOR	servivor

[a] + = correctly spelled

As was expected, the distributions of errors produced for oral and written
spelling were almost identical, a finding that is consistent with the view
that oral and written spelling of words are tasks that rely on the same
lexical processing mechanisms for accurate performance. Hence, a lexical

Table 4. Breakdown of error types produced by JG for oral and written
spelling of dictated words.

	Oral Spelling	Written Spelling
PPEs	74/84=88%	99/114=87%
PINs	5/84=6%	6/114=5%
Other	5/84=6%	9/114=8%

deficit should in principle elicit the same patterns of performance in terms of accuracy levels obtained and error types produced for these two tasks.

If the lexical deficit is at the level of addressing graphemic representations in the Graphemic Output Lexicon, we expect to observe the same pattern of errors for the other written spelling tasks as was observed for the auditorily presented tasks, all of which require an intact output lexicon for accurate performance. An analysis of the error corpus indicates that the great majority of errors produced for the other written spelling tasks (i.e., definitions of the meaning/writing to dictation, written naming, written picture description) took the form of PPEs (80% (107/134)) followed by the production of PINs (4% (5/134)) and "Other" (16% (22/134)) responses.

Issues Related to the General Architecture of the Spelling Model
The fact that it has been possible to postulate a functional lesion in the model of spelling which can readily account for our patient's overall pattern of spelling performance is taken as evidence for the general structure of the proposed model. In this section of the paper, we attempt to provide more detail about the general architecture of the spelling system through further analysis and testing of our patient's spelling deficit. One area, in particular, in which this patient's performance may be of use is with regard to issues concerning the mechanism of lexical access in the Graphemic Output Lexicon.

The model of spelling we have described assumes that entries from the Phonological Input Lexicon activate lexical-semantic representations which in turn address whole-word spelling representations in the Graphemic Output Lexicon. Is this the only means by which the spelling system operates? More specifically, is it possible to access graphemic representations in the output lexicon directly from the Phonological Input Lexicon or must a speller *always* use lexical-semantic mediation in order to access a graphemic representation in the output lexicon? By analogy to theories of word reading where it has been argued that the Phonological Output Lexicon can be addressed directly from the Graphemic Input Lexicon (e.g., see Schwartz, Saffran, & Marin, 1980; Bub, Cancelliere, & Kertesz, 1986), it could be assumed that spelling can be accomplished via a direct connection between the Phonological Input Lexicon and the Graphemic Output Lexicon.[5]

In order to explore this possibility, we took advantage of the fact that the English language contains many nonhomographic homophones, words that have the same pronunciation but different spellings (e.g., 'sun' and 'son') and are associated with different meanings. Presumably, when the phonological representation for /sʌn/ is activated in the Phonological

Input Lexicon, it addresses all meanings associated with that auditory input in the Lexical-Semantic Component (e.g., Seidenberg & Tanenhaus, 1979). Although all of the different meanings of a word are fleetingly available to the language processing system, only one meaning--that determined by contextual factors (both subjective and objective)--will become dominant and determine the course of further processing. We can speak of this process as instantiating the selection of the specific lexical-semantic representation that will direct further processing. This process is referred to here as a "selection mechanism." Once the selection mechanism has been used to activate the intended semantic representation (over the other possible representation(s)), this representation is then used to access the corresponding graphemic entry in the Graphemic Output Lexicon. Thus, the semantic code representing 'a male offspring' will access the whole-word spelling representation for 'son' but never for 'sun' since this latter code is not at all related to the former in meaning.

If there is a lexical, nonsemantic link such that the phonological representation for /sʌn/ activates both 'son' and 'sun' in the Graphemic Output Lexicon directly from the Phonological Input Lexicon, then, at least on occasion, we should observe homophone confusion errors (i.e., producing the spelling of a word with the same pronunciation but a different meaning) even when the meaning of the intended word is specified and readily understood by the speller. However, although it is in principle possible to accurately spell most English words just by use of such a link (e.g., /lʌv/ would activate 'love' in the output lexicon), bypassing lexical-semantic mediation, it is apparent that accurate spelling of homophonic words cannot be achieved solely by use of this link since multiple representations in the output lexicon could be addressed from phonological input. In this latter case, there is no guarantee that the correct spelling for a word would be produced but instead the spelling produced would depend on whichever representation had reached threshold for output. Obviously, then, if we want the system to spell homophones correctly, activation from the lexical-semantic representation is needed to determine which graphemic representation should be used for output.

The issue under consideration here is whether graphemic representations can be activated directly from phonological input (the Direct, Nonsemantic Access Hypothesis), or whether the only means of addressing these output representations is through activation from the Lexical-Semantic Component (the Indirect Access Only Hypothesis). In order to try to discriminate between the Direct, Nonsemantic Access Hypothesis and the Indirect Access Only Hypothesis, we administered the following homophone task to our patient: First, JG was auditorily presented a homophonic word (e.g., /nʌn/) immediately followed by a short definition ('a woman devoted to religious life') and finally again by the presentation of the homophonic word. JG was instructed to write only the target word and not the definition. Analyses were performed on her spelling of 60 homophone pairs; 26 of which contain one high frequency member (e.g., 'none' is a high frequency word) and one low frequency member ('nun' is a low frequency word) (HL); 17 of which contain two high frequency members (HH) (e.g., 'threw' and 'through'); and 17 of which contain two low frequency members (LL) (e.g., 'steak' and 'stake') (see Appendix I).

The Direct, Nonsemantic Access Hypothesis and the Indirect Access Only Hypothesis allow different predictions regarding JG's expected pattern of performance for the three different types of homophone pairs (i.e., HL, HH, and LL). The predictions that have been derived for the two hypotheses depend on specific background assumptions about the structure of the Graphemic Output Lexicon and the nature of the deficit in our patient JG. These assumptions must be made explicit in order to motivate differential predictions for the two hypotheses.

The first assumption is that an entry in the Graphemic Output Lexicon is activated when it has reached a set, threshold value (Morton, 1979). The threshold associated with each lexical representation is determined by the frequency of that lexical item in the language and in the modality in question. Thus, ease of access of representations in the Graphemic Output Lexicon is determined by how often their corresponding words occur in written language.[6]

A second assumption is critical for our present purposes: When inputs from different processing components converge on a lexicon the inputs summate. Thus, for the Direct, Nonsemantic Access Hypothesis the inputs from the lexical-semantic component and the Phonological Input Lexicon summate to determine which entry in the Graphemic Output Lexicon will reach threshold. We assume, however, that either input alone (from the Lexical-Semantic Component or Phonological Input Lexicon) would, under normal circumstances, be sufficient to activate representations in the Graphemic Output Lexicon. Thus, if for some reason lexical-semantic information were to be unavailable to the Graphemic Output Lexicon, the only determinant of access from this latter lexicon would be the input from the Phonological Input Lexicon. In such a case we would expect homophone errors in the direction of producing the more frequent member of a homophone pair.

A third assumption concerns the locus and nature of impairment in our patient. The evidence presented thus far suggests that JG has a deficit in gaining access to representations in the Graphemic Output Lexicon with low frequency words being especially affected. We assume that the differential ease with which graphemic representations of words of different frequency are accessed reflects the pathological elevation of activation thresholds for all lexical entries in the Graphemic Output Lexicon, thereby making representations associated with low frequency words more difficult to access. This pattern of selective lexical deficit (and associated interpretive assumptions) can be used to motivate predictions regarding the type of results we expect on the basis of the Direct, Nonsemantic Access Hypothesis and the Indirect Access Only Hypothesis for the homophone task described.

Because of JG's impairment in gaining access to graphemic representations of low frequency words in the Graphemic Output Lexicon, it is expected that for homophone pairs containing low frequency members, there is a high probability that whole-word spelling representations of that member will be unavailable for output. Given that this is the case, for the two hypotheses in question, we expect different patterns of errors to emerge:

The Direct, Nonsemantic Access Hypothesis. With direct activation of both members of a homophone pair from the Phonological Input Lexicon, when the whole-word spelling representation of a low frequency representation is unavailable for output, JG will either use as output the graphemic representation associated with the other member of the homophone pair or if that is also unavailable she will rely on the nonlexical Phoneme-Grapheme Conversion Mechanism to generate a phonologically plausible spelling. Since our expectation is that for LL homophone pairs, the graphemic representations of neither member of the pair will be accessible (a large percentage of the time), we expect JG to produce phonologically plausible errors for both members of the pair on these occasions. For pairs consisting of one low and one high frequency member, when the whole-word spelling representation for a low frequency word is unavailable for output, the graphemic representation associated with the high frequency member (if accessible in the output component) will be used instead since it may be addressed directly from the Phonological Input Lexicon. By hypothesis, this will occur even though the lexical-semantic representation associated with the *low* frequency member has been differentially selected over that associated with the high frequency member. According to this account, JG will produce homophone confusions erring in the direction of substituting the higher frequency member for the lower frequency member when that low frequency member is not available in the output lexicon. Additionally, we expect a relatively low incidence of PPEs for members of HL pairs since at least one lexical representation (presumably the high frequency one) can reach threshold in the Graphemic Output Lexicon. If both members of a homophone pair are high frequency words, we expect JG to produce few if any errors since the correct entries in the Graphemic Output Lexicon should be available in the majority of cases. If the entry for one member, is not available in the output lexicon, however, then we do expect a homophone confusion to occur since the output code for the other member of the pair will be directly activated from the Phonological Input Lexicon.

The Indirect Access Only Hypothesis. According to this view, once JG has been given the definition of a homophone (e.g., 'a woman devoted to religious life'), the selection mechanism will differentially activate the semantic representation associated with 'nun' over 'none,' and it is this representation alone that will be used to address the corresponding graphemic representation for output. If the graphemic representation is not accessible, then JG will instead use phoneme–grapheme correspondence mappings to generate a spelling, thus producing phonologically plausible errors, regardless of whether or not the word has a high or a low frequency homophonic counterpart.

Thus, the primary empirical distinction drawn between the two hypotheses is that for HL homophone pairs, the Direct, Nonsemantic Access Hypothesis predicts the production of homophone confusions whereas the Indirect Access Only Hypothesis predicts only the production of phonologically plausible errors regardless of the pair composition. In order to provide an explanation for the production of homophone confusions, proponents of the Indirect Access Only Hypothesis would have to postulate a deficit in the selection mechanism; that is, the assumption would have to be made that the patient is impaired in using the definition provided by the experimenter to access the appropriate lexical-semantic representation, leading to the activation of the incorrect whole-word spelling representation in the Graphemic Output Lexicon. For example, '/nʌn/--a woman devoted to religious life.' will activate the semantic representation of 'not any' which will, in turn, activate the incorrect graphemic representation 'none.' Hence, the homophone confusion would be the result of an improperly working selection mechanism in the Lexical-Semantic Component. Although this Modified Indirect Access Only Hypothesis may be able to account for the occurrence of homophone confusions in the HL condition, it does so by postulating an additional impairment.   However, this hypothesis makes a strong prediction concerning the patient's performance in spelling HH homophone pairs. Specifically, if JG has a deficit in the selection mechanism, then we expect her to produce a fair number of homophone confusions, particularly since both graphemic representations will almost always be available in the output lexicon. Furthermore, the number of homophone confusions expected for the HH pairs is proportional to the number of homophone confusions produced for HL pairs. Indeed, this hypothesis predicts that the patient should produce homophone substitutions for the HH pairs at roughly *twice the rate* as she does for the HL pairs.

RESULTS

Table 5 gives the percentage of high and/or low frequency words that were spelled correctly within each type of homophone pair. High frequency words belonging to the HL pairs were spelled with the same approximate degree of accuracy as were high frequency words belonging to the HH pairs (88% (23/26) and 79% (27/34) correct for high frequency members of HL and HH pairs, respectively, $X^2 = 0.86$, NS). Likewise, low frequency words belonging to the HL and LL pairs were spelled with the same degree of accuracy (35% (9/26) and 38% (13/34) correct for low frequency members of HL and LL pairs, respectively, $X^2 = 0.08$, NS).

Table 5. Percentage correct for high and low frequency words within the three types of homophone pairs.

		Type of Pair			
		HL	HH	LL	Collapsed
	High Freq'y	(23/26) 88%	(27/34) 79%	NA[a]	(50/60) 83%
WORD FREQUENCY	Low Freq'y	(9/26) 35%	NA	(13/34) 38%	(22/60) 37%
	Collapsed	(32/52) 62%	(27/34) 79%	(13/34) 38%	(72/120) 60%

[a] NA = Not Applicable

If we compare accuracy levels for homophonic words (collapsed across pair type) to that of nonhomophonic words (reported in Section I) we see that within the high frequency class, JG was 83% (50/60) and 85% (124/146) correct for homophones and nonhomophones, respectively ($X^2 = 0.08$, NS). For low frequency words, she was 37% (22/60) and 46% (67/146) correct for homophones and nonhomophones, respectively ($X^2 = 1.47$, NS). Overall, JG was 60% (72/120) and 65% (191/292) correct for homophones and nonhomophones, respectively ($X^2 = 1.08$, NS). Thus, JG shows no advantage of nonhomophone over homophone words of the same frequency values in her spelling performance. Recall that if we accept the

A. Caramazza

Modified Indirect Access Only Hypothesis we must assume that JG has an impairment in the selection mechanism involved in activating the correct graphemic representation of a homophone pair. The assumption of such a deficit leads to the prediction that JG should spell homophonic words more poorly than nonhomophonic words since to correctly spell the former requires an intact selection mechanism. The results we have obtained do not support this prediction and hence clearly undermine the Modified Indirect Access Only Hypothesis.

Table 6 reports the percentage of errors within each pair type that took the form of homophone confusions, phonologically plausible errors, and "Other" responses (see Appendix II). These results indicate that there were more homophone confusions produced for members of HL than LL pairs ($X^2 = 7.24$, $p < .01$). In contrast, there were more phonologically plausible errors produced for members of LL than HL pairs ($X^2 = 8.85$, $p < .005$).

More specifically, when we compare the proportion of phonologically plausible errors produced for low frequency members of the HL pairs to that of low frequency members of the LL pairs, we see that the percentage of such errors is substantially higher in the LL than in the HL pairs--of the errors produced for the low frequency members of the HL and LL pairs, 36% (4/11) and 76% (16/21), respectively, were phonologically plausible errors ($X^2 = 4.89$, $p < .05$). These results provide the clearest refutation of The Indirect Access Only Hypothesis since according to this hypothesis, there should be no difference in the percentage of phonologically plausible errors produced for low frequency members of one pair type over another.

Table 6. Percentage of each error type produced for the homophone task.

	Type of Pair			
	HH	HL	LL	Collapsed
Homophone Confusions	(3/7) 43%	(12/20) 60%	(4/21) 19%	(19/48) 40%
Phonologically Plausible	(2/7) 29%	(5/20) 25%	(15/21) 71%	(22/48) 46%
Other	(2/7) 29%	(3/20) 15%	(2/21) 10%	(7/48) 15%

Table 7 shows the results obtained for each type of homophone pair in terms of how many members of that pair were correctly spelled. These results allow us to evaluate the predictions derived from the Direct,

Nonsemantic Access Hypothesis and either form of the Indirect Access Only Hypothesis.

Of the seven LL pairs in which both members were misspelled, <u>none</u> of the errors were homophone confusions; 86% (12/14) took the form of PPEs and two error were visually/phonologically similar word responses (i.e., these word responses occurred for both members of the same homophone pair, 'fail' for FOUL; 'fall' for FOWL). Of the seven LL pairs in which only one member was misspelled, 57% (4/7) of the errors were homophone confusions and 43% (3/7) were PPEs.

Table 7. Number (and proportion) of members spelled correctly within the three types of homophone pairs.

| | Type of Pair | | | |
	HH	HL	LL	Collapsed
BOTH	(12/17) 71%	(7/26) 27%	(3/17) 18%	(22/60) 37%
ONE	(3/17) 18%	(18/26) 69%	(7/17) 41%	(28/60) 47%
NONE	(2/17) 12%	(1/26) 4%	(7/17) 41%	(10/60) 17%

These results are consistent with the Direct, Nonsemantic Access Hypothesis and the Modified Indirect Access Only Hypothesis but not with the Indirect Access Only Hypothesis. JG produced homophone confusions for a low frequency word that has another low frequency word as its homophonic counterpart when the substituted word is spelled correctly (hence is available in the output lexicon) during its presentation. Although the Direct, Nonsemantic Access Hypothesis and the Modified Indirect Access Only Hypothesis allow the occurrence of homophone confusions, the Indirect Access Only Hypothesis does not.

Of the errors produced for the low frequency members (17/26) of the HL pairs, 65% (11/17) were homophone confusions and the substituted homophone had been correctly spelled in all cases during *its* presentation (i.e., 'none' had been correctly spelled when presented with the definition 'not any' and was additionally produced for the definition provided for its homophonic counterpart 'nun'); 23% (4/17) were PPE's and 12% (2/17) were visually/phonologically similar word responses (i.e., 'tall' for TALE; 'hair' for HEIR). Of the three errors produced for the high frequency members of these HL pairs, one was a homophone confusion of a word that had been correctly spelled during its presentation (i.e., 'brake' for BREAK); one was a PPE; and one was a visually/phonologically similar word response (i.e., 'tall' for TAIL).

In short, for the majority of errors, JG produced a homophone, substitution erring in the direction of producing the spelling of a high frequency member for its low frequency counterpart. These results are consistent with the Direct, Nonsemantic Access Hypothesis but not the Indirect Access Only Hypothesis. The pattern of spelling errors produced by JG for homophonic words is incompatible with the hypothesis that the Graphemic Output Lexicon can only be addressed from the Lexical-Semantic Component. It would appear, instead, that it is possible to access lexical entries in the Graphemic Output Lexicon directly in response to activation from representations in a Phonological Lexicon.

An issue we have failed to address concerns the occurrence of homophone errors in spontaneous writing by normal subjects (see Ellis, 1982; Patterson, in press). For errors such as these to occur, we must postulate that a semantic representation activates both phonological and graphemic representations in their respective output lexicons and that, in turn, the phonological representation activates the semantically inappropriate graphemic representation in the Graphemic Output Lexicon.[7] This raises the possibility that the homophone confusion errors produced by our patient result from the activation of the inappropriate graphemic representation from the Phonological *Output* Lexicon. Thus, we could assume that the semantic representation for "a woman devoted to religious life" activates the phonological representation /n∧n/ in the Phonological Output Lexicon which, in turn, activates the graphemic representations 'none' and 'nun.' If one of the latter two graphemic representations was inaccessible the other could become available as a response.[8] This hypothesis of a direct link between the Phonological Output Lexicon and the Graphemic Output Lexicon predicts the identical pattern of homophone confusion errors as that discussed for the hypothesis of a direct link between the Phonological Input Lexicon and the Graphemic Output Lexicon. Consequently, we must conclude that the results reported are consistent with the hypothesis that entries in the Graphemic Output Lexicon may be activated directly from the Phonological Input Lexicon *or* the Phonological Output Lexicon.

The Phoneme-Grapheme Conversion Mechanism
Thus far, we have provided evidence that JG has a deficit in accessing spelling representations in the Graphemic Output Lexicon. When she is unable to activate the lexical representation in response to phonological or semantic input, she relies on nonlexical, phoneme-grapheme conversion

processes in order to provide a phonologically plausible spelling for the stimulus. Although there have been several reports of patients who rely on use of the Phoneme-Grapheme Conversion Mechanism for word spelling (e.g., Beauvois & Dérouesné, 1981; Hatfield & Patterson, 1983) the structural characteristics of this mechanism remain largely unexplored. In the first part of this section, we describe results obtained with a specially designed list that was used to test a complex hypothesis about the structure of nonlexical spelling processes. Some of the results obtained in this task are reported elsewhere (Goodman & Caramazza, in press) and will be reiterated here. In the second part of this section, we examine in greater detail the structure of the Phoneme-Grapheme Conversion Mechanism through an extensive analysis of the pattern of phoneme-grapheme options used by our patient in the production of phonologically plausible errors.

On the assumption that JG spells those words for which the graphemic representations are inaccessible in the output lexicon by means of the Phoneme-Grapheme Conversion Mechanism, we expect some proportion of these words to be "inadvertently" spelled correctly. We should be able to predict which words would inadvertently be spelled accurately if we knew how the Phoneme-Grapheme Conversion Mechanism operated. That is, if we were to know how phoneme-grapheme mapping options are selected in the course of spelling, we could determine which words would have a high probability of being spelled correctly even when their graphemic representation is inaccessible in the output lexicon. A complex hypothesis about the structure of the Phoneme-Grapheme Conversion Mechanism was assessed through the patient's spelling performance of a specially designed list of words. The assumptions we make about the structure of the Phoneme-Grapheme Conversion Mechanism are the following:

1. The probability of activating a specific phoneme-grapheme mapping option is a function of the activation threshold value for that option;

2. The threshold value of a phoneme-grapheme mapping option is determined by the *relative* frequency of occurrence of that phoneme-grapheme mapping in English orthography--options that occur relatively frequently will have low activation thresholds while options that occur relatively infrequently will have high activation thresholds. Thus, for example, if for the phoneme /f/, 'f' and 'ph' occur as graphemic options 70% and 30% of the time, respectively, we assume that the 'f' graphemic option will have a lower activation threshold value and thus will be more frequently selected for /f/ than the 'ph' graphemic option;

3. The Phoneme-Grapheme Conversion Mechanism is sensitive to the position of a phoneme within a syllable. This positional constraint on

phoneme-grapheme mappings is captured directly in the activation threshold values for each phoneme-grapheme mapping option. Specifically, the activation thresholds for alternative graphemic options for each phoneme differ depending on the within-syllable position of the to-be-converted phoneme. The following example illustrates this. For the phoneme /d_3/ there are a number of graphemic options that differ in their relative frequency of occurrence in English orthography. However, the graphemic options for /d_3/ also differ depending on whether the phoneme occurs in syllable-initial or syllable-final position, as can be seen in Table 8 (from Hanna, Hanna, Hodges, & Rudorf, 1966). Thus, even though 'dg' occurs in syllable-final position for /d_3/ (as in 'judge'), it never appears in syllable-initial position. Similarly, 'j' and 'g' are graphemic options for /d_3/ but their relative frequency of occurrence differ for syllable-initial and syllable-final position. Accordingly, the activation thresholds for the options 'j,' 'g,' and 'dg' for the phoneme /d_3/ will be different for syllable-initial and syllable-final positions: The activation threshold values will be proportional to the relative frequencies of occurrence for each phoneme-grapheme mapping option for each within-syllable position.

Table 8. Graphemic options for the phoneme /d₃/; revised from Hanna, Hanna, Hodges, & Rudorf (1966, Table 18, page 77).

| | Syllable Position | | Example | |
	Initial	Final	Initial	Final
GRAPHEMIC OPTION:				
'g'	58%	78%	gem	imagine
'j'	37%	1%	judge	majesty
'dg'	0%	13%		judge
.	.	.	.	.
.	.	.	.	.
.	.	.	.	.
.	.	.	.	.

Word Probability. The variable of word probability, the probability of inadvertently spelling a word correctly by implementation of phoneme-grapheme conversion rules, was assessed by analyzing results obtained from a specially designed list--The Probability of Phoneme-Grapheme Conversion List. This list consists of 110 monosyllabic words, 30 of which are high probability words, 80 low probability words; half are high frequency words, half low frequency words, ranging from four-to-six letters in length, each word consisting of three-to-four phonemes, counterbalanced for word probability, word frequency, number of phonemes per word, and word length. Words of different grammatical classes are evenly distributed across these variables. High and low probability words are defined as those that have a greater than 50% or less than 10% chance, respectively, of being accurately spelled by implementation of the most frequently occurring phoneme-grapheme correspondence rules in English orthography (according to norms provided by Hanna, et al., 1966).[9]

The prediction for JG's pattern of performance for the Probability of Phoneme-Grapheme Conversion List is the following: If JG uses the nonlexical process for generating a phonologically plausible spelling for a word that is not available for output in the Graphemic Output Lexicon, we expect that words consisting of a combination of high frequency phoneme-grapheme correspondence mappings will have a higher probability of being accurately spelled nonlexically than words composed of low frequency phoneme-grapheme correspondence mappings. More specifically, the effect of word probability should primarily be observed in spelling of low frequency words and not high frequency words. This prediction is based on the argument that the graphemic representations of the high frequency words can be addressed in the Graphemic Output Lexicon whereas the graphemic representations of the low frequency words are not likely to be available for output in the lexicon, hence forcing JG to rely on nonlexical spelling processes for assembling spelling for the lexically inaccessible words.[10]

RESULTS

JG's performance for the Probability of Phoneme-Grapheme Conversion List under written and oral spelling to dictation conditions is shown in Tables 9 and 10. There were main effect of word frequency and word probability for written and oral spelling performance. For written spelling, high and low frequency words were spelled with 93% and 58% accuracy, respectively ($X^2 = 17.72$, $p < .001$); for oral spelling, high and low frequency words were spelled with 98% and 73% accuracy, respectively ($X^2 = 14.34$, $p < .001$). For written spelling, high and low probability words were spelled with 90% and 70% accuracy, respectively ($X^2 = 4.70$, $p < .05$); for oral spelling, high and low probability words were spelled with 97% and 81% accuracy, respectively ($X^2 = 4.17$, $p < .05$). This effect of word probability on performance, however, is due to what could be considered an interaction between word frequency and word probability. That is, while there is no significant difference between JG's ability to spell high and low probability words for the high frequency set, she is statistically more accurate in spelling high than low probability words for the low frequency set. Thus, for written spelling, JG was 100%

and 90% correct for high and low probability words, respectively, within the high frequency set (X^2 = 1.62, NS) but was 80% and 50% correct for high and low probability words, respectively, within the low frequency set (X^2 = 4.02, p < .05). For oral spelling, JG was 100% and 98% correct for high and low probability words, respectively, within the high frequency set (X^2 = 0.37, NS) but was 93% and 65% correct for high and low probability words, respectively, within the low frequency set (X^2 = 4.42, p < .05).

Table 9. Results of the Probability of Phoneme-Grapheme Conversion List in JG's written spelling.

Frequency	Phoneme-Grapheme Probability		
	High N = 30	Low 80	Collapsed 110
High (N=55)	100%	90%	93%
Low (N=55)	80%	50%	58%
Collapsed	90%	70%	75%

Word Freq'y: (HF>LF) X^2 = 17.72, p <. 001
Word Prob: (HP>LP) X^2 = 4.70, p <. 05
High Freq'y: (HP>LP) X^2 = 1.62, NS
Low Freq'y: (HP>LP) X^2 = 4.02, p <. 05

These results are consistent with the hypothesis that JG is likely to be successful in accessing whole-word spelling representations of high frequency words in the Graphemic Output Lexicon but that she most often fails in accessing whole-word spelling representations for low frequency words and must assemble a phonologically plausible spelling through the implementation of phoneme-grapheme correspondence mappings. Furthermore, since for those words in which the spelling is presumably assembled by the application of phoneme-grapheme correspondence rules, the words composed of high frequency options were more often spelled correctly than words composed of low frequency options. We have support for the hypothesized structure of the Phoneme-Grapheme Conversion Mechanism.

Distributional Characteristics. Results from the Probability of Phoneme-Grapheme Conversion List provide support for the hypothesis that the probability of activating a particular phoneme-grapheme correspondence mapping is a function of the relative frequency of that phoneme-grapheme mapping in English orthography. However, our assumption is that the distribution of mapping options selected in the process of assembling orthography closely reflects the frequency of occurrence of phoneme-grapheme mappings in the language. To investigate this issue, we first administered a large number of words to JG as a writing to dictation task so as to obtain a reasonably large corpus of phonologically plausible errors. This was done in order to insure that low frequency phoneme-grapheme correspondence mappings would have a chance of being used. Over the course of this study, JG produced 687 phonologically plausible errors in written spelling of dictated words. These errors were analyzed by counting the number of times each phoneme-grapheme mapping was used within the respective syllable positions. The resulting distribution was compared to the distribution of phoneme-grapheme mappings in English orthography provided by Hanna, et al. (1966).[11]

Table 10. Results of the Probability of Phoneme-Grapheme Conversion List in JG's oral spelling.

	Phoneme-Grapheme Probability		
Frequency	High N = 30	Low 80	Collapsed 110
High (N=55)	100%	98%	98%
Low (N=55)	93%	65%	73%
Collapsed	97%	81%	85%
Word Freq'y: (HF>LF)	$x^2 = 14.34$, p <.001		
Word Prob: (HP>LP)	$x^2 = 4.17$, p < .05		
High Freq'y: (HP>LP)	$x^2 = 0.37$, NS		
Low Freq'y: (HP>LP)	$x^2 = 4.42$, p < .05		

An analysis of the percentage of usage of the various phoneme- grapheme mappings within their respective syllable positions for JG as compared to the norms was performed with the following criterion. We chose to include for analysis only those phoneme by syllable-position cells that included a minimum of 10 observations so as to ensure that various phoneme-grapheme mapping options would have a chance of being represented in the analysis.

Table 11 presents the correlations observed between JG's distribution and that for English orthography for vowels and consonants within each syllable position. These results indicate that the two distributions are highly correlated. Since the observations within each phoneme by syllable-position cell are not independent and one of the underlying assumptions of the statistic used is independence, the correlations may be slightly inflated. Nevertheless, the robustness of the correlations indicates that JG's selection of phoneme-grapheme mappings follows closely the frequency of occurrence of the mapping by syllable-position options of the language.

An important observation is that JG never produced an error in which a graphemic option was selected that was a viable option within another syllable position but that does not occur within the intended syllable position. For example, she did not produce errors of the sort provided by George Bernard Shaw in the often cited example 'ghoti' for FISH, in which 'gh' is an option for /f/ but only in syllable-final position, and so forth. Thus, we can assume that, for JG, the nonlexical mechanism responsible for keeping track of which distribution of options (i.e., syllable-initial, medial, or final) is to be used in the Phoneme-Grapheme Conversion Mechanism is intact.[12]

Table 11. Correlations for phoneme-grapheme mappings; JG as compared to English orthography norms.

		Syllable Position				
	Initial		Medial		Final	
	#Cases	Correlation	#Cases	Correlation	#Cases	Correlation
Vowels	(46)	.9103[a]	(163)	.8746	(83)	.9446
Consonants	(83)	.9797	(14)	.9965	(84)	.9553
Collapsed	(129)	.9651	(177)	.9285	(167)	.9522

[a] All correlations exceeded the .001 value.

A final observation relevant to the hypothesis that the selection of mapping options in the Phoneme-Grapheme Conversion Mechanism follows the relative frequencies of mapping options in the language is provided by an analysis of the errors made by the patient in successive attempts to spell a word. On the hypothesis entertained here, our expectation is that multiple misspellings of a word should *not* always result in the same pattern of errors if different mapping options are possible for the phonemes that comprise a word. Thus, for example, misspellings of the word /grif/ (GRIEF) should not lead to a consistent PPE misspelling since the phoneme /i/ and /f/ allow various mapping options. In order to address this issue, JG was administered for spelling to dictation 185 words on four different occasions.

Table 12 includes just those words that were misspelled on all four occasions (options that are spelled in more than one way on a different occasion are underlined; although more than one such option exists in several of these examples, only one has been underlined). Of the 46 words that were misspelled all times, 87% (40/46) elicited more than one spelling

Table 12. Words that were misspelled on all four trials.

STIMULUS	RESPONSE 1	RESPONSE 2	RESPONSE 3	RESPONSE 4
SENATE	cenit	cenout	cenet	senite
FIELD	feld	feild	feild	feild
SEVERE	saveer	savere	savere	savier
ANCIENT	aintchant	antchant	aintchent	anchant
MORAL	moreal	morral	marole	morel
CONQUER	conkore	concore	concor	councer
COLUMN	colum	collum	coilumn	collaum
BROAD	broud	brouid	brod	brode
JOURNEY	jurney	jurney	jerney	jernie
CANAL	kanow	canow	canaw	canow
THEORY	therough	thery	therry	therey
LEGEND	ledgeoned	ledgone	ledgoned	ledgoned
USELESS	yousless	usless	usless	usless
ODOR	oder	odar	odar	oder
CHORUS	courress	couras	course	kourase
SLEEVE	sleave	sleve	sleve	sleve
DEBT	dete	dept	deet	dept
STATUS	statos	statice	statice	stattice
LUNAR	lunnor	lunnor	looner	looner
GRIEF	greef	greif	greef	greef
MERCY	mercey	merse	mursy	mursey
FRAGILE	fragle	fradgil	fragel	fragial
DENY	denie	deni	deni	deni
LICENSE	lycince	licence	licence	licence
NUISANCE	newcence	newcence	newence	nusence
MYTH	meith	meith	mith	midth
URGE	earge	erge	erg	eruge
JOURNAL	jernal	jerneal	gernal	jernal
DIGIT	diggit	diget	degit	diget
CUSHION	cousion	coushin	cossin	coushin
YAWN	yoan	yoann	yon	yone
INJURE	enjor	ingor	enjor	enjor
KAYAK	cyact	couake	kiact	kiact
JEALOUS	jellis	jellous	jelous	jellous
CLIENT	cliant	clyent	cliant	claint
ANNOY	anoy	anoye	anoy	anoye
HALO	haylow	haylow	hylow	hallow
VULGAR	vougar	valgure	volgur	valgor
RATION	rashion	rasson	rachion	rassion
CLEANSE	klenze	clence	clenze	clense
COLLEGE	colledge	colledge	colledge	colledge
RATHER	rathor	rathor	rathor	rathor
FURTHER	ferther	ferther	ferther	ferther
DOUBT	dought	dought	dought	dought
DOLLAR	dallor	dallor	dallor	dallor
PITY	pitty	pitty	pitty	pitty

A. Caramazza

pattern. This result is consistent with the hypothesis that the phoneme-grapheme mapping option selected is *not always* the most frequent option but instead the various mapping options for a phoneme are selected with probabilities roughly equivalent to their relative frequency of occurrence in the language.

These results give rise to a critical question. Does the selection of a particular phoneme-grapheme mapping option in a syllable position occur independently of the selection of a phoneme-grapheme mapping option in the adjacent syllable position or, on the contrary, is there context sensitive information coded with the options? An analysis of the corpus of PPEs produced by JG reveals very few instances (less than 0.5%) of responses that 'violated' contextual rules of English. This is well illustrated by the following example.

Table 13. Distributions for the phoneme /s/; JG versus the norms.

	Initial			Syllable Position Medial			Final		
	#times[a] JG	%[b] JG	NM[c]	#times JG	% JG	NM	#times JG	% JG	NM
/S/									
S	90	77.6	77.8	25	100.0	96.9	64	61.0	62.3
C	23	19.8	15.9		0.0	2.6	36	34.3	20.3
SS	2	1.7	2.1		0.0	0.5	5	4.8	14.5
SC	1	0.1	1.1				0.0	1.5	
X		0.0	2.3						
ST							0.0	0.3	
PS		0.0	0.6						
Z		0.0	0.1				0.0	0.2	
SW		0.0	0.1						
SCH		0.0	0.1						

[a] Raw scores for the selection of particular graphemic options.
[b] Percentage that each graphemic option was chosen relative to all other possible mapping options with the respective within-syllable position (column percentages, thus, add up to 100%).
[c] NM=norms, taken from Hanna et al. (1966, page 79).

For /s/, the graphemic options for syllable initial position are shown in Table 13. This particular phoneme-within-syllable position leads to specific predictions regarding context sensitivity. If the Phoneme-Grapheme Conversion Mechanism is *not* sensitive to contextual constraints in the language, then the selection of 's' or 'c' as an option for /s/ in syllable initial position should not be affected by whether the following phoneme is a vowel or a consonant. The selection should, instead, only be based on the frequency of occurrence of the options in the language. If contextual constraints are built into the mechanism, however, there will be an obvious difference in the selection of the 's' or 'c' option for /s/ in syllable-initial position depending on whether the following phoneme is a vowel or a consonant. If the following phoneme is a consonant, only the 's' grapheme may occur in the initial position. Although 'c' does occur in English in blends (e.g., clown) and, hence, is orthographically legal, its pronunciation in the blends is never /s/ but is instead /k/. In contrast, if /s/ is followed by a vowel, then 's' as well as 'c' may occur.

The breakdown of performance for the phoneme /s/ with respect to the choice of graphemes 's' and 'c' before a vowel or a consonant is shown in Table 14. JG only selected 's' as a graphemic option for the phoneme /s/ when the following grapheme was a consonant. In contrast, the selection of 's' as compared to 'c' was distributed according to the norms when the following phoneme was a vowel. This finding is consistent with the hypothesis of context sensitivity in the phoneme-grapheme mapping mechanism. However, there is an alternative explanation that could easily account for the result. What we have observed need not reflect a general context sensitivity in the phoneme-grapheme mapping mechanism but may reflect no more than the fact that blends are stored separately in the Phoneme-Grapheme Conversion Mechanism.

Table 14. Distribution of the letters 's' and 'c' for /s/ in syllable initial position.

/s/ Grapheme	Vowel	Following Letter Consonant	Combined
s	56	34	90
c	23	0	23

In order to assess whether or not local constraints are observed, we need to consider specifically the options selected when the following grapheme is a vowel. Even though the letter 's' may precede any vowel and still be pronounced /s/, the letter 'c' may only precede the vowels 'e,' 'i,' and 'y' to maintain the /s/ pronunciation, as in the words 'cedar,' 'cigar,' and 'cycle.' When 'c' precedes the vowels 'a,' 'o,' and 'u,' it takes on a /k/ pronunciation. The critical question, then, is whether these local constraints are observed in JG's production of phonologically plausible responses.

Table 15. Distribution of the use of the letters 'c' and 's' for /s/ before vowels.

	c	s
N=	(23)	(56)
A	0	18
E	18	20
I	2	8
O	0	5
U	1	3
Y	2	2

Table 15 shows the distribution of 's' and 'c' realizations for /s/ (in syllable initial position) when they preceded each of the six vowels. The distributions of responses for 'c' versus 's' when both graphemes could legally occur in the context of the following vowel (i.e., 'i, e, y') and when *only one* grapheme (i.e., 's') could legally occur (i.e., 'a, o, u') is shown in Table 16. The distributions are significantly different ($X^2 = 13.30$, $p < .01$). Thus, when both graphemic options are permitted according to the rules of local constraints, JG uses 'c' 42% of the time and 's' 58% of the time. When, however, only the use of 's' is permitted, JG uses 'c' 4% of the time and 's' 96% of the time. This finding provides strong support for the view that the selection of phoneme-grapheme mapping options is sensitive to the dimension of local constraints.

Table 16. Distribution of the letters 's' and 'c' for /s/ for (il)legal combinations.

	c	s
Both are legal	22	30
Only 'S' is legal	1	26

The results reported in this section have been discussed in terms of a model of spelling that distinguishes between processing components for spelling familiar and unfamiliar words. And, we have considered the pattern of phonologically plausible errors as a reflection of the normal processing structure of the Phoneme-Grapheme Conversion Mechanism. We should consider, however, whether or not the pattern of errors reported might not receive an equally plausible interpretation within an analogy-based account of assembled spelling (e.g., Campbell, 1983).

Unfortunately, this is not an easy matter since this latter class of models is not sufficiently explicit to permit adequate evaluation.

The central characteristic of analogy-based models of spelling is that they do not distinguish between lexical and nonlexical processes for spelling. Instead, it is assumed that a single mechanism is involved in spelling both familiar and unfamiliar words--in both cases a graphemic representation is assembled from a set of lexical-graphemic representations that is activated in response to a phonological input. Thus, for example, given as input /grem/ the graphemic representations associated with this phonological sequence--GRAIN, BLAME, CLAIM, TAME, GREAT, and so forth--are activated and a specific graphemic representation is "synthesized" for the given input. How a specific representation is synthesized remains computationally opaque. More important for our present purposes, however, is the lack of specificity concerning the set of graphemic representations that is activated in response to a given phonological input. Since the graphemic representation that is synthesized for a phonological sequence depends on the set of graphemic representations that is activated, we must know what this set consists of in order to predict (if we knew the "synthesizing rule") the spelling response for a given stimulus. But, we know neither the synthesizing rule nor the principle underlying the activation of a particular set of graphemic representations over which the synthesis is carried out. In other words, this class of models has no quantitative predictive power with respect to expected spelling patterns for unfamiliar words nor with respect to the spelling errors produced by dysgraphic patients such as JG. Until sufficient constraints are proposed for this class of models they cannot be considered viable alternatives to the two process models we have adopted.

CONCLUSION

We have reported an extensive study of a patient with an acquired spelling disorder. The converging pattern of results, in terms of accuracy levels and error types produced for written and oral spelling of words and nonwords, clearly supports the hypothesis that this patient has a selective deficit at the level of the Graphemic Output Lexicon.[13] Because of the selective nature of the patient's spelling impairment, it has been possible to address issues relevant to the general architecture of a proposed model of spelling as well as issues relevant to the internal structure of one of the processing components that is critical to the process of assembling orthography.

The first issue addressed is whether or not whole-word representations in the Graphemic Output Lexicon can be accessed directly in response to input from phonological representations. We were able to use to advantage our patient's pattern of performance--implicating a selective impairment to the Graphemic Output Lexicon, particularly affecting her ability to access low frequency words--and a characteristic of English orthography --the presence of a number of homophones--to address this issue. JG's spelling performance of homophonic words that vary along the dimension of word frequency was examined. Although the combination of results for spelling of each member of a homophone pair consisting of either two high frequency members (e.g., weight, wait), two low frequency members (e.g., bury, berry), or one high and one low frequency member (e.g., sweet, suite) presents strong empirical support for the existence of a lexical, nonsemantic means of spelling, we will only restate the critical findings for the low frequency members of the latter two pairs of homophones.

Accuracy of performance for the low frequency members of LL and LH homophone pairs is almost identical (e.g., 35% and 38% for low frequency words in the HL and LL pairs, respectively). Thus, there is no advantage to being a low frequency member of either pair type. What becomes critical is the error pattern produced for a low frequency word as a function of its homophone partner. When the low frequency word is paired with *another* low frequency word as its homophone counterpart, 71% of JG's errors took the form of phonologically plausible responses while 19% of the errors were homophone confusions. The high incidence of PPEs in this task was interpreted as support for the view that the graphemic representation of neither member of these homophone pairs is accessible in the output lexicon and, hence, JG must rely on use of phoneme-grapheme conversion rules for generating a graphemic representation. In fact, for the LL pairs in which neither word was correctly spelled, *none* of the errors were homophone confusions and 86% of the errors took the form of PPEs. This pattern of results for low frequency words with low frequency homophone partners is in sharp contrast to results obtained for low frequency words with high frequency homophone partners. Of the errors produced for the low frequency member of a HL homophone pair, 65% took the form of homophone confusions while 23% were phonologically plausible responses. The high incidence of homophone confusion errors in this task was interpreted as support for the view that the graphemic representation of the high frequency member is available in the output lexicon and can be activated directly from a Phonological Lexicon.

Other investigators (Ellis, 1982; Morton, 1982; Patterson, in press) have postulated the existence of a link from a phonological lexicon to the Graphemic Output Lexicon. However, while we assume that this means of access to the Graphemic Output Lexicon is from the Phonological *Input* Lexicon, Ellis, Morton, and Patterson claim that the means of access is from the Phonological *Output* Lexicon. It is impossible to determine from the present case study which phonological lexicon may in fact be providing the representation that is processed by the Graphemic Output Lexicon. But, suffice it to say that it is clear that phonological information alone is sufficient to activate graphemic representations in the Graphemic Output Lexicon.

The second issue addressed in this report concerns the structure of the nonlexical, Phoneme-Grapheme Conversion Mechanism. When a graphemic representation is not available for output (in response to semantic or a phonological input), JG relies on the Phoneme-Grapheme Conversion Mechanism for assembling a candidate spelling. We assume that, like access to entries in the lexicon, access to entries in the Phoneme-Grapheme Conversion Mechanism is determined by the frequency of usage of mapping options in the language. The claim that the selection of a particular phoneme-grapheme mapping option is a function of the occurrence of that option in the language was tested by evaluating JG's performance for spelling words that only differed along the dimension of 'word probability.' Results show that high probability words--words that are 'fairly' likely to be inadvertently spelled correctly via implementation of phoneme-grapheme rules--were spelled more accurately than low probability words. This replicates other reported findings for patient RG (Beauvois & Dérouesné, 1981) and patient MW (Goodman & Caramazza, 1986). However, the dimension of word probability should not affect spelling performance for lexically inaccessible words for patients with severely impaired nonlexical spelling processes. This is the case for our patient MO, who, like JG and MW, has disruption to a lexical spelling component(s), but who, unlike JG and MW, has a severely disrupted nonlexical spelling mechanism (see Goodman & Caramazza, in press).

Table 17 summarizes results obtained for these three patients for nonwords and for words from the Probability of Phoneme-Grapheme Conversion subset. As can be seen, for JG and MW, who have an intact nonlexical, Phoneme-Grapheme Conversion Mechanism, the factor of word probability plays a major role in word spelling (see Beauvois & Dérouesné, 1981). However, for MO, a patient who has a severely impaired nonlexical spelling mechanism, the factor of word probability had no significant effect on word spelling performance.

Further analyses were carried out to evaluate the hypothesis that access to representations in the Phoneme-Grapheme Conversion Mechanism is influenced by the within-syllable frequency of occurrence of phoneme-grapheme mappings. This was accomplished by performing an extensive analysis of the pattern of phoneme-grapheme mapping options selected for syllable initial, medial, and final positions in a large corpus of our patient's phonologically plausible errors. Very high correlations were found between the distribution of our patient's usage of phoneme-grapheme mapping options and population norms provided by Hanna, et al. (1966). When the composition of phoneme-grapheme mappings that characterize JG's PPEs was analyzed in greater detail, support was obtained for the hypothesis that there are local contextual constraints on the selection of mapping options. Thus, the selection of the grapheme 's' or 'c' for syllable-initial position /s/ was influenced by whether the following grapheme was a consonant (i.e., only 's' was produced) and by which vowel followed the phoneme /s/ (i.e., 'c' can only precede the vowels 'i,' 'e,' and 'y' in order to maintain the /s/ pronunciation). There was only one instance in which there was a rule violation for syllable-initial position /s/--JG produced the response 'curcule' for CIRCLE. These results provide strong support for the hypothesis that the selection of a phoneme-grapheme option is determined not only by how frequently that option occurs within that syllable position in the language but also by the selection of adjacent mapping options.

Table 17. Results of the Probability of Phoneme-Grapheme Conversion List for patients JG, MW, and MO.

	JG	MW[a]	MO
Nonwords	100%	100%	0%
Words	(75%)	(91%)	(71%)
High Prob.	90%	100%	63%
Low Prob.	70%	88%	74%

[a] Results obtained for oral spelling

Word Probability

$$JG: x^2=4.70, p<.05$$
$$MW: x^2=4.12, p<.05$$
$$MO: x^2=1.14, NS$$

ACKNOWLEDGMENTS

We thank Brian Butterworth, Andrew Ellis, Michael McCloskey, Andrew Olson, Stacie Raymer, Scott Sokol, and an anonymous reviewer for comments on earlier drafts of this paper. We also thank Steven Breckler for his help in statistical analyses. This research was conducted as part of R.A.G.'s doctoral dissertation, and was supported by NIH grant Nos. 1 R01 NS222015 F3 NS 07851-02 to the Johns Hopkins University and by Biomedical Research Support Grant S07RR07041, Division of Research Resources, National Institutes of Health.

REFERENCES

Baxter, D. M. & Warrington, E. (in press). Ideational agraphia: A single case study. Journal of Neurology, Neurosurgery and Psychiatry.

Beauvois, M. F. & Dérouesné, J. (1981). Lexical or orthographic agraphia. Brain, 104, 21-49.

Bub, D. N., Cancelliere, A. & Kertesz, A. (1986). Whole-word and analytic translation of spelling to sound in a non-semantic reader. In K. E. Patterson, J. C. Marshall & M. Coltheart (Eds.), Surface dyslexia: Neuropsychological and cognitive studies of phonological reading. London: Lawrence Erlbaum.

Bub, D. N. & Kertesz, A. (1982). Deep agraphia. Brain and Language, 17, 147-166.

Burani, C., Salmaso, D. & Caramazza, A. (1984). Morphological structure and lexical access. Visible Language, 4, 342-352.

Campbell, R. (1983). Writing nonwords to dictation. Brain and Language, 19, 153-178.

Caramazza, A., Miceli, G. & Villa, G. (1986). The role of the (output) phonological buffer in reading, writing, and repetition. Cognitive Neuropsychology.

Caramazza, A., Miceli, G., Villa, G. & Romani, C. (in press). The role of the Graphemic Buffer in Spelling: Evidence from a case of acquired dysgraphia. Cognition.

Dunn, J. M. & Dunn, L. M. (1981). The Peabody Picture Vocabulary Test-revised. Circle Pines, MN: American Guidance Service.

Ellis, A. W. (1982). Spelling and writing (and reading and speaking). In A. W. Ellis (Ed.), Normality and pathology in cognitive functions. London: Academic Press.

Ellis, A. W. (in press). Modelling the writing process. In G. Denes, C. Semenza, P. Bisiacchi & E. Andreewsky (Eds.), Perspectives in cognitive neuropsychology. London: Lawrence Erlbaum.

Glushko, R. J. (1979). The organization and activation of orthographic knowledge in reading aloud. Journal of Experimental Psychology: Human Perception and Performance, 5, 674-691.

Glushko, R. J. (1981). Principles of pronouncing print: The psychology of phonography. In A. M. Lesgold & C. A. Perfetti (Eds.), Interactive processes in reading. Hillsdale, NJ: Lawrence Erlbaum Associates.

Goodglass, H. & Kaplan, E. (1972). The assessment of aphasia and related disorders. Philadelphia, PA: Lea and Febiger.

Goodglass, H. & Kaplan, E. (1983). The Boston Naming Test. Philadelphia, PA: Lea and Febiger.

Goodman, R. A. & Caramazza, A. (1984). The Johns Hopkins University Dyslexia Battery. The Johns Hopkins University, Baltimore, MD.

Goodman, R. A. & Caramazza, A. (1985). The Johns Hopkins University Dysgraphia Battery. The Johns Hopkins University, Baltimore, MD.

Goodman, R. A. & Caramazza, A. (1986). Dissociation of spelling errors in written and oral spelling: The role of allographic conversion in writing. Cognitive Neuropsychology, 3, 179-206.

Goodman, R. A. & Caramazza, A. (in press). Patterns of dysgraphia and the nonlexical spelling process. Cortex.

Hanna, R. R., Hanna, J. S., Hodges, R. E. & Rudorf, E. H. (1966). Phoneme-grapheme correspondences as cues to spelling improvement. U.S. Department of Health, Education, and Welfare, Office of Education, Washington, DC: U.S. Government Printing Office.

Hatfield, F. M. & Patterson, K. E. (1983). Phonological spelling. Quarterly Journal of Experimental Psychology, 35A, 451-468.

Hatfield, F. M. & Patterson, K. E. (1984). Interpretation of spelling in aphasia: The impact of recent developments in cognitive psychology. In F. C. Rose (Ed.), Progress in aphasiology. New York, NY: Raven Press.

Henderson, L. (1982). Orthography and word recognition in reading. London: Academic Press.

Hier, D. B. & Mohr, J. P. (1977). Incongruous oral and written naming: Evidence for a subdivision of the syndrome of Wernicke's aphasia. Brain and Language, 4, 115-126.

Kay, J. & Marcel, T. (1981). One process, not two, in reading aloud: Lexical analogies do the work of non-lexical rules. Quarterly Journal of Experimental Psychology, 33A, 397-413.

Kinsbourne, M. & Rosenfield, D. B. (1974). Agraphia selective for written spelling: An experimental case study. Brain and Language, 1, 215-225.

Kinsbourne, M. & Warrington, E. K. (1965). A case showing selectively impaired oral spelling. Journal of Neurology, Neurosurgery, and Psychiatry, 28, 59-64.

Marcel, T. (1980). Surface dyslexia and beginning reading: A revised hypothesis of the pronunciation of print and its impairments. In

M. Coltheart, K. E. Patterson & J. C. Marshall (Eds.), Deep dyslexia. London: Routledge & Kegan Paul.

Margolin, D. I. (1984). The neuropsychology of writing and spelling: Semantic, phonological, motor, and perceptual processes. Quarterly Journal of Experimental Psychology, 36A, 459-489.

Margolin, D. I. & Wing, A. M. (1983). Agraphia and micrographia: Clinical manifestations of motor programming and performance disorders. Acta Psychologica, 54, 263-283.

Miceli, G., Silveri, M. C. & Caramazza, A. (1985). Cognitive analysis of a case of pure agraphia. Brain and Language, 25, 187-212.

Morton, J. (1979). Word recognition. In J. Morton & J. Marshall (Eds.), Psycholinguistics 2: Structures and processes. Cambridge, MA: MIT Press.

Morton, J. (1982). Disintegrating the lexicon: An information processing approach. In J. Mehler, E. C. T. Walker & M. Garrett (Eds.), Perspectives on mental representation. Hillsdale, NJ: Lawrence Erlbaum.

Newcombe, F. & Marshall, J. C. (1980). Transcoding and lexical stabilization in deep dyslexia. In M. Coltheart, K. E. Patterson & J. C. Marshall, (Eds.), Deep dyslexia. London: Routledge & Kegan Paul.

Patterson, K. E. (in press). Acquired disorders of spelling. In G. Denes, C. Semenza, P. Bisiacchi & E. Andreewsky (Eds.), Perspectives in cognitive neuropsychology. London: Erlbaum.

Roeltgen, D. P. & Heilman, K. M. (1983). Apractic agraphia in a patient with normal praxis. Brain and Language, 18, 35-46.

Rothi, L. J. & Heilman, K. M. (1981). Alexia and agraphia with spared spelling and letter recognition abilities. Brain and Language, 12, 1-13.

Schwartz, M. F., Saffran, E. M. & Marin, O. S. M. (1980). Fractionating the reading process in dementia: Evidence for word specific print-to-sound associations. In M. Coltheart, K. E. Patterson & J. C. Marshall, (Eds.), Deep dyslexia. London: Routledge & Kegan Paul.

Seidenberg, M. S. & Tanenhaus, M. K. (1979). Orthographic effects on rhyme monitoring. Journal of Experimental Psychology: Human Learning and Memory, 5, 546-554.

Shallice, T. (1981). Phonological agraphia and the lexical route in writing. Brain, 104, 413-429.

Van Galen, G. P. (1980). Handwriting and drawing: A two-stage model of complex motor behaviour. In G. Stelmach & J. Requin (Eds.), Tutorials in motor behaviour. Amsterdam: North Holland.

Viviani, P. & Terzuolo, C. (1983). The organization of movement in handwriting and typing. In B. Butterworth (Ed.), Language production,

Vol 2, Development, writing and other language processes. London: Academic Press.

APPENDIX I

Stimuli for the homophone task
(Abbreviation key: HH=High-High; HL=High-Low; LL-Low-Low; HF=high frequency; LF=low frequency)

HH Pairs(N=17)		*HL Pairs(n=26)*		*LL Pairs(N=17)*	
		HF	LF		
		Member:	Member:		
I	eye	him	hymn	toe	toe
one	won	made	maid	stair	stare
would	wood	great	grate	loan	lone
see	sea	air	heir	profit	prophet
no	know	boy	buoy	steak	stake
through	threw	feet	feat	heal	heel
our	hour	need	knead	flee	flea
here	hear	course	coarse	berry	bury
sun	son	oh	owe	sore	soar
close	clothes	horse	hoarse	idol	idle
war	wore	rain	reign	colonel	kernel
piece	peace	real	reel	core	corps
plane	plain	hair	hare	foul	fowl
eight	ate	seem	seam	hostile	hostel
meet	meat	tail	tale	surf	serf
weight	wait	break	brake	alter	altar
dear	deer	fair	fare	gorilla	guerilla
		steel	steal		
		none	nun		
		hall	haul		
		pole	poll		
		symbol	cymbal		
		sweet	suite		
		rough	ruff		
		manner	manor		
		beat	beet		

APPENDIX II

Errors produced for the homophone task
A. Stimuli for which homophone confusions were produced:

STIMULUS	RESPONSE (Hom Conf)	WORD FREQ'Y (Stim vs Resp)
1. CLOSE	clothes	249 vs 104
2. PIECE	peace	206 vs 58
3. THREW	through	54 vs 1054
4. BREAK	brake	97 vs 10
5. BUOY	boy	4 vs 484
6. FEAT	feet	2 vs 463
7. HOARSE	horse	3 vs 213
8. REIGN	rain	4 vs 169
9. REEL	real	1 vs 168
10. FARE	fair	8 vs 77
11. STEAL	steel	13 vs 76
12. NUN	none	0.4 vs 73
13. POLL	pole	1 vs 63
14. CYMBAL	symbol	0.1 vs 58
15. SUITE	sweet	3 vs 55
16. PROPHET	profit	1 vs 9
17. STAKE	steak	5 vs 4
18. FLEA	flee	4 vs 4
19. HEEL	heal	5 vs 1

B. Stimuli for which phonologically plausible errors were produced:

STIMULUS	RESPONSE (PPEs)	WORD FREQ'Y (Stimulus)
1. WAIT	waite	109
2. PEACE	pease	58
3. MANNER	mannor	50
4. COLONEL	cernal	19
5. CORE	kore	10
6. HAUL	hawl	9
7. COARSE	korse	9
8. BURY	beary	7
9. CORPS	kore	6
10. HOSTILE	hostal	5
11. IDLE	idel	5
12. KERNEL	kurnol	5
13. HYMN	hym	4

14. SURF	searf	4
15. SOAR	soure	3
16. ALTER	altor	3
17. ALTAR	altor	3
18. GORILLA	gerrilla	1
19. GUERRILLA	gerreila	1
20. SERF	searf	0.3
21. KNEAD	kneed	0.2
22. HOSTEL	hostal	unrated

C. Stimuli for which miscellaneous responses were produced:

STIMULUS	RESPONSE (Miscellaneous)	WORD FREQ'Y (Stimulus)
1. TAIL	tall	110
2. WEIGHT	weaght	103
3. ATE	eat	75
4. TALE	tall	15
5. FOUL	fall	5
6. FOWL	fall	3
7. HEIR	hair	3

NOTES

[1] See Glushko (1979, 1981), Marcel (1980), Kay & Marcel (1981), Campbell (1983), and Henderson (1982) for an alternative view to nonlexical orthographic processes.

[2] The construction of the stimulus lists is discussed in Goodman & Caramazza (1986).

[3] Although JG exhibits a word frequency effect both in reading and spelling performance, it is not clear what the significance of this co-occurrence of impairments reflects. Given that there are reports of dissociations of lexical processing impairments for reading and spelling (e.g., Bub & Kertesz, 1982), we consider the co-occurrence of lexical impairments in JG to reflect no more that the accidental co-occurrence of deficits to lexical processes involved in reading and those involved in spelling.

[4] A corpus of errors produced for all spelling tasks is available from the authors upon request.

[5] At a later point in this paper we consider the possibility of a link between the Phonological Output Lexicon and the Graphemic Output Lexicon.

[6] The precise relationship between surface frequency of words (e.g., walked) and the morpheme frequency (e.g., walk- and -ed) and how these frequencies affect lexical access has not been worked out completely although there are clear indications that both types of frequency affect lexical access (Taft, 1979; Burani, Salmaso, & Caramazza, 1984).

[7] We would like to thank Andrew Ellis for drawing our attention to this possibility.

[8] One possibility is that the pattern of homophone confusion errors resulted from phoneme-grapheme conversion. That is, homophone confusion errors may have occurred when JG inadvertently produced the spelling of the homophone through the use of the Phoneme-Grapheme Conversion Mechanism. On this hypothesis, the higher proportion of homophone confusion errors for the low-frequency members of the HL pairs (65% of the errors) than for the LL pairs (19% of the errors) occurred because the probability of producing the homophone by phoneme-grapheme conversion was much higher for the former than for the latter. We evaluated this alternative hypothesis by calculating for each low-frequency word in the HL and LL pairs the probability of producing the homophone by phoneme-grapheme conversion. For the low-frequency words in the HL pairs, the probability was 22%, whereas for the LL pairs the probability was 14%. Clearly, the 22% probability for the HL pairs is too low to explain the finding that 65% of the errors for the low-frequency members of these pairs were homophone confusions. Further, the difference between the HL and LL pairs in phoneme-grapheme conversion probability seems insufficient to account for the very large difference between the two sets in the proportion of homophone confusion errors.

[9] Probabilities were computed by obtaining the frequency (in percent) of occurrence of the particular graphemic option associated with each phoneme of a word and calculating the joint probability of these options.

[10] The probability with which a patient spells a word correctly is determined by (at least) two factors: the probability that a whole-word graphemic representation is accessible in the Graphemic Output Lexicon and the probability of spelling a word correctly via nonlexical processes given that its graphemic representation is inaccessible in the Graphemic Output Lexicon. In principle, we should be able to compute these probabilities with a reasonable degree of accuracy. In practice, however, it is difficult to obtain the probability with which a particular word is inaccessible in the graphemic output lexicon. Hence, the only prediction

we can make is that, everything else being equal, high probability words should be correctly spelled more frequently than low probability words.

[11] The distributions of phoneme-grapheme correspondence mappings used by JG and for English orthography are available from the authors upon request.

[12] One feature of the Phoneme-Grapheme Conversion Mechanism we have not discussed concerns the use of word- versus syllable-position information. This positional information plays a role in determining whether a grapheme is an appropriate option for a phoneme. Thus, consider the following example: 't' is a graphemic option for the phoneme /t∫/ in syllable initial position (as in the word nature) but not in word initial position. Consequently, we must assume that the selection of phoneme-grapheme correspondence options is constrained by this type of positional information.

[13] There was a certain proportion of errors not directly dealt with in our discussion of JG's spelling performance. Thus, for example, 5% and 6% of her errors in written and oral spelling of dictated words, respectively, took the form of phonologically *im*plausible errors. We cannot completely rule out the possibility that these errors may, in fact, reflect a deficit of a spelling mechanism other than the Graphemic Output Lexicon.

DISSOCIATION OF SPELLING ERRORS IN WRITTEN AND ORAL SPELLING: THE ROLE OF ALLOGRAPHIC CONVERSION IN WRITING

INTRODUCTION

What are the cognitive/linguistic mechanisms necessary for the literate adult to spell a familiar word accurately or to attempt to spell an unfamiliar word or pronounceable nonword? In developing a model of single word/nonword spelling, one might postulate that accurate spelling can be accomplished solely by means of access to a system of rules specifying which graphemic units are assigned to component phonemic units of a phonological sequence. This phoneme-grapheme conversion system, used for phonologically assembled spelling, would, however, only allow for accurate spelling of pronounceable nonwords since any phonologically plausible spelling on a nonword is considered accurate. Reliance on this system for assembling spelling of words, however, is quite problematic. This is due to the opaque relationship between phonemes and their graphemic realisations in English. Thus, for example, the word /kot/ could be misspelled as "cote," "kote," "koat," etc. by use of phoneme-grapheme correspondence mappings (see Morton, 1980; Ellis, 1982). The point is that while any phonologically plausible spelling for a nonword is considered accurate, any phonologically plausible spelling for a word just won't do. In order to spell all English words accurately, one needs to have access to a lexical system containing whole-word spelling representations (i.e., a graphemic output lexicon). That is, the unique spelling for each word must be addressed in this system. Since pronounceable nonwords do not have entries in the graphemic output lexicon, they can *only* be provided a phonologically plausible spelling (in this type of cognitive architecture) by use of the nonlexical phoneme-grapheme conversion system.

This dual route model, therefore, provides the basis for accurate spelling of both words and nonwords. Accuracy with nonword spelling is dependent on a system which allows for segmentation of a phonemic code and transcoding between phonemic and graphemic units by use of phoneme-grapheme conversion rules. (An alternative view is offered by Glushko (1979; 1981), Marcel (1980), Kay & Marcel (1981), and

Henderson (1982), who have proposed lexical analogy models for nonword spelling.) Accuracy with word spelling, on the contrary, is dependent on a system which allows for lexical access to whole-word spelling representations (graphemic output lexicon); an addressed, as opposed to an assembled, spelling system.

Once we have obtained an abstract graphemic representation, what post-graphemic processes are involved in oral and written spelling? For oral spelling (i.e., saying aloud the letter names comprised in the stimulus), we might postulate the existence of a mechanism for converting graphemic units to letter names and an articulatory process for the production of the letter names. For written spelling, we might postulate the existence of a system that enables us to transcode an abstract graphemic representation (either obtained through use of an addressed or phonologically assembled system) into specific letter form prior to use of more peripheral motor processes for written production. This system must be able to specify the case (upper versus lower), type (print versus script), and finally the actual visual shape associated with each combination of case and type for each graphemic unit of a sequence. For example, the visual shape of each letter associated with the word "big" would be different for upper case print (BIG) versus lower case print (big), and so forth. In this paper, we refer to the set of processes thought to be responsible for providing the physical letter code for written spelling in terms of the visual shape, case, and type as an allographic conversion system. We are differentiating between this system and a set of processes responsible for providing the "graphic motor pattern" (Ellis, 1979; 1982), that is, the sequence of strokes corresponding to the physical letter code generated from the allographic conversion system. While the addressed or assembled abstract graphemic representation is being transcoded into a usable form for oral or written spelling, we assume that the information is temporarily held in a working memory system (i.e., output graphemic buffer). In this view, then, it is assumed that oral and written spelling are accomplished by use of the same processing mechanisms up to the point at which the letter name versus the letter shape must be specified for output. That is, for both oral and written spelling, the same lexical and nonlexical conversion processes are implemented and only at a level of post-graphemic processing beyond the output graphemic buffer is there a divergence in the set of functional components required for accurate performance. (For further discussion see Ellis (1982) and Margolin (1984).)

In sum, the major components of a model of single word/nonword spelling include nonlexical processes (phoneme-grapheme conversion system), lexical processes (e.g., graphemic output lexicon), and post-graphemic processes that operate over abstract graphemic representations to obtain specific articulatory letter forms (letter naming system) or visual letter forms (allographic conversion system), as depicted schematically in Figure 1.

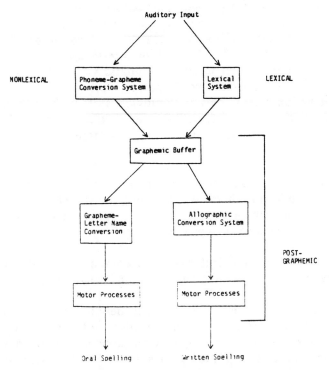

Figure 1. Schematic representation of spelling systems.

Given this general structure of the spelling system, what are the predicted patterns of performance given a functional lesion to either the lexical or nonlexical route? If the nonlexical route (e.g., phoneme-grapheme conversion system) is damaged, we expect nonword spelling to be impaired relative to word spelling. Empirical support for this distinction has been provided in case reports by Shallice (1981), Bub and Kertesz (1982), and Roeltgen, Sevush, and Heilman (1983). If, on the contrary, the lexical route is damaged, we expect word spelling to be impaired relative to nonword spelling. Empirical support for this distinction has been obtained in case reports by Beauvois and Dérouesné (1981) and Roeltgen and Heilman (1984). Thus, the double dissociation between word and nonword spelling abilities can be taken to support the theoretical distinction between at least two processing routes for spelling. Note, however, that this argument is based on just one aspect of patients' performance: the relative success in spelling words versus nonwords. A consideration of other aspects of patients' spelling performances contributes to a further characterisation of the structure of the spelling system.

Consider in this regard a patient who spells nonwords more accurately than words. This pattern of performance can be taken to suggest an impairment at some level of lexical processing and we can use the specific pattern of word spelling difficulty to draw inferences about the structure of the lexical system. That is, any systematic variation in the type of lexical factors that influence word spelling ability can be assumed to reflect organisational principles of the lexical system. For example, if a patient spells nonwords and high frequency words correctly but makes phonologically plausible errors in spelling low frequency words, we are able to conclude that:

1. some words (low frequency words) are spelled through an intact nonlexical, phoneme-grapheme conversion process; and
2. the lexical processing component that is damaged in this patient is sensitive to the dimension of word frequency.

In order to specify which lexical processing component is damaged in this patient, however, we need information beyond what we have considered thus far.

Specification of the precise locus of impairment to the lexical processing component hypothesised to underlie the observed pattern of impaired performance is dependent on the particular assumptions we make about the functional architecture of the lexical system. Further, our assumptions about the internal structure of the processing components that comprise the lexical system will govern the types of errors and pattern of performance we expect to observe given damage to a particular lexical processing mechanism. For example, in the case of a patient who produces phonologically plausible errors, we might hypothsise that there is a deficit in addressing phonological representations in the phonological input lexicon. If access to the phonological input lexicon is disrupted, then we expect to observe phonologically plausible errors only for writing to dictation, for example, but not for writing tasks that do not use the phonological input lexicon to address lexical-graphemic representations (in the graphemic output lexicon). Thus, written naming and spontaneous written narrative tasks should be error free. If, however, we observe phonologically plausible errors in these latter tasks, then the lexical processing impairment would have to be at a level of processing beyond the phonological input lexicon--perhaps a deficit in the graphemic output lexicon.[1]

Consider further the predicted pattern of performance given a deficit to the allographic conversion system. Since, in the proposed functional architecture, this system is employed only for *written* spelling of addressed (words) and assembled (nonwords) orthography, and not for *oral* spelling of words and nonwords, we expect spelling of both words and nonwords to be impaired and oral spelling of these stimuli to be intact. We do not expect lexical factors (e.g., word frequency, form class, etc.) to affect spelling performance, nor do we expect to observe phonologically plausible errors if damage were restricted to the allographic conversion system. Since this system is hypothesised to be responsible for generating case (upper versus lower), type (script versus print), and the actual letter shapes for abstract graphemic representations, we expect spelling errors in all writing tasks requiring transcoding between abstract graphemic information and a code usable for written production (e.g., written naming, writing to dictation, etc.).

In this paper, we describe a patient who produced phonologically plausible errors and "spelling" errors (i.e., substitution of a letter for a targeted letter where the response letter does not have the same phonetic value as the stimulus letter, as is the case with phonologically plausible errors).[2] More specifically, the patient produces phonologically plausible errors in written and oral spelling tasks. Through different sources of converging evidence, we hypothesise that the impairment implicated in the production of phonologically plausible errors is at the level of the graphemic output lexicon. The patient also produced spelling errors for all written spelling tasks but not for oral spelling tests. We interpret this dissociation between oral and written spelling as reflecting damage to the allographic conversion system. This patient's spelling performance, therefore, allows us to address theoretical issues relevant to the structure of the graphemic output lexicon, the organisation of the phoneme-grapheme conversion system, and the role of the allographic conversion system in writing.

CASE HISTORY

MW, a 69-year-old male, suffered a left cerebrovascular accident in February, 1983. CT-scan revealed left hemisphere infarctions in the distribution of the middle cerebral artery and occipital lobe. At that time, MW presented with a mild anomic aphasia. His reading rate was reportedly very slow and he had poor letter and word recognition skills. Neurological assessment indicated a right spastic hemiparesis and a mild right facial palsy.

MW was referred to the Cognitive Neuropsychology Laboratory of the Johns Hopkins University in March, 1984 for an assessment of his reading and writing abilities. He reportedly was reading at a very slow rate and was producing errors in writing. MW has a D.S.W. (Doctor of Social

Welfare) qualification. He was employed as the director of a social work training programme for a government agency and reportedly had excellent reading, writing, and spelling skills prior to his cerebrovascular accident.

MW was tested over a six-month period. During this time, his reading and writing deficits remained highly stable. Administration of the Boston Diagnostic Aphasia Examination (Goodglass & Kaplan, 1972) indicated the following: Spontaneous speech was fluent, with occasional literal paraphasias and some word finding difficulty. MW exhibited a rich vocabulary and used a variety of syntactic constructions. Repetition of single words and high- and low-probability sentences was perfect. Although reading comprehension of single words and sentences was perfect and oral reading of single words and sentences was relatively preserved, MW performed these tasks at an abnormally slow rate. He produced errors for all spelling tasks. Mechanics of writing, however, were intact (a sample of his writing performance is shown in Fig. 2). MW had some difficulty in confrontation naming. In further assessing this problem, the Boston Naming Test (Goodglass & Kaplan, 1983) was administered. MW received a score of 30 correct (out of 60), and he responded well to phonemic cuing. He received a score of 164 correct (out of 175) for auditory presentation of the Peabody Picture Vocabulary Test-Revised--Form M (Dunn & Dunn, 1981) indicating a high-average single-word vocabulary score.

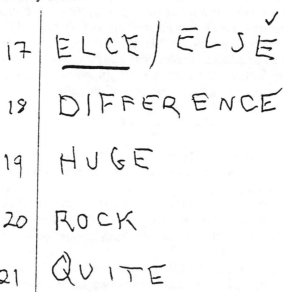

Figure 2. Sample of MW's writing.

EXPERIMENTAL TASKS

MW was administered a number of reading, writing, and oral spelling tests.

Reading

Results of the reading assessment will be discussed only briefly. MW read words with 92% accuracy (X^2 = 30.18, p < .001). The factors of grammatical word class, concreteness, word frequency, stimulus length, and orthographic regularity did not significantly affect accuracy of performance. Errors for oral reading of words and nonwords included the production of visually-similar word (e.g., "bake for *boke*) and nonword (e.g., "trisp" for *crisp*) responses. For words, a few morphologically-related (or visually-similar) words (e.g., "noise" for *noisy*; "rose" for *roses*) were also produced.

Lexical Decision

MW was administered an auditory version of the Gordon (1983) Lexical Decision Task containing 204 words (one-third of which are high frequency, one-third mid frequency, and one-third low frequency) and 204 matched nonwords. He performed almost perfectly, scoring 202/204 (99% accuracy) for words and 204/204 (100% accuracy) for nonwords. MW's excellent performance for discrimination of auditorily-presented words from nonwords indicates that his acoustic-phonemic system is intact.

Writing

MW was administered a variety of written spelling tests as described in the following sections.[3]

Writing to Dictation. Over the course of the investigation, MW was administered a number of lists to be written to dictation. (The composition of several of these lists will be discussed in a later section.) Altogether, he wrote 530 words and 242 nonwords to dictation.

Results indicate that nonwords were written more accurately than words. MW wrote 229/242 nonwords correctly (95%), in contrast to 442/530 (83%) words (X^2 = 19.01, p < .001). For nonword writing, the only type of error produced involved the substitution of one letter for another letter with a different phonetic value (e.g., *hagrib* for "hagrid"). In this paper, we refer to such errors as "spelling errors" (SEs). For word writing, MW produced two basic error types: SEs (i.e., letter substitutions) and "phonologically-plausible errors" (PPEs), errors that are explicable in terms of the application of phoneme-grapheme correspondence rules in generating the response (e.g., *groce* for "gross"). The errors in word writing were distributed as follows: 4% (21/530) SEs, 12% (65/530) PPEs, and 0.4% (2/530) mixed errors--that is, misspellings containing both phonologically-plausible and spelling-error components (e.g., *trity* for "pretty"). See Appendix I for a corpus of errors for writing to dictation tests.) Thus, MW produced SEs both in word and nonword writing at approximately the same rate of production--4% and 5%, respectively-and additionally produced PPEs and mixed errors in word writing.

The pattern of writing performance described allows us to reach some general conclusions regarding the locus or loci of impairment in MW's writing system which, although tentative, can serve as a guide in the formulation of more precise hypotheses about the loci of impairment and a directed detailed analysis of the patient's spelling performance. Thus, the fact that MW could write nonwords relatively well and produced mostly PPEs in word writing suggests that he has an intact (relatively) phoneme-grapheme conversion system. However, the presence of the small but consistent pattern of SEs produced in writing words and nonwords could reflect a deficit to the phoneme-grapheme conversion system. This possibility will be considered at a later point in this paper when we focus our attention specifically on the source of the SEs in this patient. The other tentative conclusion we can reach on the basis of the patient's performance described thus far is that he has a deficit at some level of lexical processing as evidenced by his poor performance in spelling words relative to nonwords. However, the precise locus of the deficit within the lexical system cannot be inferred merely from a consideration of the data reported to this point. The remainder of the paper represents an effort to identify more precisely the locus or loci of deficit within the lexical processing system for the word writing impairment and to explicate further the basis for the occurrence of SEs in word and nonword writing and of PPEs in word writing. As a first step in this effort we need to establish which, if any, lexical and nonlexical factors affected MW's spelling performance.

Of the 530 words administered to MW as a writing-to-dictation task, subsets of these stimuli were used to assess a variety of performance factors known to influence spelling accuracy in dysgraphic patients. A description of the variables (controlled for and manipulated) in each of these subsets is as follows:

A. Grammatical Word Class. This subset contains 104 words, 28 of which are pure (i.e., only belonging to one grammatical class) nouns, 28 pure verbs, 28 pure adjectives, and 20 function words. For function words, half are monosyllabic, half bisyllabic; all are high frequency and ranged in length from four to seven letters. For the remaining words, half are high frequency, half low frequency;[4] half are monosyllabic, half bisyllabic; ranging from four to seven letters in length, counterbalanced for word frequency, syllabicity, word length, and in the case of nouns, for abstractness. MW wrote 23/28 (82%) nouns correctly as compared to 21/28 (75%) verbs and 24/28% (86%) adjectives ($X^2 = .04$ for nouns versus verbs and adjectives, NS). Function words were written with approximately the same degree of accuracy as were high frequency nouns (95% [19/20] for function words, versus 86% [12/14] for high frequency nouns, $X^2 = .08$, NS). Hence, MW shows no grammatical class effects in written spelling performance.

B. Abstractness-Concreteness. This subset contains 42 bisyllabic nouns, half of which are abstract, half concrete;[8] one-third of which are high frequency, one-third mid frequency, one-third low frequency; ranging from five to seven letters in length, counterbalanced for concreteness, word frequency, and word length.

MW wrote concrete words with approximately the same degree of accuracy as abstract words. He wrote 18/21 concrete words correctly (86%) as compared to 16/21 (76%) abstract words ($X^2 = .62$, NS).

The results obtained for the grammatical word class and the abstractness-concreteness lists suggest that the locus of the deficit implicated in MW's word-writing impairment is *not* at the level of gaining access to the lexical-semantic system from the phonological input lexicon.

C. Word Length. This subset contains 70 bisyllabic words, divided equally among items of 4, 5, 6, 7, and 8 letters. Half of these words are high frequency, half low frequency; they are counterbalanced for word frequency and word length; and words of different grammatical classes are distributed evenly across these variables.

MW wrote 4-, 5-, 6-, 7-, and 8-letter words with 86% (12/14), 86% (12/14), 79% (11/14), and 79% (11/14) accuracy, respectively. Thus, 4-5 letter words were written with approximately the same degree of accuracy as were 7-8 letter words (86% (24/28) and 79% (22/28) for 4-5 and 7-8 letter words, respectively; $X^2 = .48$, NS).

D. Word Frequency. This subset consists of 292 monosyllabic and bisyllabic open-class words, half of which are high frequency, half low frequency words, ranging from 4 to 8 letters in length; they are counterbalanced for word frequency, word length, and syllabicity; and words of different grammatical classes are distributed evenly across these variables.

MW wrote 132/146 high-frequency words correctly (90%) in contrast to 108/146 low-frequency words (74%), ($X^2 = 13.48$, $p < .001$). This finding indicates that MW can access high frequency whole-word spelling representations from the graphemic output lexicon more easily than low frequency whole-word spelling representations.

Taken together, the findings that there are no effects of grammatical word class or concreteness in the face of a word-frequency effect, suggest that MW's lexical deficit (implicated by impaired word writing ability) is most likely not a result of difficulty in gaining access to lexical-semantic representations from the phonological input lexicon. These findings suggest that once MW has accessed the lexical-semantic representation, he then has difficulty in addressing the whole-word spelling specification in the graphemic output lexicon. Due to his relatively intact nonlexical phoneme-grapheme conversion system, he is able to use phoneme-grapheme correspondence rules in generating a phonologically plausible spelling for those stimuli in which the whole-word spelling representations are not available. This process results in the production of PPEs. It is not determinable from the data presented thus far if the mechanism responsible for the production of PPEs is also responsible for the occurrence of SEs in MW's written spelling performance.

Following is a discussion of each error type produced in MW's written spelling performance and the tasks administered in order to specify the locus/loci of impairment responsible for the production of these errors in conjunction with the word frequency effect.

Phonologically Plausible Errors
As discussed in the Introduction, PPEs may result from selective deficits to one of several lexical mechanisms; that is, if a patient has an impairment to either the phonological input lexicon, the lexical-semantic system, the graphemic output lexicon, or any combination thereof that does not allow for access to graphemic representations in the graphemic output lexicon, then the phoneme-grapheme conversion system will enable the patient to produce a phonologically plausible spelling for the word (given that this system is intact). In order to try to specify the level of impairment implicated in the production of PPEs, we administered a number of tasks to MW.

Written Naming. MW was shown 51 pictures of single objects and asked to write the name associated with each picture. He produced five errors, four of which were PPEs, and an SE involving a letter substitution (see Appendix 1).

If MW had a selective deficit to the phonological input lexicon, then a written naming task should not have elicited PPEs. These results, in conjunction with MW's excellent performance for auditory lexical decision judgements (described previously), indicate that the phonological input lexicon is intact (or, at least, this processing level does not contribute significantly to the observed errors).

Meaning/Writing to Dictation Task. MW was administered a list of 20 words auditorily. First, he was to provide a written definition of the word, and upon completion of this, to write the word. MW accurately defined all words. He produced three PPEs and one SE to the target words and additionally produced one PPE and three SEs in the definitions (see Appendix 1).

Written Narratives. MW was asked to provide a written description to the Cookie Theft Picture of the Boston Diagnostic Aphasia Examination (Goodglass & Kaplan, 1972). He wrote 64 words, ranging from 2 to 11 letters in length. MW produced seven errors, two of which were PPEs and five of which were SEs. All SEs involved letter substitutions (See Appendix 1).

MW was also asked to produce a short written essay about the civil war. He wrote 46 words, ranging from 2 to 11 letters in length. He produced four errors, two of which were PPEs, one an SE (e.g., "MILITARV" for "MILITARY"), and one response containing both PPE and SE components (e.g., "GETTIESDURGY" for "GETTYSBURG"--MW stated that he meant to write "B" instead of "D" and "H" instead of "Y") (see Appendix 1).

These results indicate that MW produces PPEs even when he has accessed the meaning of the word. These results, in conjunction with the previously mentioned findings that lexical-semantic factors do not affect performance, provide strong evidence that the locus of damage is not at the level of accessing lexical-semantic representations. We therefore hypothesise that MW's deficit is specifically in gaining access to whole-word spelling representations in the graphemic output lexicon.

Spelling Errors
An important issue to resolve is whether SEs arise from the same mechanism as do PPEs. As discussed in the Introduction, SEs can arise from one of several different loci of impairment in the graphemic output lexicon account not only for the ultimate production of PPEs (given that his phoneme-grapheme conversion system is relatively intact) but also for the occurrence of SEs in written spelling performance? If we postulate that a disruption in gaining access to whole-word spelling representations in the graphemic output lexicon results in SEs in our patient (see Miller & Ellis, in press), then the production of SEs for nonword spelling must be explained by an additional impairment to the phoneme-grapheme

conversion system, since nonwords do not have lexical entries and therefore would not be affected by a deficit to the graphemic output lexicon. The presence of SEs in writing nonwords to dictation is not due to occasional auditory misperceptions of the stimuli, since MW accurately repeated all stimuli prior to initiating his writing responses. Furthermore, it seems unlikely that MW has two deficits, one to the graphemic output lexicon and one to the phoneme-grapheme conversion system, that each produce SEs, and that these errors all take the form of letter substitutions. This skepticism concerning the reasonableness of postulating two functional lesions to account for the SEs in word and nonword spelling is based on the fact that SEs occur with the same approximate rate for word and nonword spelling (i.e., 5% and 4% for total number of nonword and word responses, respectively) and *all* take the form of letter substitutions. It is more likely that a single deficit can account for the production of SEs in written spelling of these stimuli--a deficit to a post-graphemic processing mechanism. In order to try to localise the level(s) of impairment implicated in the production SEs in word and nonword written spelling performance, we administered a variety of tasks, as described in the following section.

Oral Spelling to Dictation. Over the course of the investigation, MW was administered a number of tests as an oral spelling to dictation task, four of which included the same stimuli as were administered for the writing to dictation tasks. Altogether, he orally spelled 368 words and 54 nonwords.

Results indicate that nonwords were spelled with 100% (54/54) accuracy in contrast to 86% (314/368) accuracy for words ($X^2 = 9.23$, $p < .01$). The most striking feature of MW's oral spelling performance is that SEs not only were *not* produced for nonword spelling but were *not* produced for word spelling either. The only error type produced (for word spelling) was the PPE. PPEs were produced at the same rate of production for oral spelling to dictation as for writing to dictation (i.e., 17% of the total responses were PPEs for both conditions). Table 1 depicts what percentage of each error type was produced for overall errors for stimuli from the same four lists that were administered under oral and written spelling conditions.

Results obtained for the oral spelling tests indicate that the production of SEs observed in writing to dictation, written naming, meaning/writing to dictation, and written narrative tasks is not due to a deficit in accessing whole-word spelling representations in the graphemic output lexicon. Likewise, the observation of SEs for written nonword spelling is not due to a deficit in the phoneme-grapheme conversion system. MW's perfect performance for oral spelling of nonwords indicates that the nonlexical phoneme-grapheme conversion system is intact. These findings suggest that the production of SEs for written spelling of both words and nonwords occurs at a post-graphemic level in the spelling system that is critical for written spelling performance of both addressed (words) and assembled (nonwords and for this patient some low frequency words in particular) orthography.

Table 1. Distribution of errors for oral written spelling.

	WORDS		NONWORDS	
	Oral Spelling	Written Spelling	Oral Spelling	Written Spelling
PPEs	100%	75%	NA	NA
SEs	0%	24%	0%	100%
Mixed	0%	2%	NA	NA

NA = Not applicable (any phonologically plausible response for a nonword is considered accurate, thus PPEs do not exist for nonword spelling).

Our data thus far already allow us to rule out the possibility that the post-graphemic deficit is at the level of the output graphemic buffer. That is, if MW has a deficit in the buffer, then both written *and* oral spelling performance would elicit SEs since both types of tasks require the use of this buffer in temporarily storing abstract graphemic representations prior to implementation of more peripheral output processes. We therefore postulate that the post-graphemic processing component implicated in the production of SEs in MW's written spelling performance is at the level of the allographic conversion system.

If MW has a deficit in accessing the correct allographic forms of letters (i.e., in particular in accessing the visual shape of a graphemic unit), then we expect performance for both writing of dictated letters and copy transcription tasks to be impaired (i.e., yielding the production of SEs) since both tasks require an intact allographic conversion system for accurate performance.

Writing Dictated Letters. For writing of dictated letters, MW was presented with single letter names auditorily and asked to write that letter. Each letter of the alphabet was given 8 times, and the 208 stimuli were presented in random order. After MW had completed each response, the response was covered and he was asked to repeat the stimulus. MW accurately repeated all of the letters. Among his written responses, he produced 9 letter substitution errors (4.3%), all to consonants (see Appendix 1).

Copy Transcription. MW was administered the same stimuli used for the oral spelling task as a delayed copy-transcription task (nonwords were spelled with a regular spelling pattern, e.g., /fin/ on the oral spelling task was presented as "feen" for this task). All stimuli were presented in upper-case print. MW first viewed each stimulus. Then, after the stimulus was covered, he transcribed it into lower case script. MW had no difficulty in transcribing from upper-case print to lower-case script. He produced eight errors: six SEs and one PPE. All SEs took the form of substitutions (five to consonants, two to vowels). MW accurately transcribed 17 of the 20 nonwords (85.0%) and 38 of the 42 words (90.5%), indicating that there was no significant word advantage for this task (X^2 = .79, NS; see Appendix 1). For five of the six SEs, MW commented that he had produced an error (the stimulus was not in view). This indicates that MW's errors are not due to visual misperception of the stimuli. MW was administered the same set of stimuli as a direct copy-transcription task. For this task, he was to transcribe from lower-case print to upper-case print. MW had each stimulus in view while performing this task. He produced three substitution errors, two for consonants, one for a vowel (see Appendix 1). Again, MW commented that he had produced an error for all three error responses. Errors produced for these additional writing tasks support the view that SEs arise at the level of the allographic conversion system with a disruption of the rules which specify the visual shape that each graphemic unit will take, prior to implementation of more peripheral motor processes.

The Organisation of the Phoneme-Grapheme Conversion System
Results obtained from a number of converging sources indicate that our patient, MW, has two functional deficits contributing to his impaired pattern of spelling performance. One deficit is in gaining access to whole-word spelling representations in the graphemic output lexicon and the other is in selecting the appropriate letter shape for graphemic units in the allographic conversion system. Hence, a deficit to the former mechanism makes whole-word specifications for low-frequency words in particular more difficult to access than those for high-frequency words. When these representations are inaccessible, MW has the phoneme-grapheme conversion system available for use and, through the implementation of phoneme-grapheme correspondence rules, he produces a phonologically plausible spelling for these words.

This hypothesis--that low-frequency words are more likely than high-frequency words to be spelled through the use of the phoneme-grapheme conversion system--leads to an empirically testable claim concerning the interaction between word frequency and the probability of correctly spelling specific words. The prediction concerns the selection of specific phoneme-grapheme correspondence mappings when the whole-word spelling representation is unavailable for output. Thus, if MW is relying on the phoneme-grapheme conversion system for spelling of some (or many) low-frequency words, then we might expect a word frequency X probability of phoneme-grapheme conversion options interaction. That is, low-frequency words which have a high probability of being accurately spelled by use of phoneme-grapheme correspondence mappings should be more likely to be spelled accurately than low-frequency words which have a low probability of being spelled accurately by use of phoneme-grapheme correspondence mappings. This should not hold true for high-frequency words, in this patient, because these words can be addressed from the graphemic output lexicon, and, thus, do not require the application of phoneme-grapheme conversion rules for assembling spelling. This hypothesis rests on the assumption that the selection of a particular phoneme-grapheme correspondence mapping is determined by the frequency with which that mapping occurs in English words--for example, if the letter "c" (as in "cake") is the most common graphemic realisation of the phoneme /k/, and "ch" (as in "chorus") is an infrequent graphemic option for /k/ in syllable initial position of English words, then "c" will have a higher weight than "ch" as a graphemic option for /k/ in syllable initial position when applying phoneme-grapheme conversion rules. On this account , then, the use of particular graphemic mappings should reflect the distribution (in terms of weights/frequency) of possible graphemic options for a particular phoneme. This "interaction" of word frequency *and* probability of phoneme-grapheme correspondence mapping options was assessed by administration of a specially constructed list of words: the Probability of Phoneme-Grapheme Conversion List.

This list contains 110 monosyllabic words. One-third have a high phoneme-grapheme conversion probability (i.e., ≥ 50% chance of being spelled correctly when applying phoneme-grapheme probability (i.e., ≤ 10% chance of being spelled correctly when applying phoneme-grapheme correspondence rules);[6] half are high-frequency words, half low-frequency words. These words range from four to six letters in length, contain three to four phonemes per word, and are counterbalanced for phoneme-grapheme conversion probability, word frequency, number of phonemes per word, and word length. Words belonging to different grammatical classes are distributed evenly across the various dimensions. Results for written and oral spelling of the stimuli from this list (administered several weeks apart) are as follows.

Written Spelling. Results (in percent correct) indicate the probabilities shown in Table 2.(7) There are significant effects of word frequency (96% (52/54) and 80% (41/51) accuracy for high- and low-frequency words, respectively, $X^2 = 6.54$, $p < .01$) and word probability (100% (27/27) and 85% (66/78) for high- and low-probability words, respectively, $X^2 = 4.70$, $p < 0.05$). This latter effect, however, is the result of an interaction between word frequency and word probability. That is, for high-frequency words, MW was 100% (14/14) and 95% (38/40) correct for high- and low-probability words, respectively ($X^2 = .73$, NS) whereas for low-frequency words, MW was 100% (13/13) and 74% (28/38) correct for high-and low- probability words, respectively ($X^2 = 4.25$, $p < .05$).

Table 2. Percent correct performance for written spelling.

		Probability of P-G Conversion		
		High	Low	High + Low
Word Frequency	High	100	95	96
	Low	100	74	80
	High + Low	100	85	89

Oral Spelling. Results obtained for oral spelling of the stimuli that comprise the Probability of Phoneme-Grapheme Conversion List are shown in Table 3 (in percent correct).

Table 3. Percent correct performance for oral spelling.

		Probability P-G Conversion		
		High	Low	High + Low
Word Frequency	High	100	100	100
	Low	100	75	82
	High + Low	100	88	91

There are significant effects of word frequency 100% (55/55) and 82% (45/55) accuracy for high-and low-frequency words, respectively, $X^2 = 4.12$, $p < .05$). These effects are entirely due to a word frequency X phoneme-grapheme probability interaction (for high-frequency words, both high-and low-probability words were spelled with 100% accuracy, whereas for low-frequency words, MW obtained 100% (15/15) and 75%

(30/40) accuracy for high- and low-probability options, respectively, X^2 = 4.59, $p < .05$).

The word frequency X probability of phoneme-grapheme conversion options interaction observed in written and oral spelling indicates that when MW is using the phoneme-grapheme conversion system in assembling spelling sequences, he is more accurate at assembling spellings for low-frequency words with a high probability of phoneme-grapheme correspondence mappings than for low-frequency words with a low probability of phoneme-grapheme correspondence mappings. The finding of no difference in spelling performance for high-frequency words with a high versus low probability of phoneme-grapheme options supports the view that, for this patient, spelling of high-frequency words, in general, is accomplished by addressing whole-word spelling representations in the graphemic output lexicon and not by application of phoneme-grapheme conversion rules.

The reported interaction is important for two reasons. First, it supports the general hypothesis that lexical and nonlexical writing mechanisms are autonomous and that the nonlexical, phoneme-grapheme conversion system is involved in word writing when access to the graphemic output lexicon is impaired. Second, and more specifically, the reported results support the thesis that the selection of phoneme-grapheme mapping options reflects the statistical distribution of phoneme-grapheme mappings in words.

DISCUSSION

Results obtained for written and oral spelling tasks indicate that our patient, MW, has a deficit in addressing whole-word spelling representations in the graphemic output lexicon, making low-frequency words less accessible than high-frequency words. When whole-word spelling representations for words (typically low-frequency words) are not accessible, MW relies on the phoneme-grapheme conversion system for assembling spellings, thus producing PPEs under written and oral spelling conditions (Hatfield & Patterson, 1983).[8] This is further supported by findings of a word frequency X phoneme-grapheme probability options interaction (for written and oral spelling), where high-frequency words are spelled equally well irrespective of whether they have a high or a low probability of phoneme-grapheme correspondence mappings as compared to spelling of low-frequency words for which high-probability words are spelled more accurately than are low-probability words. (This result parallels results obtained for a patient with an acquired reading disorder in which the patient produced phonological regularization errors in oral reading (e.g., /trid/ for "tread") more often for irregular low-frequency words than for regular low-frequency words whereas regular and irregular high-frequency words were read with the same degree of accuracy--Bub, Cancelliere, & Kertesz, in press.) These findings indicate that access to whole-word spelling representations in the graphemic output lexicon is sensitive to the dimension of word frequency. Damage to the access system presumably elevates the activation threshold levels of all words, subsequently making the threshold levels of some (or many) low-frequency words too high to allow for access of these entries (see Nolan & Caramazza, 1982).

Although MW produced PPEs for written and oral spelling of words, he additionally produced SEs in all tasks involving written spelling of words *and* nonwords, but not for oral spelling of these stimuli. (See Kinsbourne & Rosenfield (1974) and Kinsbourne & Warrington (1965) and references therein for discussion of other cases showing a dissociation between oral and written spelling.) The dissociation between written and oral spelling in the production of SEs was used to motivate an account of the level of impairment responsible for this particular type of spelling error in this patient. Evidence from a variety of converging sources (i.e., SEs occurring in writing words and nonwords to dictation, written naming, spontaneous written narratives, direct and delayed copying, writing of dictated single letters) indicates that these particular spelling errors arise from a deficit in the allographic conversion system, a system responsible for assigning the case, type, and visual shape to each graphemic unit of an abstract graphemic representation.

Since MW is able to transcribe from print to script, from upper to lower case (and vice versa), and uses the appropriate case for written narratives of either type (e.g., capitalises when appropriate in print or script format), we can assume that the processes within the allographic conversion system used for assigning case and type information are intact. By contrast, the fact that MW's production of substitution errors for words and nonwords was unaffected by the case-type format to be used (i.e., upper-case print, lower-case print, lower-case script) suggests that the allographic process for assigning the visual shape to a graphemic unit is impaired. It is suggested here that one level of impairment in MW's writing system is to an allographic process as opposed to subsequently-employed processes that assign the sequence of strokes to the specific visual shapes (i.e., the processes referred to as "graphic motor patterns" by Ellis, 1979; 1982). This conclusion is supported by the fact that MW always produces legible, correctly shaped letters. According to a number of researchers (e.g., Ellis, 1979, in press; Margolin & Wing, 1983; Margolin, 1984), an impairment at the level of assigning the graphic motor pattern will result, at least on occasion, in a nonletter. For example, a subject might add an additional loop to the letter "m," creating '𝗆𝗆.' Since MW does not produce such errors and produces only correctly shaped and legible letters, we can assume that the selection and execution of the graphic motor pattern that corresponds to the (correctly or incorrectly) selected allograph is intact.

Our findings also rule out the possibility that MW's SEs can be accounted for by a deficit to the output graphemic buffer as opposed to an impairment in the allographic conversion system. If MW has a deficit to the output graphemic buffer, then we would have expected to observe the presence of SEs for written *and* oral spelling of words and nonwords since both tasks require an intact output graphemic buffer for accurate performance. Our finding of a dissociation between written and oral spelling tasks in MW's performance with respect to the production of SEs rules out the possibility of an output graphemic buffer deficit. In addition, MW's spelling performance was not affected by stimulus length, a variable that has been correlated with disruption to this working memory system, as in the case of a previously described patient, FV (Miceli, Silveri, & Caramazza, 1985). Thus, the production of SEs can only be accounted for by a deficit to a processing mechanism used after the computation of graphemic representations and after this information has been stored in the output graphemic buffer prior to implementation of other processes used for oral or written spelling of stimuli.

In our discussion of MW's pattern of spelling performance, we have placed much emphasis on the dissociation between the production of a certain kind of spelling error, SEs, for different tasks (i.e., oral versus written spelling) in order to specify the locus of the deficit implicated in the production of such errors. Although an analysis of patterns of dissociations for different types of (spelling) errors is one approach to discerning the level(s) of impairment implicated in a patient's overall performance, we can also look at converging patterns of performance regarding the nature of the errors in order to specify the locus of impairment responsible for the production of each error type. A case in point is provided by Caramazza et al. (in press). They hypothesise that the functional locus of impairment contributing to the SEs exhibited by their patient, IGR, is in the output phonological buffer. IGR produced SEs which had a strong phonological relationship to the target letters (but which did not have the same phonetic value and were therefore not phonologically plausible errors) in all writing tasks involving use of the output phonological buffer system. Further, the same pattern of errors involving phonological principles was observed for reading and repetition tasks, (both of which require an intact output phonological buffer in order to be performed accurately), providing empirical support for the claim

that the SEs observed in writing were manifestations of a deficit in the
output phonological buffer.

The findings we have reported for patient MW together with other
results we have reviewed provide evidence for the independent
functioning of two processing mechanisms for written spelling that operate
subsequent to the computation of graphemic representations--the output
graphemic buffer and the allographic conversion system. Disruption to
each of these systems results in different patterns of spelling performance
and in different combinations of types of SEs. A schematic representation
of the functional architecture of the spelling system that has emerged from
the analysis presented here is shown in Fig. 3.

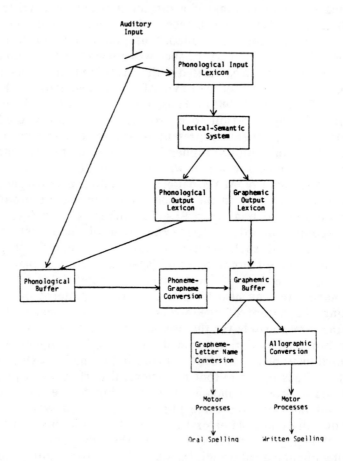

Figure 3. Extended schematic representation of written and oral
systems.

In conclusion, at least four possible processing components in the spelling system have thus far been implicated in the production of phonologically *im*plausible visually similar spelling errors--the graphemic output lexicon (Miller & Ellis, in press), the output graphemic buffer (patient FV; Miceli et al., 1985), the output phonological buffer (patient IGR; Caramazza et al., in press) and the allographic conversion system (patient MW). It is evident that SEs do not represent a homogeneous set of responses in terms of being explicable by a functional lesion to only *one* processing component of the writing system. The heterogeneity in the nature of the SEs and associated patterns of impairments provides the basis for the development of an increasingly articulated functional architecture of the spelling system which, in turn, provides the basis for a principled account of patterns of dysgraphia.

ACKNOWLEDGMENTS

The research reported here was supported by NIH grant NS22201 to The Johns Hopkins University, and by Biomedical Research grant S07-RR07041, Division of Research Resources, National Institutes of Health. This research is part of the first author's doctoral dissertation of the University of Maryland, College Park. We thank William Badecker and Michael McCloskey for their suggestions and comments in various phases of the reported research and Andy Ellis, Alan Wing, and an anonymous referee for constructive criticisms of an earlier version of this paper. We also thank Kathy Sporney for her help in various stages of the preparation of this manuscript.

REFERENCES

Beauvois, M. F. & Dérouesné, J. (1981). Lexical or orthographic agraphia. Brain, 104, 21-49.

Bub, D. N., Cancelliere, A. & Kertesz, A. (in press). Whole word and analytic translation of spelling to sound in a non-semantic reader. In K. Patterson, J. C. Marshall & M. Coltheart, (Eds.), Surface dyslexia: Neuropsychological and cognitive studies of phonological reading. London: Lawrence Erlbaum Associates Ltd.

Bub, D. & Kertesz, A. (1982). Evidence for lexicographic processing in a patient with preserved written over oral single word naming. Brain, 105, 697-717.

Caramazza, A., Miceli, G. & Villa, G. (in press). The role of the (output) phonological buffer in reading, writing, and repetition. Cognitive Neuropsychology.

A. Caramazza

Carroll, J. B., Davies, P. & Richman, B. (1971). Word frequency book. New York, NY: American Heritage Publishing Co., Inc.

Dunn, L. M. & Dunn, L. M. (1981). The Peabody Picture Vocabulary Test-revised. Circle Pines, MN: American Guidance Service.

Ellis, A. W. (1079). Slips of the pen. Visible Language, 13, 265-282.

Ellis, A. W. (1982). Spelling and writing (and reading and speaking). In A. W. Ellis (Ed.), Normality and pathology in cognitive functions. London: Academic Press.

Ellis, A. W. (in press). Modelling the writing process. In G. Denes, C. Semenza, P. Bisiacchi & E. Andreewsky (Eds.), Perspectives in cognitive neuropsychology. London: Lawrence Erlbaum Associates Ltd.

Friendly, M., Franklin, P. E., Hoffman, D. & Rubin, D. C. (1982). The Toronto Word Pool: Norms for imagery, concreteness, orthographic variables, and grammatical usage for 1,080 words. Behaviour Research Methods and Instrumentation, 14, 375-399.

Glushko, R. J. (1979). The organisation and activation of orthographic knowledge in reading aloud. Journal of Experimental Psychology: Human Perception and Performance, 5, 674-691.

Glushko, R. J. (1981). Principles for pronouncing print: The psychology of phonography. In A. M. Lesgold & C. A. Perfetti (Eds.), Interactive processes in reading. Hillsdale, NJ: Lawrence Erlbaum Associates Inc.

Goodglass, H. & Kaplan, E. (1972). The assessment of aphasia and related disorders. Philadelphia, PA: Lea and Febiger.

Goodglass, H. & Kaplan, E. (1983). The Boston Naming Test. Philadelphia, PA: Lea and Febiger.

Gordon, B. (1983). Lexical access and lexical decision: Mechanisms of frequency sensitivity. Journal of Verbal Learning and Verbal Behaviour, 22, 146-160.

Hanna, R. R., Hanna, J. S., Hodges, R. E. & Rudorf, E. H. (1966). Phoneme-grapheme correspondences as cues to spelling improvement. U.S. Department of Health, Education, and Welfare, Office of Education, Washington, DC: U.S. Government Printing Office.

Hatfield, M. & Patterson, K. E. (1983). Phonological spelling. Quarterly Journal of Experimental Psychology, 35, 451-468.

Henderson, L. (1982). Orthography and word recognition in reading. New York, NY/London: Academic Press.

Kay, J. & Marcel, T. (1981). One process, not two, in reading aloud: Lexical analogies do the work of non-lexical rules. Quarterly Journal of Experimental Psychology, 33(A), 397-413.

Kinsbourne, M. & Rosenfield, D. B. (1974). Agraphia selective for written spelling. Brain and Language, 1, 215-225.

Kinsbourne, M. & Warrington, E. K. (1965). A case showing selectively impaired oral spelling. Journal of Neurology, Neurosurgery and Psychiatry, 28, 563-566.

Marcel, T. (1980). Surface dyslexia and beginning reading: A revised hypothesis of the pronunciation of print and its impairments. In M. Coltheart, K. E. Patterson & J. C. Marshall (Eds.), Deep dyslexia. London: Routledge and Kegan Paul.

Margolin, D. I. (1984). The neuropsychology of writing and spelling: Semantic, phonological, motor, and perceptual processes. Quarterly Journal of Experimental Psychology, 36(A), 459-489.

Margolin, D. I. & Wing, A. M. (1983). Agraphia and micrographia: Clinical manifestations of motor programming and performance disorders. Acta Psychologica, 54, 263-283.

Miceli, G., Silveri, M. C. & Caramazza, A. (1985). Cognitive analysis of a case of pure agraphia. Brain and Language, 25, 187-212.

Miller, D. & Ellis, A. W. (in press). Speech and writing errors in "neologistic jargon aphasia": A lexical activation hypothesis. In M. Coltheart, R. Job, & G. Sartori, (Eds.), Cognitive neuropsychology of language.

Morton, J. (1980). The logogen model and orthographic structure. In U. Frith (Ed.), Cognitive processes in spelling. London: Academic Press.

Nolan, K. & Caramazza, A. (1982). Modality independent impairments in processing in a deep dyslexic patient. Brain and Language, 16, 237-266.

Roeltgen, D. P. & Heilman, K. M. (1984). Lexical agraphia: Further support for the two-system hypothesis of linguistic agraphia. Brain, 107, 811-827.

Roeltgen, D. P., Sevush, S. & Heilman, K. M. (1983). Phonological agraphia: Writing by the lexical-semantic route. Neurology, 33, 755-765.

Shallice, T. (1981). Phonological agraphia and the lexical route in writing. Brain, 104, 413-429.

APPENDIX 1 CORPUS OF ERRORS
WRITTEN SPELLING TASKS

(Note: a "+" indicates that MW self-corrected.)

1. Writing to Dictation

(a) Single Word/Nonword Dictation
(i) Words
Phonologically Plausible Errors

STIMULUS	RESPONSE	STIMULUS	RESPONSE
space	spaice, +	palace	palece
merge	murge	belief	beliefe
while	wile, whyle, +	pursuit	purcuit, persute
solve	sav		persuit
cheap	cheep	bullet	bullit
vulgar	vulger, +	poem	powen, +
common	commin, commen	cushion	cushen
digit	didgit, diget, +	pirate	piret, +, pyrate
column	columm, +	cable	cabel, cabil
caught	cought	rooster	ruster
speak	speek	nuisance	nusence
grief	greafe, greaf	pigeon	pigion
success	succes, +	igloo	iglu
horror	horrer	complete	complite
fabric	fabrick	odor	odur, oder
offense	offence	jerk	jirk, jurk
skull	scull	allure	alure
group	groop, grupe	channel	chanel
rinse	rince	immense	imense, immence
learn	lern, +	ferry	fery
gross	groce, grose	splurge	splerge, +
cheer	chear	stipple	stiple, +
sauce	sause	typhoon	typhun
phase	faze	support	suport, +
shack	shake	usurp	userp, +
moose	muse	sense	sence, +
rascal	rascle	array	aray, +
torrid	torid	natty	knaty, +
whiff	whif	cement	sement, +
slouch	sloutch	arbor	arbur
tweak	tweke	balloon	baloon
verge	vurge, +	fluff	fluf, fluph
truffle	trufle, +	veneer	venier

Spelling Errors

STIMULUS	RESPONSE	STIMULUS	RESPONSE
pierce	tierce	thief	chief, +
starve	starze	yawn	yown, +
point	toint	refrain	refrail
bump	bumd	half	holf, +
sneeze	sneeve	purse	turse, +
broom	brood, +	gloss	glose

nature	mature	guitar	guiter, +
annoy	annoe, annoi	doubt	dougt, +
vivid	fifid, +	loop	look
special	speceal, +	clue	clve
frequent	prequent		

Mixed Errors

| pretty | trity, preddy, | cull | kule, kull, + |

(ii) Nonwords

STIMULUS	RESPONSE	STIMULUS	RESPONSE
/hegr d/	hagrib	/r lt/	rolt
/ri /	reech	/spag/	spob
/vand/	lond	/ d pt/	adept, adipt
/s lt/	surelt	/bil/	peal, beal
/ sp t/	aspic	/p sk/	task, pask
/garn /	gorner, garner	h n nt/	fenant

(b) Provides a Written Definition, Then the Dictated Word

(The intended target words for errors produced in the definitions are in brackets.)

Phonologically Plausible Errors

STIMULUS	DEFINITION/RESPONSE
digit	a number - didget
pierce	penetrate with knife - pearce
thief	person who takes things - thefe
engine	a machine to power a vehikle (vehicle) - engine

Spelling Errors

STIMULUS	DEFINITION/RESPONSE
sneeze	a sound made with the nose - sheeze
starve	go uithout (without) food - starve
science	method of organizing hnowledge (knowledge) - science
pretty	attraetive (attractive) - pretty

(c) Writing of Single Dictated Letters

STIMULUS	RESPONSE	STIMULUS	RESPONSE
K	Q	G	B
R	P, +	Y	V, +
V	Z (twice)	J	Q, +

H   F, +
Z   S

(d) Written Naming
Phonologically Plausibel Errors

STIMULUS	RESPONSE	STIMULUS	RESPONSE
money	mony	anchor	ancher, +
canoe	canue	doctor	docter
train			trail

(e) Spontaneous Written Narratives
(Note: the intended target word appears in brackets next to MW's error response.)

Written description of the Cookie Theft Picture (Boston Diagnostic Aphasia Examination)

Mother is washing dishes in kitchen. Two problems, water is overflowing onto *kloor*/floor. Boy *ang* (and) girl are getting *k/cookles* (cookies) from *shelp* (shelf), boy is falling off ladder; girl is observing this but not *halping* (helping). Disaster; girl has left hand up to take *cooky* (cookie); right hand is on mouth. Boy does not seem to know he is falling, kitchen is looking *owt* (out) over the back yard.

Written narrative about the Civil War

What are the major lessons of the Civil Wor (War) - US?
1. Were the basic issues understood?
    A. Unity of the central government
    B. Slavery?
2. Why the north won.
    A. More resources.
        Manpower
        Economic
    B. Good leadership
        1. Lincoln and his cabinet
        2. Militarv (Military)
        3. Naval power
    C. Ideological control
3. Handling of successive crices/creices (crises)
    1861, 1862, 1863, 1864, 1865
    gettiesdurgy (Gettysburg)

(f) Copy Transcription

(i) Direct Copying

Words		Nonwords	
STIMULUS	RESPONSE	STIMULUS	RESPONSE
talent	talant	lorn	forn
	skart		skarp, +

(ii) Delayed Copying

Words		Nonwords	
STIMULUS	RESPONSE	STIMULUS	RESPONSE
grief	griel	teeble	teebre
borrow	gorraw	dute	bute, +
bring	gring	sarcle	surcle
pursuit	persuit, +		

ORAL SPELLING

Phonologically Plausible Errors

STIMULUS	RESPONSE	STIMULUS	RESPONSE
poem	powem	success	succes, +, succes
borrow	barow	horror	horrer, +
carry	cary, +,	engine	ingine, +
severe	sevear	fabric	fabrick
priest	preast	offense	ofence
caught	cought	system	sistem, +
space	spaice, +	belief	beleaf, +
stripe	strip, +	beauty	butey
column	colum, +	tragic	trajic, +
career	carear, +	cushion	kushen, cushen
grief	greaf	pressure	preshure
decide	deside	language	languag
argue	argu, +	trouble	truble
merge	murge, +	pretty	prety
happen	hapin, hapen, +,	color	couler
hapen	rooster	ruster	
carry	cary, +, cary	nuisance	nusence
hurry	hury	pigeon	pidgen, pidgin,
caught	cought		pidgen
deny	denie	igloo	iglue
sleek	sleak	machine	michine
fierce	fearce, +, fearce	excess	exces
common	comin, comen	odor	odure
while	wile	leopard	leapord
should	should	skull	scul
shall	shal, +	rinse	rince

cattle	catle, +	pulse	puls
degree	degre, degrea, +	gross	groce

NOTES

[1] This conclusion is motivated only if a single deficit hypotheses of the locus of functional damage is entertained. Of course, it is possible for there to be multiple functional loci of damage-damage to the phonological input lexicon and damage to other processing systems involved in lexical selection for written picture naming and spontaneous written narrative.

[2] Although there are other types of phonologically *implausible* spelling errors such as semantic errors ("cat" for "dog"), and morphological errors ("run" for "running"-see Caramazza, Miceli, & Villa (in press) for further discussion), we have restricted the use of the term "spelling" error in this particular paper to refer to a subclass of errors which may include substitutions ("dat" for "cat'), deletions ("mose" for "mouse"), transpositions ("paly" for "play"), additions ("gamre" for "game"), and mixed errors (any combination of the two of the above mentioned errors).

[3] Due to MW's right-sided hemiparesis, he is unable to write with his dominant hand; hence he used the nonpreferred left hand in performing all written spelling tasks.

[4] For all lists included in our battery, frequency measures were obtained from norms provided by Carroll, Davies, and Richman (1971). Based on the range and distribution of frequencies within the U distribution of the norms, we opted to restrict the high frequency range for nouns, verbs, and adjectives to words occurring between 51 and 313 times per million ($\overline{X}$ = 141), mid frequency range to words occurring between 25 and 48 times per million ($\overline{X}$ = 35), and low frequency range to words occurring between 0.5 and 25 times per million ($\overline{X}$ = 6). The frequency range for the function words is 137 to 3350 times per million ($\overline{X}$ = 1005).

[5] Concreteness measures were obtained from norms provided by Friendly, Franklin, Hoffman, and Rubin (1982), who used a 1-7 rating scale, 1 representing the greatest degree of abstractness, 7 representing the greatest degree of concreteness. Concrete words were defined as words referring to "tangible objects, materials, or persons which can be easily perceived with the senses." (P.376.) Abstract words were defined as words referring to "abstract concepts which are not easily objectified or perceived." (P.376.) Based on the distribution of concreteness scores, we opted to select abstract words, which ranged from 2.5 to 4.0 ($\overline{X}$ = 3.34), and concrete words, which ranged from 6.1 to 7.0 ($\overline{X}$ = 6.55).

[6] Phoneme-grapheme probability measures were obtained from norms provided by Hanna, Hanna, Hodges and Rudorf (1966) who calculated the

frequency of occurrence of each phoneme-grapheme option within syllable position for English words. we opted to select as high probability words those which have ≥ 50% probability of being accurately spelled by use of phoneme-grapheme correspondence mappings ranging from 50.0%-82.9% ($\overline{X}$ = 66.3) and as low probability words those which have ≤ 10% probability of being accurately spelled by use of phoneme-grapheme correspondence mappings ranging from 0.1%-9.3% ($\overline{X}$ = 3.55).

[7] Note that the relevant observations here include only correct responses and PPEs. we have already shown that SEs do not arise at the level of the phoneme-grapheme conversion process and, therefore, these latter errors are not relevant to the hypothesis being tested.

[8] We have, for simplicity's sake (but perhaps misleadingly) argued that the graphemic representation that is ultimately used in spelling is the product either of just the lexical or just the nonlexical system. However, as has been suggested by Ellis (in press) it is possible that in some cases information from the two processing routes--lexical and nonlexical--may combine to generate a single graphemic representation. In other words, there may be cases where only partial lexical knowledge is available for a target item and the additional spelling information must be provided by the operation of the phoneme-grapheme conversion system. Possible examples of the use of this strategy in our patient's error corpus are "typhoon" → typhun and "pursuit" →purcuit.

CHAPTER EIGHT

THE ROLE OF THE GRAPHEMIC BUFFER IN SPELLING:
EVIDENCE FROM A CASE OF ACQUIRED DYSGRAPHIA

INTRODUCTION

Information processing models of spelling assume that an abstract graphemic representation of the to-be-written word must be generated at some point in the spelling process. This representation specifies the orthographic structure-the sequence of letters-that must be produced. How these graphemic representations are generated in the course of spelling is currently a much debated issue. One class of models assumes that the graphemic representations of familiar and novel words are generated by a single processing mechanism (e.g. Campbell, 1983). Another class of models assumes that the graphemic representations of familiar words are addressed directly in a graphemic lexicon whereas the graphemic representations for novel words (or nonwords) are computed through the application of a Phoneme-Grapheme Conversion Mechanism (e.g., Patterson, in press; Caramazza, Miceli, & Villa, 1986). However, independently of the class of model one adopts for the generation of graphemic representations, there is the issue of how these representations are processed further in the course of spelling. That is, we must specify the types of processes that transform an abstract graphemic representation into a form that is suitable for guiding motor output processes (see Margolin, 1984). Thus, we can consider the spelling process as consisting of two stages: First, those processes involved in the generation of a graphemic representation and, second, those processes involved in using the computed graphemic representation to generate the proper graphomotor processes for oral and written spelling.

The increasingly detailed analyses of acquired disorders of spelling (dysgraphia) in brain-damaged adults have revealed many interesting patterns of deficits. These analyses have served, on the one hand, as the basis for the development of models of the normal spelling process and, on the other hand, as the basis for characterizing the dissolution of the spelling process under conditions of brain damage (see Ellis, in press, for a review). The logic used to constrain models of the normal spelling process through the analysis of patterns of dysgraphia is relatively straightforward. We assume that patterns of dysgraphia are explicable by functionally lesioning one or more components of the cognitive system that underlies spelling. More specifically, we assume that a particular form of dysgraphia constitutes empirical support for a model of spelling (over some alternative model) if the observed pattern of spelling impairment is explicable by specifying a functional lesion to the postulated model. Thus, for example, it has been argued (e.g., Caramazza et. al., 1986; Patterson, in press) that models of spelling which postulate distinct procedures for generating graphemic representations for familiar and novel words are supported by the existence of dysgraphic patients who, in the face of considerable difficulties in spelling familiar words, present with absolutely no difficulty in spelling novel words (nonwords). In this case, it is assumed that the procedure for generating graphemic representations for familiar words has been selectively damaged.

Over the past years a number of quite detailed analyses of dysgraphic patients have been reported which have led to the formulation of a reasonably articulated functional architecture of the spelling process. A diagrammatic representation of a model of the spelling process which is compatible with extant observations of various patterns of acquired dysgraphia is depicted in Figure 1. This model, which assumes that there are distinct procedures for computing graphemic representations for familiar and novel words, can account for the reported double dissociation in spelling these two classes of stimuli. Patients have been described who present with difficulties in spelling nonwords (novel words) in the face of normal ability to spell familiar words. In one case the hypothesized locus of impairment was to the Phoneme-Grapheme Conversion Mechanism (Shallice, 1981), in the other case the hypothesized locus of impairment was to the Phonological Buffer (Caramazza, Miceli, & Villa, 1986). Patients who present with the reverse pattern of dissociation--impaired word spelling with intact nonword spelling--have also been described. In these patients the hypothesized locus of impairment was to the Graphemic Output Lexicon (Beauvois & Dérouesné, 1981; Goodman & Caramazza, 1986; Hatfield & Patterson, 1983). Other patterns of dysgraphia which locate the source of impairment to the Allographic Conversion mechanism (Goodman & Caramazza, 1986; Kinsbourne & Rosenfield, 1974) or to the Graphemic Buffer (Miceli, Silveri, & Caramazza, 1985) have also been reported. There have also been reports of patients with selective damage to relatively peripheral graphomotor processes (Baxter & Warrington, in press; Margolin, 1984). In short, diverse patterns of acquired dysgraphia are explicable by hypothesizing damage to one or more components of the postulated model of spelling and, thus, constitute evidence in favor of the model.

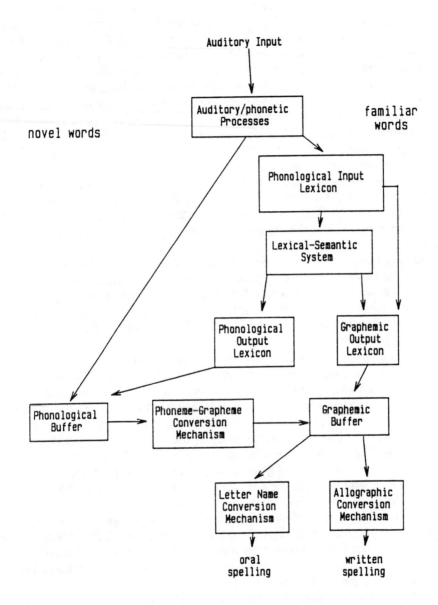

Figure 1. Schematic representation of a model of the spelling process.

Not all the cited cases are equally unequivocal in the inferences they allow about the hypothesized locus of functional impairment to the spelling process. Thus, although the patient (F.V) reported by Miceli et al.(1985) could have had a deficit to the Graphemic Buffer, there were features of his performance which resisted clear interpretation. In particular, although the patient presented with similar patterns of spelling errors in various tasks including written naming, writing to dictation, and spontaneous writing, he performed essentially flawlessly in delayed copy of words and nonwords even with a 10-s delay. Miceli et al. interpreted this dissociation in spelling performance as problematic for the hypothesis that the pattern of dysgraphia displayed by F.V might have resulted from a selective deficit to the Graphemic Buffer. In the present paper we report a case study of a dysgraphic patient (L.B.) whose pattern of spelling errors is less problematically explicable by assuming a selective deficit to the Graphemic Buffer. The detailed analysis of the patient's spelling performance provides the opportunity to explore the role and the structure of the Graphemic Buffer in the spelling process.

Many current models of the cognitive system that underlie spelling assume that a critical component of the spelling process is the Graphemic Buffer--a working memory system that temporarily stores a graphemic representation for conversion into specific letter shapes (for written spelling) or letter names (for oral spelling) (e.g., Ellis, 1982; Miceli et al., 1985). Caramazza et al. (1986) have formulated a useful criterion for motivating the inclusion of a working memory component in a cognitive system: A working memory system should be postulated whenever the computational units in a processing component are incommensurate--that is, smaller or larger--with the representations that serve as input to the processing component in question. This criterion is satisfied in the present case. The units of analysis of the Allographic Conversion Mechanism and the Letter Name Conversion Mechanism are single graphemes/letters whereas the representations generated by the Graphemic Output Lexicon and the Phoneme-Grapheme Conversion Mechanism range from whole-word units to single letters (note that the output of the Phoneme-Grapheme Conversion Mechanism may consist of single letters (e.g., /o/ → 'o') as well as several letters (e.g., /o/ → 'ough')). Consequently, the Graphemic Buffer is needed to store multi-grapheme representations temporarily while they are being converted into forms which can be used to guide more peripheral motor processes.

The model of spelling presented here assigns to the Graphemic Buffer a fairly central role. Damage to this component of the system should have clearly specifiable consequences for spelling. Specifically, since the Graphemic Buffer is strategically located in the spelling system so that it mediates between those processes needed to generate graphemic representations for the items to be spelled and the more peripheral processes needed for motor output, damage to this component of processing should affect spelling performance for familiar and novel words independently of the modality of input (i.e., writing to dictating, delayed copy, written naming, or spontaneous writing) or the modality of output (i.e., oral or written spelling or typing). Furthermore, since the representations processed by the Graphemic Buffer consist of a series of graphemic units, selective damage to this component should result in degradation of graphemic representations. In other words, spelling errors should be explicable exclusively by reference to graphemic units; we do not expect lexical (e.g., form class, morphology, etc.) or phonological factors to play a role in explicating the spelling errors produced by patients with selective damage to the Graphemic Buffer. Finally, since the hypothesized functional role of the Graphemic Buffer is to store information temporarily, damage to this storing function should result in increasingly severe spelling difficulties for longer stimuli.

Although the model we have presented allows relatively specific expectations for a range of performance in the eventuality of selective damage to the Graphemic Buffer, it is obvious that more specific predictions concerning the detailed nature of spelling errors are not possible in the absence of more richly articulated claims about the structure of the Graphemic Buffer. To be sure, there are some intuitively-driven, qualitative expectations about the type of spelling errors that may result from damage to the Graphemic Buffer. The intuition is that the Graphemic Buffer stores a spatially coded sequence of graphemes and that damage to this processing component would result in loss of specific item and/or spatial information. Consequently, errors should take the form of substitutions, insertions, deletions or transposition of letters (Miceli et at., 1985; Nolan & Caramazza, 1983).

CASE HISTORY

L.B.'s case history has been reported in detail elsewhere (see Caramazza, Miceli, Silveri, & Laudanna, 1985). The patient is a 65-year old, right-handed man who suffered a CVA in December, 1982. A CT-scan showed involvement of pre- and post-rolandic areas (both superficial and deep) in the left hemisphere. L.B. has university degrees in engineering and mathematics.

The neuropsychological evaluation at 8 months post-onset, when both the present and the above-quoted study were begun, demonstrated essentially normal results in all language tests, except for reading and spelling. Connected speech was fluent and informative, with occasional hesitations that occurred prior to the (usually successful) production of low-frequency words. Scores on oral naming and word and sentence repetition were normal. On the receptive side, discrimination of CV syllables was within normal limits. In a word-picture matching task L.B. flawlessly matched auditorily (or visually) presented words to their corresponding picture from an array that contained semantically and phonemically (or visually) related items. In an auditory sentence-to-picture matching test, the patient demonstrated normal comprehension of reversible sentences of the declarative and of the relative type (both in the active and in the passive form), and of sentences expressing reversible temporal relations (of the type before/after). L.B. obtained normal scores on the shortened version of the Token Test (30/36 correct responses) and on Raven's Colored Progressive Matrices (31/36 correct responses).

The patient presented with a mild reading disorder that impaired his ability to read nonwords, while leaving word reading unaffected. L.B.'s dyslexic disorder is described in detail in Caramazza et al. (1985). The patient's considerable difficulty in spelling is the focus of the present report.

EXPERIMENTAL STUDY

The analysis of L.B.'s performance will be organized into two parts: In the first part we consider those general features of spelling that are relevant to determining whether or not L.B.'s impairment results from damage to the Graphemic Buffer. In the second part we use L.B's pattern of spelling errors to constrain hypotheses about the computational structure of the Graphemic Buffer.

Overall results for a number of spelling tasks
In the Introduction we proposed a set of criteria for determining whether or not the locus of damage, for a particular functional architecture of the spelling process, is at the level of the Graphemic Buffer. One expected feature of spelling performance under conditions of selective damage to the Graphemic Buffer is spelling difficulties for both familiar and novel words(nonwords), independently of modality of input or output. L.B's spelling performance satisfies this criterion. As can be seen in Table 1, he encountered difficulties in spelling words and nonwords in oral and written spelling, both in dictation and delayed copy; he also had difficulties in spelling when the stimulus input consisted of line drawings of objects (i.e., in a written naming task).[1] This configuration of spelling

performance is consistent with the hypothesis of selective damage to the Graphemic Buffer. More detailed analyses where we consider the contribution of stimulus dimensions on performance in each of the spelling tasks are discussed below.

Table 1. Spelling errors for words and nonwords in various tasks (percentages are in parentheses).

	Words	Nonwords
Written spelling-to-dictation	305/743 (41)	246/425 (58)
Oral spelling-to-dictation	44/64 (69)	49/64 (77)
Written naming	65/124 (52)	--
Copy from model	5/57 (9)	2/56 (4)
Delayed copy	21/59 (36)	38/60 (63)

(1) Written spelling to dictation. L.B. was asked to spell to dictation 743 words and 425 nonwords, presented in random order over several sessions. The word sample included sublists controlled for grammatical class, abstractness/concreteness, word frequency and length. The nonword sample included sublists controlled for length and morphological decomposability (the possibility of parsing a nonword stimulus into a real root and a real suffix, not permissible for that particular root (e.g., walken), Word and nonword stimuli ranged in length from 4 to 12 letters.

In this task, as well as in all other tasks of written spelling, L.B. produced his responses to word and nonword stimuli at a normal rate, without any noticeable delay after stimulus presentation. His written output was smooth and fluent. On occasion, he would pause in the middle of a response in order to correct a just-produced letter, or would reconsider his just-completed response, in order to try to identify incorrect letters. some of these attempts succeeded, but most of them failed. Although he was never explicitly asked, L.B. never mentioned trying to visualize internally to-be-written stimulus prior to or during response production.

L.B. made 305 errors on words (41%) and 246 on nonwords (57.9%). Results for controlled sublists of words and nonwords are shown in Table 2. None of the lexical factors considered affected spelling performance: There was no effect of grammatical class, abstractness/concreteness nor word frequency. Stimulus length, by contrast, exerted a major influence on performance: L.B. spelled incorrectly only 5/40 (12.5%) short stimuli, ranging from 4 to 6 letters, but made 24/60 (60%) errors on stimuli ranging from 7 to 9 letters. Nonword spelling was not influenced by the morphological decomposability of a stimulus; however, stimulus length was a major factor on performance (8/30 (26.7%) errors on short stimuli and 16/30 (53.3%) errors on long stimuli). The effect of stimulus length on L.B.'s spelling performance is even more striking when the entire stimulus sample is considered. A monotonic (roughly linear) relationship exists between stimulus length, for both word and nonword stimuli, and number of spelling errors (see Table 3). This effect of stimulus length remain seven when we scale the probability of an error on a word by the number of letters in that word.[2] Furthermore, the mean length of words spelled correctly (5.93 letters) is significantly shorter than the mean length of words spelled incorrectly (8 letters): t=15.0 (741), p<.001. The analogous comparison for nonwords also showed a significant length effect (mean length of nonwords spelled correctly: 5.79; mean length of nonwords spelled incorrectly: 8.11; t=3.906 (423), p<.001).

Table 2. Written spelling-to-dictation: Errors made by L.B on controlled sublists.

Words	
Sublist 1. (Concreteness/abstractness x frequency; N-40)	
Concrete words	2/20
Abstract words	2/20
High-frequency words	3/20
Low-frequency	1/20
Sublist 2. (Grammatical class x frequency x length; N=80)	
Nouns	7/20
Adjectives	7/20
Verbs	7/20
Function words	9/20
High-frequency words	14/40
Low-frequency words	15/40
Short words	5/40
Long words	24/40
Nonwords	
Sublist 1. (Morphological decomposability; N=40)	
Morphologically decomposable nonwords	10/20
Morphologically non-decomposable nonwords	11/20
Sublist 2. (Length; N=60)	
Short nonwords	8/30
Long nonwords	16/30

Although a detailed error analysis will be reported in a later section of the paper, we wish to note here that the spelling errors produced by L.B. took the form of substitution, insertion, deletion, or transposition of letters or combinations of these single error types.

Oral spelling to dictation. L.B. was asked to spell orally 128 stimuli (64 words, 64 nonwords). Word and nonword stimuli were exactly matched in length, and ranged from 4 to 11 letters.

Performance on this test was poorer than performance on the written spelling task; L.B. incorrectly spelled 44/64 (68.7%) words and 49/64 (76.5%) nonwords. However, at a qualitative level the patient's performance is identical for the two tasks: There was a clear length effect (see Table 3) for both words (mean length of correctly spelled words: 5.43; mean length of incorrectly spelled words: 8.51; t=6.418 (62), p<.001) and nonwords (mean length of correctly spelled nonwords: 5.13; mean length of incorrectly spelled nonwords: 8.22; t=8.22 (62), p<.001). Furthermore, the same type of errors were produced in this task as in the written spelling task; that is, errors consisted of substitution, deletion, insertion and transposition of letters.

Table 3. Spelling errors as a function of stimulus length produced by L.B. in various spelling tests (percentages are in parentheses).

Stimulus length	Writing-to dictation	Oral spelling	Written naming	Copy from a model	Delayed copy
			Words		
4-5	37/242(15.3)	4/16 (25.0)	9/36 (25.0)	2/16(12.6)	2/15 (13.3)
6-7	90/264(34.1)	11/16 (68.7)	14/33 (42.4)	2/29 (6.9)	9/23 (39.1)
8-9	100/150(66.7)	13/16 (81.2)	23/34 (67.6)	1/12 (8.3)	10/21 (47.6)
10/12	78/87 (89.7)	16/16(100)	19/21 (90.5)	---- ----	---- ----
Total	305/743(41.0)	44/64 (68.7)	65/124(52.4)	5/57 (8.8)	21/59 (35.6)
			Nonwords		
4-5	31/113(27.4)	5/16(31.2)	---- ----	0/15 (0)	5/15 (33.3)
6-7	79/155(51.0)	14/16(87.5)	---- ----	1/29 (3.5)	12/24 (50.0)
8-9	64/85 (75.3)	14/16(87.5)	---- ----	1/12 (8.3)	21/21(100)
10/12	74/74(100)	16/16(100)	---- ----	---- ----	---- ----
Total	246/425(57.9)	49/64 (76.6)	---- ----	2/56 (3.6)	38/60 (63.3)

The overall level of performance obtained by our patient on this test must be interpreted very cautiously. It must be stressed that Italian speakers are totally unfamiliar with oral spelling. Oral spelling is not taught in school, and is never practiced in adult life–in fact, L.B. claimed that he had never orally spelled before we asked him to.[3] Thus, the discrepancy in overall level of performance between written and oral spelling should not be given undue importance. The primary value of the oral spelling performance is to rule out the hypothesis that L.B.'s dysgraphia results from selective damage to the Allographic Conversation Mechanism--a mechanism that

converts graphemic representations into specific letter forms for graphomotor output (see Ellis, in press; Goodman & Caramazza, 1986).
Written naming. L.B. was asked to write the names of 124 black-and-white pictures of objects. The target responses covered a wide frequency range, and varied in length from 4 to 12 letters.

The patient responded correctly to 56 stimuli (45.2%). He also produced 3 responses that, although orthographically correct, could be considered as visual-perceptual (i.e., misperception of the picture stimuli) or semantic errors (gallo (rooster) → gallina (chicken); cigno (swan) → oca (duck); ciliegia (cherry) → mela (apple)), and 65 orthographically incorrect responses. All but one of the errors consisted of substitution, insertion, deletion, or transposition of letters in the target response (39 (60%) errors) or combinations of two of these error types (25 (38.5%) errors). The only 'anomalous' error consisted of the written response 'fiscocima,' produced for 'armonica' (harmonica)--presumably a combined semantic/spelling error ('fisarmonica' (accordion)).   Errors were not influenced by frequency, but a highly significant length effect was observed (mean length of correctly written words: 6.13; mean length of incorrectly written words: 8.22; $t = 5.726$ (122), $p < .001$). The distribution of errors as a function of stimulus length is shown in Table 3.

Copying tests. L.B. was asked to copy/transcode from upper to lower case words and nonwords under two conditions: copying with and without the model in view. In both tests, stimuli ranged from 4 to 9 letters in length. Words were drawn from all grammatical classes; half of the words were of high frequency, half were of low frequency. Nonwords were exactly matched in length to words.

(a) Copying from a model. In this experimental condition, L.B. produced the response while freely looking at the stimulus, typed in large characters and left in view.

He made errors on 5/57 (8.8%) words and on 2/56 (3.6%) nonwords.[4] Lexical factors did not influence his performance, and no length effect was observed (words: $t = 0.601$ (55), p = n.s.; nonwords: $t = 0.113$ (55), p = n.s.). All the errors were close approximations to the target response, and always differed from it by one letter.

(b) Delayed copy. The patient was allowed to look at the stimulus for as long as he wished to, until he felt that he could reproduce it. At this point, he removed the stimulus and after 3 seconds had elapsed he would write his response.

L.B. incorrectly wrote 21/59 (35.6%) words and 38/60 (62.3%) nonwords (see Table 3). Neither grammatical class nor frequency affected word spelling performance. However, stimulus length significantly affected performance both for words (mean length of correctly reproduced words: 6.45; mean length of incorrectly reproduced words: 7.14; $t = 1.720$ (57), $p < .05$) and nonwords (mean length of correctly reproduced nonwords: 5.94; mean length of incorrectly reproduced nonwords: 7.30; $t = 4.511$ (58), $p < .001$). All incorrect responses to words were orthographically related to the target, deviating from target responses by the substitution, deletion, addition, or transposition of letters; that is, spelling errors were qualitatively identical to those produced in the dictation and naming tasks.

The overall pattern of results obtained for L.B., in the various spelling tasks, is consistent with the hypothesis of selective damage to the Graphemic Buffer in the proposed model of spelling. The patient's roughly comparable difficulty in oral and written spelling for words and nonwords rules out the hypotheses of selective damage to either the Allographic Conversion Mechanism or the Letter Name Conversion Mechanism; the presence of comparable spelling difficulties in written naming, delayed copy, and spelling to dictation rules out the hypothesis of selective damage to input mechanisms; furthermore, since none of the lexical factors manipulated in the spelling to dictation and copying tasks affected spelling performance, we can infer that the Graphemic Output Lexicon as well as other lexical components are intact in this patient. This configuration of spelling performance together with the fact that both words and nonwords were misspelled, that stimulus length was a major determinant of spelling performance, and that spelling errors were qualitatively identical across tasks and explicable in terms of degradation of graphemic representations, all point to a selective deficit to the Graphemic Buffer.

The one discordant note to the coherent story we have developed concerns the discrepancy in level of spelling performance for words and nonwords: Words were consistently spelled more accurately than nonwords. This difference in level of performance for words and nonwords is not predicted by the hypothesis of a selective deficit to the Graphemic Buffer which, instead, predicts comparable levels of difficulty for the two classes of stimuli. This prediction is motivated by the assumption that the Graphemic Buffer merely stores graphemic representations and, therefore, should be insensitive to lexical factors, including lexicality. Consequently, the consistent and sizeable differences in spelling performance for words and nonwords that have been obtained for L.B. suggest that either this assumption is wrong or that an additional, subtle deficit to some other mechanism is responsible for the patient's relatively poorer performance in spelling nonwords. Unfortunately, however, it has not been possible to obtain evidence to unequivocally distinguish between these two possibilities, although as we shall see shortly the latter possibility is the more likely one.

We should not neglect yet another possibility--that the hypothesis of a selective deficit to the Graphemic Buffer is false. However, the overall pattern of performance obtained for L.B. makes this last possibility quite unlikely, at least for the model of spelling proposed here. We have argued that the reported pattern of performance is most readily explicable by assuming a deficit to a post-lexical, centrally located mechanism that is involved in processing both familiar and novel words. In the model proposed in the Introduction the only mechanism that meets these requirements and is compatible with the obtained pattern of results is the Graphemic Buffer. Thus, if we are to reject the hypothesis of a selective deficit to the Graphemic Buffer we must turn to an alternative functional architecture of the spelling process.

Two alternative functional architectures of the spelling process, both of which reject the assumption that distinct mechanisms are involved in spelling familiar and novel words may be entertained. We have already briefly alluded to one such alternative: The lexical analogy model of spelling (e.g., Campbell, 1983) assumes that a single mechanism is responsible for generating graphemic representations of both familiar and novel words. The other "single-route" model of spelling capitalized on an important feature of Italian orthography; namely, that Italian orthography is highly transparent. That is, sound-to-print mappings in Italian are almost perfectly predictable.[5] This property of Italian orthography suggests the possibility that spelling familiar and novel Italian words may be accomplished by converting phonological representations (both lexical and nonlexical) into graphemic representations through the application of phoneme-grapheme conversion rules (Miceli et al., 1985). Even though there is recent evidence (Caramazza et al., 1986) which disconfirms a strong version of this hypothesis, the possibility remains that because of the transparency of Italian orthography some speakers of the language may rely on the Phoneme-Grapheme Conversion Mechanism in spelling familiar and novel words. For this reason we thought it necessary to attempt to rule out the possibility that L.B.'s spelling difficulties arise from selective damage to either the Phonological Buffer or the Phoneme-Grapheme Conversion Mechanism in this type of 'single-route' model-- mechanisms which if damaged could give rise to the constellation of symptoms thus far reported for out patient. To this end, we administered to L.B. several repetition and spelling tests.

Spelling CV syllables to dictation. In order to rule out damage to the Phoneme-Grapheme Conversion Mechanism, L.B. was asked to spell to dictation 20 meaningless CV syllables. Each stimulus was repeated five times and the whole list of 100 syllables was presented in random order. L.B. performed this test flawlessly. If the Phoneme-Grapheme Conversion Mechanisms were damaged in this patient, he should have produced spelling errors in this task. The results indicate that L.B. has an intact Phoneme-Grapheme Conversion Mechanism.

Spelling words with ambiguous phoneme-grapheme mappings. Although Italian orthography is virtually totally transparent there are a few words in the language that contain ambiguous sound-to-print mappings. For example, the word /kwɔkɔ/ (chef) could be spelled as 'cuoco' or 'quoco' by the application of phoneme-grapheme conversion rules, but only the former spelling is a word in Italian. If L.B. is relying on the Phoneme-Grapheme Conversion Mechanism to spell words, then we expect him to make a significant number of phonologically plausible errors in spelling such words.

L.B. was asked to spell to dictation a list of 80 words; forty words contained ambiguous phoneme-grapheme segments, the other forty words were completely unambiguous. The two sets of words were matched for frequency and length. The patient made 23/40 (57.5%) errors for the ambiguous words and 21/40 (52.5%) errors for the unambiguous words. Only one error for the ambiguous words could be scored as phonologically plausible--he wrote 'squotere' for 'scuotere' (to shake). The remaining errors were qualitatively identical to those he produced for unambiguous words and consisted of substitutions, additions, deletions, and transposition of letters. The performance obtained by L.B. on this task, in terms of proportion of phonologically plausible errors, is comparable to that obtained by 8 matched controls who produced two or three phonologically plausible errors in spelling the ambiguous words. We can conclude, therefore, that L.B. is not using phoneme-grapheme conversion rules to spell words.

Repetition of words and nonwords. In order to evaluate the possibility of damage to the Phonological Buffer the patient was asked to repeat single words and nonwords. Seventy-two stimuli of each type were presented in random order. The stimuli ranged in length from 4 to 12 phonemes. L.B. repeated all words flawlessly and made three errors on nonwords (4.2%). If the spelling difficulties encountered by our patient arose from damage to the Phonological Buffer, we would have expected our patient to present with difficulties in repetition (especially for nonwords) *comparable* to those he presents in spelling (see Caramazza et al., 1986, for discussion on this issue).

Spelling and repetition of words and nonwords. L.B. was asked to spell to dictation a list of words and nonwords ranging in length from 4 to 11 letters. The words and nonwords were intermixed and presented in random order. The patient was instructed to first spell the auditorily presented stimulus and immediately upon completion of that task to repeat the presented stimulus. L.B.'s performance on this task is shown in Table 4. As in previous tasks, the patient produced spelling errors for words and nonwords. A striking effect of stimulus length was again present--longer stimuli being much more difficult to spell than shorter stimuli. The important result here, however, is the marked dissociation between spelling and repetition performance; repetition is essentially intact while spelling is severely impaired. Obviously, L.B.'s spelling difficulty cannot be attributed to an impairment to the Phonological Buffer or other phonological processes since, as revealed by repetition performance, these processes are relatively intact in this patient.

Table 4. Spelling and repetition errors in response to auditorily presented word and nonword stimuli (percentages are in parentheses).

Stimulus length (in letters)	Words		Nonwords	
	Spelling	Repetition	Spelling	Repetition
4-5	1/16 (6.3)	0/16(0)	6/16 (37.5)	0/16 (0)
6-7	10/16 (62.5)	0/16(0)	8/16 (50.0)	2/16 (12.5)
8-9	16/16 (100)	0/16(0)	15/16 (93.8)	5/16 (31.3)
10-11	16/16 (100)	0/16(0)	15/16 (93.8)	4/16 (25.0)
Total	43/64 (67.0)	0/64(0)	44/64 (68.8)	11/64 (17.2)

The results reported in this section of the paper argue against the hypothesis that L.B.'s spelling difficulties are due to a deficit to the Phoneme-Grapheme Conversion Mechanism or to the Phonological Buffer. The repetition results suggest, however, that L.B. has a subtle phonological processing deficit that affects his performance in processing nonwords. The precise nature of this deficit has not been determined but, whatever its source, it is likely to be the basis for the discrepancy in overall error rate in spelling familiar and novel words. Finally, whether or not L.B.'s pattern of performance can be accommodated within a Lexical Analogy Model is not clear; this latter possibility can only be evaluated against a more articulated view of this type of model of the spelling process than is currently available in the literature.

Error analysis

Our analysis of L.B.'s spelling difficulties has focused, thus far, on gross features of performance: We have considered the distribution of errors as a function of stimulus length and type of task. We have argued that the configuration of results obtained is consistent with the hypothesis of damage to the Graphemic Buffer in the proposed model of spelling. A consideration of the type of spelling errors produced by L.B. reinforces this conclusion and provides a data base for speculation about the structure of the Graphemic Buffer. For this purpose we analyzed the total corpus of errors produced by L.B. in the written spelling-to-dictation task. This corpus consists of 305 and 204 errors produced in spelling words and nonwords, respectively.

The functional role assigned to the Graphemic Buffer in the proposed model of spelling is sufficiently explicit to permit predictions about the type and distribution of spelling errors that are expected to result from damage to this processing component. The predictions are primarily qualitative in nature, but not the less important for this. These predictions are evaluated in this section.

A critical prediction concerns the type and distribution of errors that are expected to result for words and nonwords as a consequence of damage to the Graphemic Buffer. The role of the Graphemic Buffer is to store graphemic representations temporarily in preparation for conversion into letter names (oral spelling) or specific letter shapes (written spelling). Representations for words and nonwords are indistinguishable at this level of the cognitive system--they are merely spatially coded strings of graphemic units. Therefore, damage to this processing component should lead to the same type and distribution of errors for the two classes of stimuli. Furthermore, since the form of representations held in the Graphemic Buffer consists of graphemic units, damage to this system should result in degradation of graphemic representations; that is, in substitution, deletion, addition, and transposition of graphemic units. The behavioral manifestation of these degradations of graphemic representations should be the substitution, deletion, addition, and transposition of letters. These expectations were borne out by our analyses of L.B.'s performance in the written spelling to dictation task.

The total corpus of errors, for word and nonword stimuli, produced by L.B. in the written spelling to dictation task were classified into one of the following error categories: substitution, deletion, addition, or transposition of letters. Since each response might contain more than a single error, we distinguished between responses that contained single errors, responses with multiple errors of the same type (e.g., two substitution errors), and mixed errors (i.e., responses containing at least two errors of different type, e.g., a substitution and a deletion error). Some errors could not be classified by this scheme and were scored as unclassifiable. Examples of each of these types of errors are shown in Table 5.

Table 5. Examples of the various error types produced by L.B.

---

(1) Single errors
   Substitutions   giovane (young) → giogane   femasto → famanto
   Insertions   violento (voilent) → violeneto   tenomato → tentomato
   Deletions   semplice (single) → sempice   mansot → masote
   Transpositions recenti (recent) → renceti   serepa → resepa

(2) Multiple errors
   Substitutions   passare (to pass) → rasiare   arguage → arguece
   Insertions   amerai (you will love) → amerirai none
   Deletions   racontare (to tell) → racconae   altiande → atinde
   Transpositions none   none

(3) Mixed errors
   Subst. + Insert. signora (lady) → signiona   esentute → esensunte
   Subst. + Delet. provvedo (I take care of) → povveto ondaso → adaso
   Subst. + Transp. discreto (discreet) → disrteto   imieto → iemeto
   Insert.+ Delet. finestre (windows) → frinetre   none
   Insert.+ Transp. concime (manure) → comicine   none

(4) Unclassifiable errors
              decaduto (decayed) → sedecuto   gotadepo → gattepo
              fradicio (soaking) → friagio   toglieri → terlele

---

The distribution of single, multiple, mixed, and unclassifiable errors for word and nonword stimuli as a function of stimulus length are shown in Table 6. As can readily be seen, only a relatively small proportion of errors could not be classified (7.5% and 16.5% of words and nonwords, respectively).

Two aspects of these data are worth stressing. First, and most important, the distribution of error types for words and nonwords is remarkably similar, not only when we consider overall percentage of each error type but also when we consider the distribution of error types as a function of stimulus length. The striking similarity in distribution of error types for words and nonwords is consistent with the hypothesis that the patient's difficulties in spelling words and nonwords have a common source. The other aspect of these data worth noting is the distribution of Single versus

Mixed and Unclassifiable errors as a function of stimulus length (for both words and nonwords): Single errors predominantly occur for short stimuli; Mixed and Unclassifiable errors mostly occur for long stimuli. This result suggests that the degradation of graphemic representations in our patient are more severe for longer than shorter stimuli, as might be expected if the Graphemic Buffer were damaged.

Table 6. Distribution of Single, Multiple, Mixed and Unclassifiable Errors as a function of stimulus length for words and nonwords (percentages are in parentheses).

Stimulus length	Single	Multiple	Mixed	Unclassifiable	Total
		Words			
4-5	34 (91.9)	---	3 (8.1)	---	37
6-7	54 (60.0)	6 (6.7)	30 (33.3)	---	90
8-9	54 (54.0)	7 (7.0)	31 (31.0)	8 (8.0)	100
10-12	8 (10.3)	15 (19.2)	40 (51.3)	15 (19.2)	78
Total	150 (49.2)	28 (9.2)	104 (34.1)	23 (7.5)	305
		Nonwords			
4-5	27 (87.1)	---	4 (12.9)	---	31
6-7	46 (58.2)	3 (3.8)	22 (27.8)	8 (10.1)	79
8-9	16 (25.0)	11 (17.2)	25 (39.1)	12 (18.7)	64
10-12	2 (2.7)	9 (12.2)	42 (56.8)	21 (28.4)	74
Total	91 (36.7)	23 (9.3)	93 (37.5)	41 (16.5)	248

Table 7. Distribution of substitution, insertion, deletion and transposition errors in writing words and nonwords to dictation (percentages are in parentheses).

	Words	Nonwords
Substitutions	65 (36.5)	41 (36.0)
Insertions	14 (7.9)	10 (8.8)
Deletions	61 (34.3)	42 (36.8)
Transpositions	38 (21.3)	21 (18.4)
Total	178	114

A finer-grained analysis of the distribution of error types for words and nonwords provides even stronger evidence that the spelling difficulties encountered by L.B. for these two classes of stimuli have a common source. For this analysis we considered only Single and Multiple errors, which were combined to make a set of 178 errors for words and a set of 114 errors for nonwords. The distributions of substitution, insertion, deletion, and transposition errors for words and nonwords are shown in

Table 7. The two distributions are virtually identical[6] and remain highly similar even when error types are presented as a function of stimulus length (see Table 8). Worthy of special note in this latter Table is the contrasting pattern of deletion and transposition errors as a function of stimulus length. It is quite clear that deletions increase as a function of stimulus length while transpositions have the opposite pattern. These contrasting patterns, once again, suggest that the degradation of graphemic representations is much greater for longer than shorter stimuli. Thus, for long stimuli, errors frequently take the form of deletions presumable because their graphemic representation is so deformed as to be unusable for guiding the selection of specific letter forms. Contrastively, transposition errors can only occur when the graphemic representation is sufficiently spared to contain information about specific graphemes even if their respective order is not retained. Thus, this latter error type is only likely to occur for short stimuli.[7]

Table 8. Distribution of the various error types as a function of stimulus length (percentages are in parentheses).

Stimulus length	Substitutions	Insertions	Deletions	Transpositions	Total
		Words			
4-5	10 (29.4)	2 (5.9)	2 (5.9)	20 (58.8)	34
6-7	29 (49.1)	3 (3.4)	15 (25.4)	13 (22.0)	60
8-9	22 (36.1)	7 (11.5)	27 (44.3)	5 (8.2)	61
10-12	4 (18.2)	2 (4.5)	17 (77.3)	---	23
Total	65 (36.5)	14 (7.9)	61 (34.3)	38 (21.3)	178
		Nonwords			
4-5	10 (37.0)	5 (18.5)	---	12 (44.4)	27
6-7	19 (38.8)	2 (4.1)	20 (40.8)	8 (16.3)	49
8-9	8 (29.6)	2 (7.4)	16 (59.3)	1 (3.7)	27
10-12	4 (36.4)	1 (9.1)	6 (54.5)	---	11
Total	41 (36.0)	10 (8.8)	42 (36.8)	21 (18.4)	114

Other aspects of the error data are also consistent with the hypothesis of a selective deficit to the Graphemic Buffer. Since the hypothesized deficit is to a post-lexical mechanism, we do not expect errors to be sensitive to lexical dimensions such as grammatical class, for example. This is indeed the case as already noted. Furthermore, however, neither do we expect errors to result in word responses (e.g., producing 'chair' for 'chain' or 'chair' for 'table,' or 'chairs' for 'chair,' respectively visual/phonological, semantic, and morphological errors). L.B. produced only one response (1/305) that could be construed as a morphological error--he spelled 'gioco' (I play) for 'gioca' (he plays)--and no semantic errors. He did produce a few word errors both in response to word (16/305 (5.7%)) and nonword (12/248 (4.8%)) stimuli. The distribution of these errors for words and nonwords as a function of stimulus length is shown in Table 9. We note that the very few errors produced are more likely to occur for shorter than longer stimuli and that most (20/28) of these error responses differed from target responses by only one letter. These observations suggest that word errors were most likely chance occurrences that resulted when a letter substitution error occurred, and not lexically induced errors.

Table 9. Incidence of incorrect word responses as a function of stimulus length for word and non-word stimuli (percentages are in parentheses).

Stimulus length	Words	Nonwords
4-5	6/37 (16.2)	3/31 (9.7)
6-7	8/90 (8.9)	7/79 (8.9)
8-9	2/100 (2.0)	2/64 (3.1)
10-12	0/78 (0)	0/74 (0)
Total	16/305 (5.7)	12/248 (4.8)

Finally, if the spelling errors produced by L.B. reflect degradation of graphemic representations that result from damage to the Graphemic Buffer, we expect that a fair number of these errors should result in violations of orthographic constraints of Italian (e.g., tempo → tempto*; ultimo → utmilmo*). In the total corpus of errors under consideration, 57 of the errors (10.3%) contained at least one violation of Italian orthography. The distribution of errors containing violations of orthographic rules for word and nonword stimuli is shown in Table 10. The occurrence of violations of orthographic rules can be taken as further support for the hypothesis that L.B.'s spelling deficit results from damage to the Graphemic Buffer.[8]

Table 10. Incidence of incorrect responses containing violations of orthographic rules (percentages are in parentheses).

Stimulus length	Words	Nonwords
4-5	3/34 (8.8)	5/31 (16.1)
6-7	7/90 (7.8)	6/79 (7.6)
8-9	14/100 (14.0)	4/64 (6.2)
10-12	7/78 (9.0)	12/74 (16.2)
Total	31/305 (10.2)	27/248 (10.9)

The analyses of the type and distribution of errors we have undertaken thus far have focused on two factors: lexicality (word vs. nonword) and stimulus length. There is, however, another stimulus dimension that has been proposed as being relevant to considerations of the processing structure of the Graphemic Buffer--letter position within a word (or nonword). Wing and Baddeley (1980) have suggested that a source of spelling errors, at least for normal spellers, involves 'read-out' failure from the Graphemic Buffer. Specifically, they have proposed that 'read-out' errors from the Graphemic Buffer are more likely to occur for the medial positions of a word than for the flanking positions (both initial and final). The primary impetus for this proposal was the observation that 'slips of the pen' occur more frequently for medial than flanking positions. Unfortunately, however, the proposal of a 'read-out' failure from the Graphemic Buffer is not computationally motivated but is derived instead by analogy to read-out limitations from a visual array in perceptual recognition experiments. That is, it is not obvious what computational characteristic of the Graphemic Buffer might serve to motivate the speculation that medial positions of the graphemic representations stored in this system should be relatively inaccessible. Nonetheless, this intuitively derived property of the Graphemic Buffer can be subjected to test by considering the positional distribution of errors produced by out patient.

The reasoning underlying our contention that L.B.'s spelling performance can serve as a test of the proposal that 'read-out' from the Graphemic Buffer is relatively less accurate from medial than flanking positions is based on two assumptions: that the patient has a selective deficit to the Graphemic Buffer and that this deficit takes the form of a reduction in capacity or processing efficiency of the Graphemic Buffer. If these assumptions are correct and the proposal of relatively inefficient 'read-out' from the graphemic Buffer for medial positions of a graphemic representations is true, then L.B. should present with a higher incidence of errors for medial than flanking positions for words and nonwords. This complex hypothesis was evaluated by analyzing the distribution of 'single' errors produced by L.B. in the written spelling-to-dictation task.

Since stimuli varied in length we used a procedure proposed by Wing and Baddeley to 'normalize' the distribution of errors across all stimulus length. That is, we collapsed performance for stimuli of different lengths into a single, arbitrary stimulus length. In this procedure, each stimulus is divided into five letter 'positions' (four-letter stimuli were excluded from analysis). Each 'position' contains one or more letters, depending on the number of letters that, for each stimulus, exceed 5 or multiples of 5. The letters in excess are distributed across the 5 'positions' so as to maintain a symmetrical structure in the arbitrarily reconstructed stimulus. Table 11 shows the number of letters assigned to each 'position' for stimuli of various lengths. Using this procedure we were able to include in the analysis 207 word and 146 nonword errors.

Table 11. Number of letters assigned to each stimulus position for the analysis of letter position effect.

Stimulus length	A	B	C	D	E
5	1	2	3	4	5
6	1	2	3-4	5	6
7	1	2-3	4	5-6	7
8	1-2	3	4-5	6	7-8
9	1-2	3-4	5	6-7	8-9
10	1-2	3-4	5-6	7-8	9-10
11	1-2	3-4	5-6-7	8-9	10-11
12	1-2	3-4-5	6-7	8-9-10	11-12

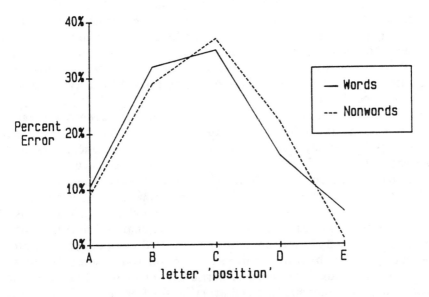

Figure 2. Distribution of errors as a function of letter 'position' in a letter string.

The distribution of errors for words and nonwords as a function of letter 'position' in a stimulus is depicted in Figure 2. The results are striking in two regards: First, the two distributions of errors are virtually identical; and, second, the bow-shaped function predicted on the basis of Wing and Baddeley's proposal about the 'read-out' limitation from the Graphemic Buffer is clearly supported. Thus, it would appear that a property of the Graphemic Buffer is that information from this system is not homogeneously accessible but, instead, medially located graphemes are 'read-out' less efficiently than flanking graphemes.

CONCLUSION

The pattern of results we have reported allows us to determine the locus of damage to the proposed functional architecture of the spelling system. The virtually identical distribution of errors for words and nonwords implies that damage to a single mechanism is responsible for L.B.'s spelling difficulties for the two classes of stimuli. Furthermore, since we were able to rule out deficits to shared input or output mechanisms as the locus of damage, and since the types of errors produced are most reasonably explicated by reference to the degradation of graphemic representations, we must locate the source of damage to the Graphemic Buffer. Consequently, we are justified in considering the results of this analysis as support for the proposed model of spelling: We assume that a pattern of impaired performance constitutes evidence in support of a model of a cognitive system (over alternative formulations) if it is possible to explain the observed pattern of impairment by hypothesizing a functional lesion(s) to the proposed model.

The degree of confidence we have in a model depends on various factors. A critical one is the extent to which the model allows us to make sense of progressively finer details of relevant performance, presumable because it becomes increasingly more difficult to construct alternative explanations for richly articulated sets of observations. To state this point differently, the degree of detail of performance we are able to account for depends on the richness of detail of our theories of cognitive systems. If we are content to remain at the level of functional architecture without specifying the algorithmic content of postulated components of a model we must be content with explanations of relatively gross features of performance. Thus, for example, a particular model may allow predictions about whether or not spelling performance for familiar and novel words may dissociate, but remain completely silent about the particular types of spelling errors that are expected when the predicted dissociation obtains. In such a case the existence of two patients, both of whom present with a specific dissociation but a different pattern of error types, would be uninformative with respect to such a model. In order to make sense of this latter set of observations the model must be articulated in greater detail, perhaps at the level of specifying the algorithmic content of hypothesized components of the model. It is obvious that this effort may fail, and, thereby, undermine our confidence in the model. Thus, concern for the details of performance is not a luxury we can afford to do without.

What are the implications of this argument for the case under consideration? Under ideal conditions we would have been able to articulate in some detail the computational structure of the Graphemic Buffer. This would have allowed a theoretically motivated account of the relevant details of our patient's performance--that is, we would have been able to make explicit links between such features of the patient's performance and the distribution of error types (e.g., substitution errors) and processing features of the Graphemic Buffer. Unfortunately, as we have noted, we are far from being able to do so. Instead we relied on an intuitive characterization of the processing structure of the Graphemic Buffer to guide our analysis of the patient's performance. In this regard, we exploited the notion of graphemic degradation, a vague one to be sure, to predict the qualitative nature of the expected error types in the case where the Graphemic Buffer is selectively damaged. Thus, although our account of the algorithmic content of the Graphemic Buffer remains unpleasantly underspecified, we have, nonetheless, provided a general framework within which to begin serious discussion of the structure of this component of the spelling system

We also provided support for an empirical generalization about a feature of the processing structure of the Graphemic Buffer which does not, at this time, have an explicit theoretical justification. Wing and Baddeley (1980) have proposed that a property of the Graphemic Buffer is that it has a 'read-out' procedure which is characterized by nonhomogeneous accessibility of the graphemic string stored in the system. Specifically, they suggested that there is interference between adjacent graphemic units in the Buffer and that, therefore, the medial graphemes in a string will be relatively inaccessible. No clear theoretical justification is provided for this claim. Nonetheless, they report 'slips of the pen' data which are characterized by a bow-shaped function, with a higher incidence of errors in the medial positions. We evaluated the hypothesis of nonhomogeneous accessibility of graphemes form the Graphemic Buffer through an analysis of the effect of letter position on the distribution of errors produced by L.B. We obtained clear evidence in support of the stated hypothesis. In other words, we have provided evidence which empirically, though not yet theoretically, links the bow-shaped function of errors for letter positions in a word to some processing aspect of the Graphemic Buffer.

To conclude, the analysis of L.B.'s spelling performance has provided support for the functional architecture of the spelling system proposed in the Introduction of this paper. Equally, if not more importantly, we have provided evidence in support of some intuitively and empirically driven hypotheses about the computational structure of the Graphemic Buffer.

ACKNOWLEDGEMENTS

The research reported in this paper was supported by NIH grant NS22201 to The Johns Hopkins University and by a grant from the CNR, Italy. We would like to thank Bill Badecker, Roberta Goodman, Brenda Martin, Tim Shallice and an anonymous referee for their comments on an earlier version of this paper. We also thank Kathy Sporney for her assistance in the preparation of this manuscript.

REFERENCES

Baxter, D. M. & Warrington, E. K. (in press). Ideational agraphia: A single case study. Journal of Neurology, Neurosurgery & Psychiatry.

Beauvois, M. F. & Dérouesné, J. (1981). Lexical or orthographic agraphia. Brain, 104, 21–49.

Campbell, R. (1983). Writing nonwords to dictation. Brain and Language, 19, 153–178.

Caramazza, A., Miceli, G., Silveri, M. C. & Laudanna, A. (1985). Reading mechanisms and the organization of the lexicon: Evidence from acquired dyslexia. Cognitive Neuropsychology, 2, 81–114.

Caramazza, A., Miceli, G. & Villa, G. (1986). The role of the (output) phonological buffer in reading, writing, and repetition. Cognitive Neuropsychology, 3(1), 37–76.

Ellis, A. W. (1982). Spelling and writing (and reading and speaking). In A. W. Ellis (Ed.), Normality and pathology in cognitive functions. London: Academic Press.

Ellis, A. W. (in press). Modeling the writing process. In G. Denes, C. Semenza, P. Bisiacchi & E. Andreewsky (Eds.), Perspectives in cognitive neuropsychology. London: Lawrence Erlbaum.

Goodman, R. A. & Caramazza, A. (1986). Dissociation of spelling errors in written and oral spelling: The role of allographic conversion in writing. Cognitive Neuropsychology, 3, 179–206.

Hatfield, M. & Patterson, K. E. (1983). Phonological spelling. Quarterly Journal of Experimental Psychology, 35, 451–468.

Kinsbourne, M. & Rosenfield, D. B. (1974). Agraphia selective for written spelling. Brain and Language, 1, 215-225.

Margolin, D. I. (1984). The neuropsychology of writing and spelling: Semantic, phonological, motor and perceptual processes. Quarterly Journal of Experimental Psychology, 316(A), 459-489.

Miceli, G., Silveri, M. C. & Caramazza, A. (1985). Cognitive analysis of a case of pure dysgraphia. Brain and Language, 25, 187-196.

Nolan, K. A. & Caramazza, A. (1983). An analysis of writing in a case of deep dyslexia. Brain and Language, 20, 305-328.

Patterson, K. E. (in press). Acquired disorders of spelling. In G. Denes, C. Semenza, P. Bisiacchi & E. Andreewsky (Eds.), Perspectives in cognitive neuropsychology. London: Lawrence Erlbaum.

Shallice, T. (1981). Phonological agraphia and the lexical route in writing. Brain, 104, 413-429.

Wing, A. M. & Baddeley, A. D. (1980). Spelling errors in handwriting: A corpus and a distributional analysis. In U. Frith (Ed.), Cognitive processes in spelling. London: Academic Press.

NOTES

[1] We wish to note that the absolute level of performance across tasks is not easily interpretable for two reasons. First, because we did not use the same stimuli across different tasks and, therefore, we cannot make quantitative predictions about absolute levels of performance. Second, because there could be subtle deficits to cognitive mechanisms required for the normal execution of one task that are not implicated in other tasks (e.g., written naming involves perceptual and cognitive mechanisms needed for processing pictures which are not involved in spelling-to-dictation). In this latter case, too, absolute levels of performance cannot be predicted. Hence the emphasis in this report is on qualitative and grossly quantitative features of performance.

[2] Arbitrarily setting a word length of 4.5 letters as unity and scaling the probability of an error on a word by the discrepancy of word length from unity

$$\frac{\text{probability of an error} \times 4.5}{\text{word length}},$$

we obtained new (scaled) error probabilities for words and nonwords of different lengths. These are: 15.3%, 23.6%, 35.3%, and 36.7% for words of 4-5, 6-7, 8-9, and 10-12 letters long, respectively, and 27.4%, 35.3%, 39.4%, and 40.9% for nonwords of 4-5, 6-7, 8-9, and 10-12 letter long respectively. As is quite apparent, more errors were made for longer words even when correcting for the number of letters in a word.

[3] Italian has a highly transparent orthography which renders oral spelling unnecessary as a teaching strategy. Indeed, the translation of "spelling" into Italian is "scrivere" which means *written* spelling. For this reason, we even had difficulty finding words to describe the oral spelling task to our patient. We had to use words such as "scandire" (to parse) and locutions such as "dire a voce le lettere che compongono la parola" (say aloud the letters that comprise a word) to communicate the task requirements.

[4] This seemingly paradoxical result--more accurate performance (though not statistically so, $X^2 = 1.36$, $p < .30$) with nonwords than words in copying from a model--can be readily explained if one considers the constellation of symptoms shown by L.B. The patient has a reading deficit that impairs his ability to read nonwords, but spares his ability to read words. (Caramazza et al., 1985). This deficit led the patient to use different strategies when copying words and nonwords. When copying a nonword stimulus, L.B. read it repeatedly and tended to reproduce it letter by letter, frequently checking his production with the printed stimulus; by contrast, in copying a word he would read it without effort and reproduced it quickly and confidently without checking his spelling response against the target stimulus. This difference in the strategies used to perform the copying task may account for the counterintuitive result obtained for this task.

[5] The regularity of print-to-sound mappings in Italian is almost perfect. There are, however, a few words in the language that contain phonologically ambiguous segments and, therefore, their correct spelling cannot simply be determined by phoneme-grapheme conversion rules. For example, the correct spelling of the phoneme /k/ in the stimulus /kwɔcɔ/ (cuoco = cook) and in the stimulus /kwɔtə/ (quota = share or quote) is lexically determined, as is the spelling of the segment /č/ in /nɔče/ (walnut) and /speče/ (species)--compare *c*uoco vs. *q*uota, and no*c*e vs. spe*c*ie. However, in Italian there are no truly unpredictable spellings, such as /jɑt/ 'yacht' in English.

[6] The hypothesis being evaluated here predicts a similar pattern of error distribution for words and nonwords in the oral spelling task. We did not have a large enough corpus of errors on this task for detailed analysis due in part to the fact that oral spelling is a strange task in Italian and our patient was unwilling to be tested extensively on this task. Nonetheless, even with the limited data at our disposal the distribution of errors for words and nonwords in consistent with theoretical expectations. The distribution of errors for words and nonwords was as follows: Words--5 (27.8%) substitutions, 1 (5.5%) insertions, 9 (50.0%) deletions, 3 (16.7%)

transpositions; Nonwords--7 (24.6%) substitutions, 0 insertions, 18 (69.2%) deletions, 1 (7.2%) transpositions.

[7] Tim Shallice has drawn our attention to the fact that if we wish to maintain that the reason for the higher level of errors for nonwords results from an additional deficit to the processing mechanisms involved in processing nonwords, then we should not expect to have such a close correspondence in the distribution of error types for words and nonwords. If this observation is correct, we are forced to reconsider the assumption that the Graphemic Buffer is insensitive to lexicality. However, we remain unclear as to how lexicality exerts its effects at the level of the Graphemic Buffer.

[8] It should be noted that although violations of orthographic rules are not a common feature of 'slips of the pen' this does not mean that normal 'slips of the pen' (in some cases) reflect processing errors at the level of the Graphemic Buffer. The errors produced by our patient occur in the context of a severe limitation of processing capacity of the Graphemic Buffer presumably resulting in a grossly degraded graphemic representation while for normal spellers the graphemic representation is, by definition, unimpaired.

CHAPTER NINE

ORTHOGRAPHIC STRUCTURE, THE GRAPHEMIC BUFFER
AND THE SPELLING PROCESS

The notion of representation plays a fundamental role in information processing theories of the functioning of the brain. Theories of this type attempt to characterize cognitive abilities in terms of the sorts of representations that are computed in the course of intelligent behavior (e.g., reading). The flow of information through the cognitive system may be represented as $I \rightarrow R1 \rightarrow R2 \rightarrow R3 ... \rightarrow Rn \rightarrow O$, where I and O stand for input and output, respectively, R stands for representation, and '$\rightarrow$' stands for some type of process that transforms Ri into Ri+1 (or, alternatively, computes Ri+1 from Ri). The core claim in this theoretical framework is that a cognitive process may be thought of as a set of operations carried out over different types of representations. Nontrivial theoretical claims in this framework require that we specify in some detail the structure of the hypothesized representations and the nature of the operations that are applied to these representations in the course of processing.

The task of developing reasonably well-articulated theories of cognitive processing has proven to be very difficult. Most information processing models of cognitive tasks go no further than the mere identification of the several levels of representation suggested by a "common sense" analysis of those tasks. This is no less (nor more) true for models of spelling than it is for models of other cognitive processes. Thus, models of spelling typically, though not always, assume a cognitive architecture roughly as that shown in Figure 1, but do not provide any more information about the nature of the hypothesized processes and representations than that which is suggested by the flow diagram itself. For example, there is no more detailed theory about the structure of the orthographic lexicon than the nominal fact that the information processed at that level of the system consists of orthographic representations.

Still, if a measure of a model's adequacy were the success it has when used as the basis for making sense of the various forms of cognitive disorders that result from brain-damage, then the model of spelling schematically depicted in Figure 1 should be considered a reasonable first approximation of the cognitive mechanisms involved in spelling. This model provides an adequate explanatory framework for the various types of acquired dysgraphias, so long as we restrict attention to relatively general features of patients' performance--e.g., presence or not of semantic errors (writing 'chair' in response to the stimulus /teybl/), whether or not spelling errors consist principally of phonologically plausible responses (writing 'taybel'in response to the stimulus /teybl/), and so forth. The various patterns of dissociation and association of symptoms in dysgraphic patients can adequately be explained as resulting from damage to one or more of the components of processing that comprise the proposed model of spelling. For example, patients have been described whose performance can be explained as reflecting selective damage to the orthographic output lexicon, the phoneme-to-grapheme conversion component, the semantic component, the allographic conversion component, the phonological buffer, or the graphemic buffer.

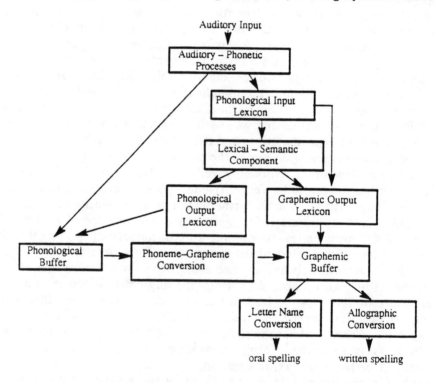

Figure 1. Schematic diagram of the spelling process.

Although the model's success in accounting for relatively gross features of dysgraphic disorders constitutes strong support for the overall architecture of the model, it remains woefully underspecified, especially with regard to the processing structure of its component parts. Whatever the reason for this situation, it is not for lack of relevant empirical observations. Indeed, as we hope to show for at least one component of the spelling system, the detailed analysis of dysgraphic patients' performance allows us to articulate considerably stronger claims about the structure of orthographic representations than are made by current information processing models of the spelling process.

In this paper we will address two interrelated issues. First, we will briefly review recent research which shows that the graphemic buffer may be damaged selectively. Second, we will show that a detailed consideration of the spelling errors produced by a patient with apparently selective damage to the graphemic buffer reveals important properties of the lexical-orthographic representations that are temporarily held in the graphemic buffer.

THE GRAPHEMIC BUFFER AND ITS SELECTIVE IMPAIRMENT

The motivation for proposing the existence of a buffer in an information processing system is relatively straightforward: storage in a temporary memory is postulated at that point in the flow of information where a representation contains sub-units that must be processed sequentially (or, alternatively, where a set of independent representations must be processed simultaneously). In the spelling process a graphemic buffer is postulated because the graphemic representations activated in the orthographic lexicon as well those computed by the phoneme/grapheme conversion component consist of sets of graphemes (abstract letter representations) which must be processed sequentially for conversion into specific visuo-spatial patterns for written spelling, or into letter names for oral spelling. The graphemic buffer occupies a central position in the spelling process (see Figure 1): it mediates between the processes that compute graphemic representations (the orthographic lexicon and the phoneme/grapheme conversion component) and more peripheral output processes (letter name and allographic conversion component). Selective damage to the graphemic buffer should have widespread but clearly identifiable consequences for spelling.

The strategic location of the graphemic buffer in the spelling process and the fact that the buffer stores graphemic representations severely constrain the type of errors that may be expected to result from damage to this component of the spelling system. Damage to the graphemic buffer should result in the following pattern of performance: 1) there should be errors in all spelling tasks, independently of modality of input (e.g., spelling-to-dictation vs. written naming) or modality of output (written vs. oral spelling); 2) spelling performance should not be affected by lexical factors (e.g., grammatical class, word frequency, etc.) or lexicality (familiar vs. unfamiliar words/nonwords) since the damage is at a point beyond which these factors play a role in processing; 3) errors should only reflect properties of the representation that is affected by the damage: graphemic structure; 4) errors should be qualitatively (and quantitatively?) similar for familiar and unfamiliar words; and, finally, 5) there should be a marked effect of word length on performance--longer words being more difficult to spell than shorter words.

This richly articulated pattern of performance was first clearly documented by Caramazza et al. (1987; but, see also Hillis & Caramazza, in press; Miceli et al., 1985; Posteraro et al., in press). Their patient L.B. made spelling errors in all tasks, independently of modality of input or output; his errors were exclusively transparent deformations of the graphemic structure of the stimulus and were unaffected by lexical factors; he showed a healthy word length effect, being able to spell correctly all two-letter stimuli but only 30% of 8/9-letter words; and, the pattern of errors for word and nonword stimuli (operationally standing in for unfamiliar words) was essentially identical. To better appreciate the strength of the results, it may be useful to present some of them here.

L.B.'s errors consisted almost entirely of letter substitutions (svolta → svonta), additions (taglio → tatglio), deletions (nostro → nosro), and transpositions (stadio → sdatio). This fact is in itself already quite important since dysgraphic errors may take distinctly different forms: some patients make semantic or other lexical errors, some make phonological errors, while others make various combinations of these error types. In other words, the exclusively orthographic nature of the error types in L.B.'s performance indicates that the locus of impairment in the spelling system is at a level where graphemic structure is represented. An equally striking feature of L.B.'s performance is the distribution of error types for words and nonwords: the proportion of substitution, deletion, addition, and transposition errors were identical for words and nonwords (see Figure 2). The distribution of errors as a function of relative position of letters in words and nonwords was also identical for the two types of stimuli (see Figure 3).

These results, showing that the representation type affected by the damage is graphemic in nature and that familiar and unfamiliar words are affected identically by the damage, together with the other results showing a marked length effect and impaired performance independently of modality of input or output, strongly invite the conclusion that L.B. has a selective "functional lesion" to the graphemic buffer. Since L.B.'s spelling performance is explicable by hypothesizing a specific transformation of (functional lesion to) the proposed model of spelling, we may take the reported results as support for this model. We are reinforced in this conclusion by the observation that the model of spelling proposed here can also account for other well-documented patterns of dysgraphia by assuming damage to other parts of the system. In other words, our confidence in the "correctness" (or usefulness) of a model does not depend only on whether it can serve to explain a specific form of impairment but, crucially, on whether it can account for the diverse patterns of deficits found in different patients.

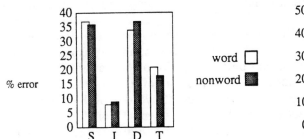

Figure 2. Distribution of substitution (S), insertion (I), deletion (D), and transposition (T) errors for words and nonwords.

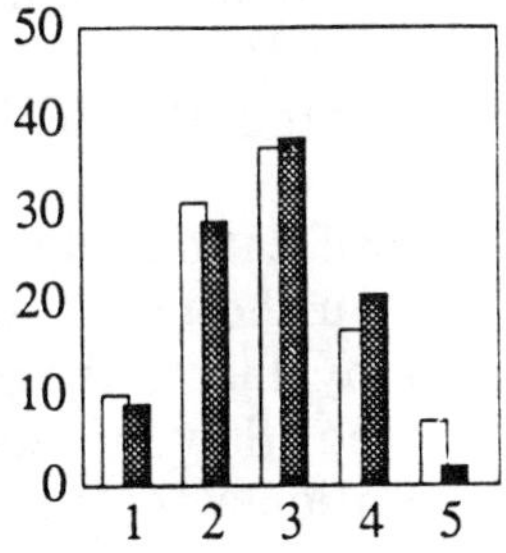

Figure 3. Distribution of errors for words and non-words as a function of relative position in letter string.

Still, if we want the component processes that comprise the model of spelling proposed here to be more than the maligned "black boxes" of the critics of the information processing paradigm, we will have to articulate in greater detail the nature of the processes and representations that characterize the components of the system. We can be helped in this difficult task by attempting to explain not only relatively general features of patients' performance, but also increasingly finer details of their performance. In this latter task, we will have no choice but to articulate ever more detailed hypotheses about the nature of cognitive representations and the processes that support them. An example of such a development is provided by our effort to explain certain features of the spelling performance of patients with putative damage to the graphemic buffer.

THE STRUCTURE OF GRAPHEMIC REPRESENTATIONS

Let us suppose that the analysis presented for L.B. is correct; that is, let us suppose that he has suffered selective damage to the graphemic buffer. On this hypothesis, we may take the distribution of spelling errors produced by L.B. to reflect properties of (only?) the abstract letter sequences that are temporarily held in the graphemic buffer. Consequently, if we can explain the distribution of spelling errors produced by L.B. by appeal to damage-induced perturbations of hypothesized structural properties of graphemic representations, we will have provided empirical support for the hypothesized structural properties; that is, we will have provided empirical support for some hypothesis about the nature of the graphemic representations computed in the course of spelling.

Recall that L.B.'s spelling errors could be exhaustively described in terms of letter substitutions, deletions, additions, and transpositions--an error classification scheme that only appeals to orthographic features of words. Furthermore, since the distribution of these errors was only affected by the "orthographic" parameter of word length and by the relative position of letters in words, we may conclude that the representation affected by the deficit concerns an ordered set of abstract letter representations.

If graphemic representations were assumed to specify only the identity and the order of letters that comprise a word, then the only variation in the distribution of errors resulting from damage to graphemic representations should concern these two parameters--letter identity and order. That is, damage to the graphemic representation should result either in the loss of letter identity or order information, or both. On this view, and without additional constraints, we would predict that damage to the graphemic representation should result in errors such as those we have reported for L.B.--letter substitutions, deletions, additions, and transpositions. Furthermore, on this impoverished view of graphemic representations we would also expect, for example, that errors should just as likely result in the substitution of consonants for vowels or vowels for consonants as to result in the substitution of vowels for vowels or consonants for consonants. Thus, we should not only find errors such as 'tavolo' (table) → 'tasolo' or 'tavelo' but also errors such as 'tavolo'→ 'tavslo' or 'taeolo. This expectation is based on the fact that the conception of graphemic representation developed to this point fails to distinguish between consonants and vowels--the only information specified is individual letter identities and their order. However, as it turns out, L.B. (but also other patients with putative damage to the graphemic buffer) appears not to substitute consonants for vowels or vowels for consonants. In fact, upon close scrutiny his performance reveals a rich set of orthographic constraints on the distribution of spelling errors.

In the course of preparing an earlier report of L.B.'s spelling impairment (Caramazza, et al., 1987), we had noted several apparently inexplicable features in his performance. The most obvious was a remarkable consistency in substitution errors: consonants were substituted for consonants and vowels were substituted for vowels. Other features discordant with our simple view about the structure of graphemic representations were the fact that transposition errors appeared to involve exclusively either consonants or vowels (e.g., 'tavolo' → 'talovo') and that there appeared to be disproportionately fewer errors on double-consonant (geminate) words (e.g., canna (cane)) than words of the same length but without double letters (e.g., canta (sing)). None of these features in L.B.'s performance was consistent with the view that the representations held in the graphemic buffer specified only letter identities and their order. We decided to explore this issue in greater detail.

To obtain a reliable corpus of errors we asked L.B. to spell several thousand words (>4000) over a period of several months. Here we will focus on just a few aspects of the results, enough to motivate the claim that graphemic representations share many structural properties with phonological representations (a detailed discussion of the results is available in Caramazza & Miceli, in preparation). Specifically, our data strongly suggest that graphemic representations, just like phonological representations (see for example, Clements & Keyser, 1983), should be considered as linked, tiered structures: one tier each for abstract letter identities or graphemes, consonant/vowel (CV) structure, and ortho-syllabic structure, respectively.

THE CV LEVEL OF REPRESENTATION

There are several aspects of L.B.'s performance which would remain inexplicable unless we assume that graphemic representations specify an autonomous level for CV structure.

1. *Substitution errors.* One important source of evidence concerns the distribution of substitution errors. L.B. made 643 substitutions, 276 involving vowels and 367 involving consonants. Essentially all substitutions respected CV structure--in 640 of the 643 errors (99.5%), consonants were substituted for consonants and vowels for vowels. To explain this pattern of performance we must assume that L.B. had access to information about CV structure even when information about a specific abstract letter identity was unavailable. With this assumption, we would then be able to explain substitution errors as 'repairs'[2] of representations in which the CV tier correctly specifies the CV structure, but the letter identity tier fails to specify one or more of the graphemes in the representation. Thus, for example, if the damaged representation of

'tavolo' failed to specify the identity of the third letter but correctly specified that it is a consonant, subsequent components of processing (letter name or allographic conversion) could use the CV level information to produce a consonant: the 'repair' is constrained by CV level information.[1] A schematic representation of this process is shown in Figure 4. Were we not to assume an autonomous CV level of representation, the striking regularity in L.B.'s substitution errors would remain unexplained.

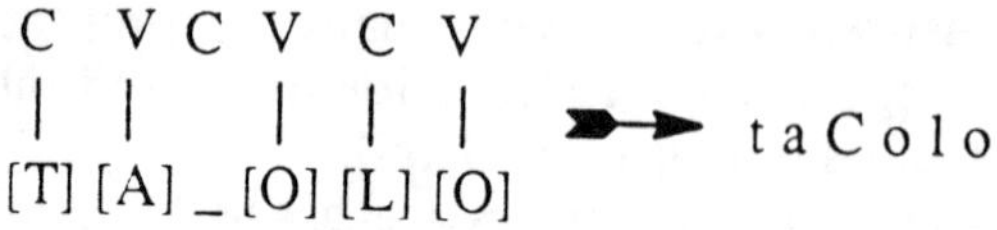

$$C \quad V \; C \quad V \; C \quad V$$
$$| \quad | \quad | \quad | \quad | \qquad \blacktriangleright\!\!\rightarrow \quad t\,a\,C\,o\,l\,o$$
$$[T]\,[A]\,\_\,[O]\,[L]\,[O]$$

Figure 4. In this figure the substitution of a consonant, C, in the third letter position is driven by information at the CV tier.

2. *Transposition errors.* Another aspect of L.B.'s performance which strongly argues for a multidimensional graphemic structure that includes a CV level of representation is the distribution of transposition errors. These errors also appear to be influenced by CV structure. Restricting attention, for the moment, to the subset of stimuli with regularly alternating CV structure (e.g., tavolo, cugino (cousin), etc., but not sedia (chair)), L.B. made 75 transposition errors in spelling these words. All the errors involved exchanging consonants for consonants (e.g., denaro → derano) or vowels for vowels (e.g., decine → dicene). As in the case of letter substitutions, this constraint on the distribution of errors can only be explained by assuming that CV structure is specified autonomously. With this assumption, if the letter identity level failed to specify correctly the order of some letters, the 'repair' resulting from subsequent processes would have available the CV structure information to order the letter identities. Thus, for example, if the graphemic representation for the word 'tavolo' were damaged so that the letter identities [T], [V], [L], [A], [O], and [O] were correctly specified, but the only order information available was that the first two positions were occupied by [T] and [A], then the possible 'repairs' that could result given information about CV structure are the correct response 'tavolo' and the transposition error 'talovo.'

3. *Double-letter word errors.* There is approximately a 20% difference between L.B.'s spelling accuracy for double-letter words (78%; 114/146) and non double-letter words (57%; 579/1024). To explain this difference

in spelling accuracy, as well as qualitative features of spelling errors for double-letter words, we may have to assume that CV structure is represented autonomously in the graphemic representation.

With respect to the quantitative difference in performance, a possible explanation is that letter identity information for double letters is specified only once. Letter doubling would then be represented by associating the single letter identity with two positions at the CV level. In this representational format there are fewer letter identities represented for double-letter words than comparable non double-letter words; for example, the respective representations for stella and stanco are:

As is apparent, the representation for stella specifies only 5 letter identities ([S], [T], [E], [L], and [A]), whereas stanco specifies 6 letter identities ([S], [T], [A], [N], [C], and [O]). And, since L.B.'s performance is strongly influenced by the parameter of word length, we may attribute the discrepancy in levels of spelling accuracy for the two types of words to the number of letter identities that are specified in their respective graphemic representations--5 vs. 6 graphemes. If, however, we are going to explain the discrepancy in performance for these two types of stimuli by appealing to differences in the size of their corresponding abstract letter representations in the buffer, we will then have to assume that the doubling of the letter is indicated by specifying two CV units or timing slots at the CV level--that is, we would be committed to the hypothesis that graphemic representations contain an autonomous CV level.

Qualitative aspects of error performance with double-letter words also generally support the proposed representational format. Although not exceptionless, transposition errors involving double letters behaved just like transposition errors with single letter exchanges; that is, consonants were exchanged with consonants. For example, we found errors such as crollo (crumble) → clorro and scappa (run away) → sacca. This type of error suggests that information about letter identities has been damaged independently of information about the CV structure of the word, which for this patient appears to be relatively spared. Consistent with this interpretation is the fact that in this corpus of errors we did not find errors such as crollo → crrolo, where the letter identities remain in their relative word position and the doubling occurs at some other part of the word. The occurrence of this latter type of error would have required, contrary to what seems to be the case for L.B., that information about the

CV structure of the word was damaged while information about letter identities and their order was spared.

THE ORTHO-SYLLABIC LEVEL OF REPRESENTATION

The results we very briefly reviewed in this last section focused on features of L.B.'s performance which show that separate CV and letter identity tiers are needed in order to account for some aspects of the distribution of errors in his spelling performance. Other aspects of L.B.'s performance, as we will see below, show that a theory of graphemic representation that specifies only CV and letter identity tiers leaves unexplained a substantial part of his performance. A further level of representation--the ortho-syllabic tier, which specifies the syllabic organization of the graphemes that comprise a word--must be added to the graphemic representation in order to account for these other aspects of L.B.'s performance. Several aspects of L.B.'s performance are relevant to this issue. Here we discuss just one source of evidence for the hypothesis (see Caramazza & Miceli, in preparation, for detailed description).

The distribution of errors as a function of the orthographic structure of words
L.B. was asked to spell two sets of 6-letter words: one set consisted of regularly alternating CV sequences (e.g., tavolo), "regular CV" for short, and the other set consisted of various other orderings of CV sequences (e.g., intero, stanco, nostro, onesto, and so forth), "nonregular CV" for short. On the assumption that a graphemic buffer deficit results in the underspecification of graphemic representations, in our patient affecting primarily but not exclusively the letter identity tier, and on the further assumption that the only structure specified at the graphemic level is CV and letter identity information, we would expect spelling performance to be unaffected by the syllabic structure of a word. That is, we would not expect the syllabic structure of a word, whether it is "regular" or "nonregular," to affect either the overall level of spelling accuracy or the distribution of error types. For both types of CV strings, the 'repair' of underspecified letter identity information would proceed under the control of the CV tier information leading, where this information is available, to the replacement of consonants for consonants and vowels for vowels for both the "regular CV" and "nonregular CV" strings. Our results disconfirm this overly simple hypothesis.

The overall levels of accuracy for "regular CV" and "nonregular CV" words were significantly different--73% (1300/1777) and 57% (579/1024), respectively. This large difference in accuracy levels is accompanied by an even more striking difference in terms of the distribution of error types associated with the two orthographic structures. The only errors made for the "regular CV" words consisted of letter substitutions and (non-adjacent) exchanges (e.g., 'tavolo' → 'talovo'); there were (almost) no deletion, insertion, or (adjacent) exchange errors (for "regular CV" words the latter type of error would have required exchanging a consonant for a vowel as in, for example, 'tavolo' → 'taovlo,' violating CV structure information specified at the CV tier level). In marked contrast, "nonregular CV" words in addition to substitution and (non-adjacent) exchange errors also led to insertion, deletion and (adjacent) exchange errors. These results are summarized in Figure 5, where it may be seen that the two distributions of errors are markedly different. What can account for these striking differences in error distributions?

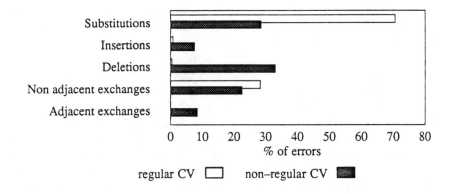

Figure 5. The effect of orthographic structure on writing performance: Incidence of various error types in incorrect responses to regular and non-regular CV stimuli.

As already noted, a two-tier hypothesis of the structure of graphemic representations cannot account for the reported results. To account for our results we must assume, at the very least, that graphemic representations specify syllabic boundaries in addition to CV and letter identity information. We can schematize the structure of graphemic representations as follows, where σ stands for syllable (for a similar proposal see Badecker, 1988):[2]

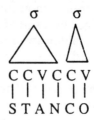

Damage to this type of representation, when it principally affects the letter identity level but also, though less severely, the CV and ortho-syllabic levels, would have less drastic consequences for "regular CV" structures than "nonregular CV" structures.[3] That is, given local under-specification of a representation, it is easier to reconstruct "regular CV" sequences than "nonregular CV" sequences if graphemic representations specify syllabic structure. An example will help clarify this claim.

Suppose that the representations for 'tavolo' and 'stanco' were to be damaged in identical ways at the CV and letter identity levels, as schematically shown in Figure 6. In the case of the "regular CV" word, 'repair' of the damaged representation with the constraint that it respect information specified at the syllabic level can only lead to a "regular CV" structure. This is because the only default location for the obligatory vowel demanded by information at the syllabic tier is the fourth position. With the default vowel in this position, the default CV value for the third position is a consonant, leading to a "regular CV" sequence. By contrast, the damaged "nonregular CV" sequence allows different default solutions in 'repair.' A default vowel may be placed either in the third or fourth position, allowing 'repair' solutions that violate the original CV structure; another 'repair' solution available for this graphemic string is to leave the non-vowel position blank--that is, produce a consonant deletion error. In other words, there are major differences between "regular CV" and "nonregular CV" words in terms of the types of 'repair' solutions that are possible when defaults are driven by ortho-syllabic information--syllabic level information helps recover more of the "regular CV" structure than "nonregular CV" structure.

Consider along these lines the case of deletion errors in L.B.'s spelling performance. Why are there no deletion errors for "regular CV" words? And, when deletion errors occur for "nonregular CV" words, what gets deleted?

Vowel deletions may only occur when letter identity information about a vowel is unavailable and 'repair' fails to insert a vowel in the appropriate location. For "regular CV" sequences, a "repair" failure to insert a vowel can only occur when vowel information is damaged at the letter identity and CV tiers and syllable information is missing. This entails that vowel deletion errors for this type of word can only occur in the context of deletion of a whole syllable. Indeed, the only deletion error produced by L.B. involved the deletion of a whole syllable (cugino → gino). If vowels are not deleted in "regular CV" words, a consonant will be introduced by default in non word-initial positions. Since there were essentially no errors in word initial position, there were no opportunities for L.B. to make consonant deletion errors either.

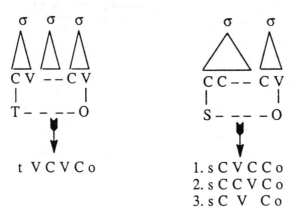

Figure 6. This figure shows the default solutions obtained for equally impaired "regular CV" and "nonregular CV" words when defaults are driven by syllabic structure.

The situation is quite different for "nonregular CV" words. L.B. produced a large number of deletion errors (see Figure 4). However, by the hypothesis developed above, these deletions should not involve vowels when they are the only vowel in a syllable. The data strongly confirm the hypothesis. As predicted, of the 141 deletion errors the great majority were consonant deletions (91%; 128/141). Of the 13 vowel deletion errors, only one (stagno → stgno) violates the vowel insertion default solution predicted by the hypothesis. The remaining vowel deletion errors involved two-vowel contexts (e.g., compie → compe; giugno → gugno) where deletion of one of the two vowels is a permissible default in the 'repair' process. That is, our hypothesis allows us to provide a motivated account for 140 of the 141 deletion errors produced by L.B. in spelling 6-letter words! The hypothesis that there is an ortho-syllabic tier in the graphemic representation is strongly supported by the results we have briefly reviewed.

CONCLUSIONS

When results are very clear, conclusions may be brief.

It has been shown in a series of empirical reports on the structure of certain dysgraphic disorders that a plausible model of the spelling process will have to include a working memory component or buffer which temporarily stores graphemic representations. The further detailed analysis of the spelling performance of patients with selective damage to the graphemic buffer has allowed us to constrain, in highly specific and important ways, claims about the structure of graphemic representations-- graphemic representations are highly structured, specifying not only an ordered set of abstract letter identities, but also CV and syllabic structure. This theory of the structure of the orthographic representations that are computed in the course of spelling is a natural extension of the proposed cognitive architecture of the spelling process. Therefore, we may interpret our success in providing a motivated explanation of the fine details of L.B.'s dysgraphic performance as providing the strongest support yet for the functional architecture of the spelling process schematically represented in Figure 1.

ACKNOWLEDGEMENTS

The research reported here was supported by grants from NIH (NS22202) and the Seaver Institute to the first author. This support is gratefully acknowledged. The ideas concerning orthographic representation presented here were stimulated by L.B.'s beautifully systematic performance and by discussions with members of the Cognitive Neuropsychology Laboratory, especially Bill Badecker, Caroline Carrithers, and Mike McCloskey. Andrew Olson and Jean-Roger Vergnaud explained to us some of the intricacies of computers and phonological theory, respectively. We are indebted to all of them.

REFERENCES

Badecker, W. (1988). Representational properties common to phonological and orthographic output systems. Unpublished manuscript.

Caramazza, A. & Miceli, G. (in preparation). The structure of orthographic representation.

Caramazza, A., Miceli, G., Villa, G. & Romani, C. (1987). The role of the graphemic buffer in spelling: Evidence from a case of acquired dysgraphia. Cognition, 26, 59-85.

Clements, G. & Keyser, S. (1983). Phonology: A generative theory of the syllable. Cambridge: MIT Press.

Hillis, A. & Caramazza, A. (in press). The graphemic buffer and attentional mechanisms. Brain and Language.

Miceli, G., Silveri, M. C. & Caramazza, A. (1985). Cognitive analysis of a case of pure dysgraphia. Brain and Language, 25, 187-212.

Posteraro, L., Zinelli, P. & Mazzucchi, A. (in press). Selective impairment of the graphemic buffer in acquired dysgraphia: A case study. Brain and Language.

NOTES

[1] Note that by 'repair' we simply mean the default computation that is possible given an underspecified representation. In the present case, if the letter identity information at one position in a graphemic string is, for whatever reason, not available, but the CV information is available, then the latter information will be used to compute a representation at the next level of processing. In this case, however, since the only information available concerns CV status, the letter that is produced may be any consonant for the consonant feature and any vowel for the vowel feature.

[2] Various hypotheses about the structure of the syllabic tier may be entertained. Depending on how richly structured we make the ortho-syllabic tier, we may find that the CV tier becomes totally redundant. In this latter case, the level of representation we have called the CV tier could instead correspond to a timing tier that specifies only a series of locations. Unfortunately, space limitations prevent us from considering alternative formulations in this chapter. (see Caramazza & Miceli, in preparation, for a more detailed discussion).

[3] This expectation need not go through for severely damaged representations where there may be insufficient structure for default decisions in the course of 'repairs.'

D. Speaking

Introduction to Section on Speaking

The most obvious signs of aphasia are impairments of language production. And, of these, the most celebrated and most assiduously studied is a pattern associated with a form of aphasia clinically classified as Broca's aphasia--agrammatism. The most striking features of agrammatism are the omission of function words (sometimes called free-standing grammatical morphemes or closed class words) and the omission or substitution of bound grammatical morphemes, both occurring in the context of a reduced range of syntactic constructions. Other features associated with this syndrome, but not universally accepted as part of it, are the omission of verbs and role reversal errors (e.g., producing "the girl is kissing the boy" for the boy is kissing the girl"). This production disorder is frequently (invariably, for some investigators) associated with a comprehension disorder characterized by difficulties in comprehending syntactically reversible sentences but not non-reversible sentences: asyntactic comprehension (e.g., difficulties comprehending "the boy kissed the girl" but not "the boy ate the apple"). The study of patients clinically classified as agrammatic aphasics has generated much controversy and some real insights into the nature of language production disorders. The papers included in this section consider both the controversies and the progress.

One question about the morphological errors produced in the context of the clinical picture of agrammatic production concerns their functional cause: are morphological errors the result of a deficit to sentence level, lexical-morphological, or phonological processes? Although I suspect that the answer to this question will turn out to be: all of the above, one attested case involves a deficit to specifically lexical-morphological processes (Miceli & Caramazza, 1988; Chapter 10). We have reported the performance of a brain-damaged subject, FS, whose language production performance could be classified as agrammatic. Detailed analysis of his single-word repetition performance revealed that he made many morphological as well as phonological errors. However, almost all of the morphological errors involved inflectional and not derivational substitutions. Furthermore, frank phonological errors occurred almost entirely on the stem part of a word and not on suffixes, suggesting that the phonological and morphological errors had different causes. Direct evidence for this hypothesis was obtained by comparing FS's performance on the rate and type of repetition errors across adjectival forms, which in italian are marked for number and gender (e.g., beautiful: bello, masculine singular; bella, feminine singular; belli, masculine plural; belle, feminine plural; polite: gentile, masculine or feminine singular; gentili, masculine or feminine plural). In this task, FS made relatively few errors on the masculine singular form--the morphologically unmarked form--and many errors on the other forms, which frequently resulted in the production of the unmarked form. This effect was independent of frequency, and could not be explained as resulting from a preference for one phonological form, /o/. The latter conclusion is based on the observation that the same effect of morphological markedness was obtained for two-form adjectives, but in this case the morphologically unmarked form for which better performance was obtained is phonologically realized as /e/--the phonological form most impaired for four-ending adjectives (feminine plural). We interpreted these results as evidence for the hypothesis that lexical forms represent stems and inflections independently. We also concluded that FS has an impairment specifically in morphologically processing in addition to a phonological processing deficit. Thus, at least some of the morphological errors produced by FS in spontaneous speech have a lexical-morphological.

The conclusion reached for FS does not imply that all his morphological errors have a lexical-morphological basis--some errors could arise at sentence level processes; nor does it imply that the morphological errors in other patients clinically classified as agrammatics have the same basis. Indeed, it has been shown that at least in some patients the agrammatic production impairment results from a deficit at sentence-level processes (Nespoulous, Dordain, Perron, Ska, Bub, Caplan, Mehler, Lecours, 1988; Caramazza & Hillis, 1989). Argye Hillis and I (Chapter 11) describe the performance of a brain-damaged subject, ML, whose language production, both spoken and written, could be classified as agrammatic. The patient omitted function words and bound grammatical morphemes and had a reduced "mean length of utterance"--produced short, ungrammatical sequences (e.g., ... water flowing floor ...). These problems obtained both in spontaneous production and in controlled experimental tasks where the patient had to describe simple pictures by producing a sentence. Despite these difficulties in sentence production, ML performed virtually flawlessly in all single-word production tasks. Thus, it would appear that in some cases (ML) the inability to process morphology is the result of deficit at sentence level processing, while in other cases (FS) a lexical-morphology deficit may be the cause of morphological errors.

Another interesting aspect of ML's performance is the marked dissociation between his production disorder in sentence processing and his normal ability to comprehend sentences. This result reinforces previous reports (Miceli, Mazzucchi, Menn, & Goodglass, 1983; Kolk, van Grunsven, & Keyser, 1985; Nespoulous et al., 1988) which have shown that agrammatic production is not necessarily associated with asyntactic comprehension. The implication of this result is that, as expected on strictly computational considerations, we must distinguish between those mechanisms that are devoted to the processing of syntactic/morphological structure in sentence production and those mechanisms involved in computing syntactic/morphological structure in sentence comprehension. Their independence is attested by the recorded dissociations. The computational considerations for this distinction were presented in Caramazza and Berndt (1985).

In various papers I have argued that research based on the a priori classification of patients (such as agrammatic, deep dyslexic, and so forth) cannot result in meaningful conclusions (Caramazza, 1984; 1986; Caramazza & Badecker, 1989; Caramazza & McCloskey, 1988; McCloskey & Caramazza, 1988). Badecker and I (Badecker & Caramazza, 1985), discuss the problem of patient classification in the specific case of agrammatism. We concluded that the criteria used to define this category are theoretically arbitrary and that the actual practice of classification is problematic. The practical problem concerned the manifest heterogeneity of putative cases of agrammatism. In Chapter 12 we (Miceli, Silveri, Romani, and Caramazza, 1989) document this contention through the analysis of the language production performance of 20 patients who could be classified as agrammatic aphasics. In this paper we show that the variability in the rate of omission and substitution of function words is considerable. Some patients make as many substitution errors as they make omission errors. This result is problematic because substitution errors are supposed to signal a different type of disorder-- paragrammatism. Equally problematic is the result concerning errors for bound grammatical morphemes. Here, too, there was extreme variation which was uncorrelated with problems in the production of free-standing grammatical morphemes, suggesting independent mechanisms in the processing of these two sets of elements. Finally, we found that there was extreme variation in the production of main verbs, which was also uncorrelated with production difficulties for grammatical morphemes. Given the attested variability what is to be gained by maintaining the category agrammatism? Or, which of the various patterns observed in our sample is the true pattern of agrammatic production? It would seem that the category of agrammatism is not only theoretically arbitrary but also practically problematic. It is time that we abandoned the theoretically unproductive practice of trying to explain the underlying causes of the mythical category agrammatism.

References

Badecker, W. & Caramazza, A. (1985). On considerations of method and theory governing the use of clinical categories in Neurolinguistics and Cognitive Neuropsychology: The case against Agrammatism. Cognition, 20, 97-125.

Caramazza, A. (1984). The logic neuropsychological research and the problem of patient classification in aphasia. Brain and Language, 21, 9-20.

Caramazza, A. (1986). On drawing inferences about the structure of normal cognitive systems from the analysis of patterns of impaired performance: The case for single-patient studies. Brain and Cognition, 5, 41-66.

Caramazza, A. & Berndt, R. S. (1985). A multicomponent deficit view of agrammatic Broca's aphasia. In M.-L. Kean (Ed.), Agrammatism, 27-63. New York, NY: Academic Press.

Caramazza, A. & McCloskey, M. (1988). The case for single-patient studies. Cognitive Neuropsychology, 5, 517-528.

Caramazza, A. & Badecker, W. (1989). Patient classification in neuropsychological research. Brain and Cognition, 10, 256-295.

Caramazza A. & Hillis, A. (1989). The disruption of sentence production: Some dissociations. Brain and Cognition, 36, 625-650.

Kolk, H. H. J., Van Grunsven, M. J. F. & Keyser, A. (1985). On parallelism between production and comprehension in agrammatism. In M.-L. Kean (Ed.), Agrammatism. New York, NY: Academic Press.

McCloskey, M. & Caramazza, A. (1988). Theory and methodology in cognitive neuropsychology: A response to our critics. Cognitive Neuropsychology, 5, 583-623.

Miceli, G., Mazzucchi, A., Menn, L. & Goodglass, H. (1983). Contrasting cases of Italian agrammatic aphasia without comprehension disorder. Brain and Language, 19, 65-97.

Miceli, G., Silveri, M. C., Romani, C. & Caramazza, A. (1989). Variation in the pattern of omissions and substitutions of grammatical morphemes in the spontaneous speech of so-called agrammatic patients. Brain and Language, 36, 447-492.

Nespoulous, J-L., Dordain, M., Perron, C., Ska, B., Bub, D., Caplan, D., Mehler, J., & Lecours, A. R. (1988). Agrammatism in sentence production without comprehension deficits: Reduced availability of syntactic structures and/or of grammatical morphemes? A case study. Brain and Language, 33, 273-295.

CHAPTER TEN

DISSOCIATION OF INFLECTIONAL AND DERIVATIONAL MORPHOLOGY

INTRODUCTION

A number of reports in the literature have attempted to deal with various aspects of morphological processing in brain-damaged patients. Thus, for example, Patterson (1980, 1982) has provided detailed analyses of "derivational" errors in oral reading (we place derivational in quotation marks because Patterson did not distinguish between inflectional and derivational errors in her analyses); Caplan, Kellar, & Locke (1972) analyzed the pattern of inflections in a patient who produced neologistic stems; and, Goodglass and his associates (Goodglass, 1976; Goodglass & Berko, 1960; Goodglass, Gleason, Ackerman, & Hyde, 1972), Gleason (1978), and DeVilliers (1978) have all reported detailed analyses of inflectional errors in the speech of agrammatic patients. These results (as well as others; see Caramazza, Miceli, Silveri, & Laudanna, 1985; Coltheart, 1985) converge nicely with experimental results in psycholinguistic research with normal subjects which suggest the need to represent lexical information in morphologically decomposed form (see Butterworth, 1983; Cutler, 1983; Henderson, 1985; Taft, 1985 for recent reviews of the literature - note that not all these authors endorse the view that the lexicon represents lexical information in morphologically decomposed form.). However, major issues remain unresolved, both with respect to the question of how morphological processing may be affected in various conditions of brain damage and with respect to the question of how lexical information is represented and accessed.

To properly address questions concerning morphological processing, we need a reasonable characterization of the morphological component of the language processing system. Fortunately, after a period of relative neglect, there has recently been within linguistics a strong resurgence of interest in morphology (e.g., Anderson, 1982; Aronoff, 1976; Jackendoff, 1975; Lapointe, 1979; Lieber, 1980; Matthews, 1974; Scalise, 1984; Selkirk, 1982; Siegel, 1974; Williams, 1981). Although many issues remain unresolved some general principles have emerged which can be used to guide research in morphological processing. We will assume that all morphological operations--both inflectional and derivational--are located in the lexicon (e.g., Lapointe 1979; Lieber, 1980; Scalise, 1980; Selkirk, 1982; Williams, 1981). However, following Anderson (1982), Aronoff (1976) and Scalise (1984), we will further assume that inflectional and derivational operations constitute functionally distinct processes (see Figure 1). Briefly a major distinction is drawn between the Derivational Processes Component (DPC) and the Inflectional Processes Component (IPC). Various arguments have been presented in support of this distinction. Some of these are briefly summarized here: (i) Inflections never change the syntactic category of the word to which they are applied whereas derivations may do so (e.g., *boy → boys*; *division → divisive*; inflectional and derivational, respectively); (ii) Rules of inflection are applied only after any rule of derivation may have been applied (e.g., *beauty → beautify → beautified*); (iii) Rules of the IPC and DPC are sensitive to different properties of the base to which they are applied (e.g., syntactic category and semantic features); (iv) The rules of the IPC and DPC affect the root morpheme to which they are applied in different ways (e.g., derivations always change the meaning of the root morpheme to which they are applied--*kind → kindness, boy → boyhood*--whereas inflections never do so); and, most generally, (v) "Inflectional morphology is what is relevant to syntax" (Anderson, 1982; pg.587), but the same cannot be stated for derivational morphology.

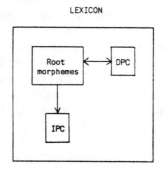

Figure 1. Organization of lexicon. The lexicon has three components: A set of root morphemes, a set of derivational affixes and associated rules of affixation (DPC), and a set of inflectional affixes with associated rules of affixation (IPC).

An important feature of the model of the lexicon adopted here is that lexical stem representations (base plus derivational affixes) and inflectional affixes interact with different kinds of information in the syntactic component of language--only the latter are sensitive to the morphosyntactic representation specified at the S-structure level (e.g., Anderson, 1982). Stating this claim in terms of a process model of sentence production (e.g., Garrett, 1980), lexical stems are accessed through their semantic specification for insertion at the Functional Level Representation while inflectional affixes are selected through morphosyntactic information for insertion at the Positional Level Representation (see also Stemberger, 1985; Dell, 1986; for alternative models of sentence production which nonetheless assume morphologically decomposed lexical representations). Given these differences in the nature of the IPC and the DPC it seems natural to consider these differences to be reflected in processing distinctions in the language system. In such a case it ought to be possible, in principle, to selectively disrupt one or the other morphological component of the lexical system.

As already noted there are some indications to suggest that the inflectional component of morphological processing may be disrupted selectively, implying the functional autonomy of this subcomponent of morphological structure. The speech of so-called "agrammatic" patients is supposed to be characterized by the selective omission (or misselection) of inflectional affixes and free-standing grammatical markers. However, it is not clear whether deficits of this general type reflect damage to a lexical or a syntactic component of the language production system--either hypothesis is consistent with the performance of the loosely-characterized category of agrammatism. One could maintain that damage to a component of the lexical system which "stores" free-standing grammatical markers and inflectional affixes could result in the pattern of speech classified as agrammatic; alternatively, one could place the locus of damage in the processing device that specifies the syntactic frame of the sentence to be produced (see Caramazza & Berndt, 1985, for discussion). Thus, although in either case the deficit is defined in terms of morphological features of language structure, the underlying cause of the impairment may be assumed to be located either in the lexicon or the syntactic processing component of language production. Of course, for any one "agrammatic" patient the underlying deficit may be to either or both components of processing.

One way to distinguish between specifically lexical and syntactic deficits in morphological processing is to consider a patient's performance in single-word processing. If the patient were to make morphological errors in single word processing, we would be able to conclude that at least one factor contributing to the patient's impairment is a deficit of the lexical processing system. In this paper we report a detailed analysis of a patient who makes morphological errors both in sentence *and* single word processing. This pattern of results and the presence of a marked dissociation between inflectional and derivational errors in the patient's single-word repetition performance are consistent with the hypothesis of a selective deficit to an autonomous Inflectional Processing Component of the lexicon.

CASE HISTORY

F.S. is a 60-year old, right-handed man. Prior to his illness he was a well-known lawyer. In March, 1978, he underwent surgery for the evacuation of an acute intracerebral hematoma. After surgery, he was severely aphasic and had marked neurological deficits. The patient was referred to one of the authors (G.M.) approximately 2 years post onset, and has been seen regularly as an outpatient since then. The study reported here was carried out between January, 1984 and February, 1985. The patient's condition remained stable throughout this period.

Neurological Exam

The patient has a right hemiplegia, with a severe spastic hypertonus. He shows extinction phenomena on the right in all modalities, but has no clinical signs of neglect. Visual extinctions are more frequent in the right inferior than in the right superior quadrant. A CT-scan, performed in 1982 (4 years post-onset), revealed a large hypodense area in the left hemisphere. The lesion involved the temporal lobe in its anterior and middle portions, the claustrum, the internal capsule and (probably) the insula, and also extended to the periventricular white matter of the parietal lobe (see Figure 2).

Neuropsychological Examination

The patient was submitted to an extensive battery of clinical tests. The results demonstrated normal visuo-perceptual and visuo-spatial abilities, and normal constructional praxis. There were very mild signs of ideomotor apraxia on verbal command, but they disappeared when the patient was asked to imitate gestures made by the examiner. A very mild buccofacial apraxia on verbal command was also present. It also disappeared on imitation, but the movements were executed slowly and with hesitations. The ability to perform sequences of meaningless movements with the buccofacial apparatus was severely impaired (F.S. scored 5/12 on the Nonverbal Agility subtest of the BDAE (Goodglass & Kaplan, 1972)).

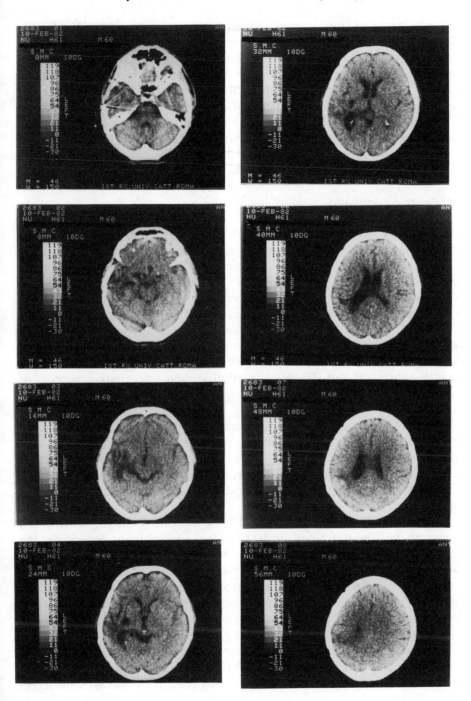

Figure 2. CT-scan of patient F.S. showing a large lesion in the left hemisphere.

Visual memory functions were well within normal limits. On Corsi's blocks, F.S.'s span was 6 forward, 4 backward. Verbal memory functions, by contrast, were impaired. On the Rey's 15 word list, the patient performed very poorly. The test consists of the auditory presentation of a list of 15 words. After each presentation the patient is asked to report as many words as possible. F.S. reported only 2/15, 5/15, 6/15, 4/15 and 5/15 items after each presentation and, 15 minutes later, he was able to recall only 5/15. Digit span was 3 forward and 3 backward. Pointing span for objects was 3. The patient scored 24/36 on Raven's Colored Matrices. A moderate acalculia was also present.

Language Examination

The motor aspects of F.S.'s verbal output were peculiar in many respects and could probably be best described as 'foreign accent' production. Articulation had an 'explosive' character, with abrupt changes in voice pitch, often within the same word. The patient showed some difficulties in producing complex consonant clusters, but no systematic simplifications were noted. Prosody was severely disturbed: Far from being flat, the poor control of pitch made it sound awkward to the listener. F.S. himself reported that people who did not know him mistook him for a foreigner (German, to be specific). Verbal agility was reduced (4/14 on the Verbal Agility subtest of the BDAE). Qualitative and quantitative aspects of F.S.'s verbal production will be discussed in the Results section of this paper.

Oral naming was mildly impaired for objects (92% correct) and moderately for actions (75% correct). Most of the errors were anomias (inability to provide a response) or phonemic paraphasias, with very few semantic substitutions. Written naming displayed essentially the same features (with spelling errors - letter substitutions - instead of phonemic paraphasias).

The performance obtained by F.S. in repeating single words and nonwords will be described in detail below. In sentence repetition, the patient demonstrated difficulties with free-standing grammatical markers (omissions and substitutions) and with bound grammatical markers (substitutions). In addition, he also produced some semantic substitution errors on major-class lexical items (for example, 'Giovanni ha comprato due macchine' (John bought two cars) → 'Giovanni acquistate (f.pl.) due auto' (John purchased (past part., f.pl.) two autos)).

Comprehension of isolated words was "normal" for both auditory and visual presentation. This was true for tests using phonemic foils (1/57 incorrect responses) and for tests employing semantic foils (3/60 incorrect responses). Auditory phoneme discrimination based on meaningless CCVC syllables was poor (41/120 incorrect responses) as was auditory-visual matching using the same material (24/120 incorrect responses).

Auditory sentence comprehension was also severely impaired. On the syntax comprehension test by Parisi & Pizzamiglio (1970), F.S. responded incorrectly to 14/80 stimuli. He made errors on declarative (1/4) and embedded active reversible sentences (2/4), on declarative passive (3/4) and locative sentences (6/36), and on sentences requiring the comprehension of verb morphology (2/8). In another test of sentence comprehension F.S. produced 21/50 incorrect responses. He made errors on declarative reversible sentences (1/10 active, 6/10 passive), on embedded reversible sentences (3/10 active, 9/10 passive), and on sentences expressing reversible temporal relations of the type before/after (3/10). The patient also had some minor difficulty in acting out sentences which required comprehension of the weak (clitic) vs. strong form of the personal pronoun, of the type: 'Dammi/Dagli la penna' (Give me/Give him the pen) vs. 'Dai la penna a me/a lui' (Give the pen to me/to him). He made 2/20 errors with sentences of the first type, but performed flawlessly with sentences of the second type. In an auditory sentence-to-picture matching task, F.S. also showed impaired comprehension of sentences containing the reflexive vs. the anaphoric forms of the clitic pronoun (e.g., 'La donna si lava' (The woman washes herself), and 'L'uomo li ferisce' (The man hurts them), respectively). The patient had to choose from two pictures, one corresponding to the stimulus sentence, the other representing the contrasting clitic personal pronoun (e.g., for the stimulus sentence 'La donna si lava' (the woman washes herself), F.S. was shown a picture representing the correct response, and a picture depicting 'La donna li lava' (The woman washes them); for the stimulus 'L'uomo li ferisce' (The man wounds them) the incorrect alternative portrayed 'L'uomo si ferisce' (The man wounds himself); and so on). F.S. made 8/48 errors on this test.

EXPERIMENTAL STUDY

1. *Spontaneous speech*

A sample of connected speech consisting of 873 words was obtained by asking F.S. to tell us about his illness, to describe some habitual daily activities, and to recount the story of Little Red Riding Hood.

F.S.'s speech displayed marked grammatical deficits as is obvious from the speech sample shown in Table 1 (see also Appendix I). The patient's speech is characterized by the omission or misselection of free-standing grammatical markers, reduced phrase length, and violation of gender, number, and tense/aspect agreement. Thus, for example, the patient produced '...poi ancora spesso *andare* [allo] studio.' where 'allo' (to the) is omitted and the verb is inappropriately inflected in the infinitive (andare) instead of the correct finite, first person, singular form (vado). We have quantified various grammatical aspects of the patient's speech; and this is shown in Table 2, together with the performance of another patient whose speech would also be clinically classified as "agrammatic" and a matched normal control subject.

Table 1.

1	ritorno a casa mia	la
2	Poi <u>ritorna</u> (a) <u>la</u> mia casa.	Poi io ascolto <u>il</u> televisione
3	Then returns the my house (f.sg.)	Then I hear the (m.sg.) television (f.sg.)
4	Then returns my house.	Then I listen to the television

1	faccio	vivo
2	o poi <u>fare</u> il pranzo	perché, caro dottore, io <u>vive</u> solo!
3	or then to make the lunch	because, dear doctor (m.sg.) I lives alone (m.sg.)
4	or then make lunch because, dear doctor, I lives alone!

1	ricevo faccio	le lunghe
2	Poi telefono, <u>riceve</u>, <u>fare</u>,	perché <u>il</u> giornate (sono) <u>lungo</u>,
3	Then (I) telephone, receives, to make	because the (m.sg.) days (f.pl.) long (m.sg.)
4	Then I telephone, receives, make (phone calls), because the days long,

1	vado	i Parioli
2	poi ancora spesso <u>andare</u> (allo) studio.	(In) via C. (a) <u>il</u> <u>Pariolo</u>
3	then still often go my office	street C. il Pariolo
4	then still often go my office. C. Street, Pariolo,

1	il mio studio
2	c'e <u>la mia studia</u> ancora aperto.
3	there is the (f.sg.) my (f.sg.) office (f.sg.) still open (m.sg.)
4	there is my office, still open.

NOTE. In this sample the patient is describing what he habitually does in the morning. The patient's speech is reported in line 2, which reproduces verbatim his spontaneous speech. Words omitted in obligatory context are in square parentheses. Words produced incorrectly are underlined. Line 1 gives the correct target words. Line 3 is the literal, word-by-word English translation of line 2. Whenever agreement is ambiguous in English, gender and number information is provided in parentheses (m=masculine; f=feminine; sg=singular; pl=plural). Finally, line 4 is a rough equivalent of line 2, to give the reader an approximate idea of how the patient's spontaneous speech would sound in English.

Table 2. Features of F.S.'s spontaneous sentence production performance.*

	F.S.	C.D.A.(agr.)**	E.B.(control)
Percentage of words out of syntactic context	4.2%	14.4%	0%
Mean phrase length (syntactic)	6.11	3.2	10.14
Mean phrase length (morphological)	3.16	2.4	10.14
Rate of omission of free-standing grammatical markers	54/242 (22.3)	62/255 (24.3)	0/227 (0)
Rate of sustitution of free-standing grammatical markers	48/242 (19.8)	19/255 (7.4)	0/277 (0)
Rates of Main to Subordinate clauses	2	14.9	1.7
NP-PP/Total NP	21/184 (11.4)	11/175 (6.3)	25/214 (11.7)
Violations of det/N agreement	19/138 (13.8)	2/91 (2.2)	(0)
Violations of N/Adj agreement	11/55 (20.0)	0/11 (0)	(0)
Violations of Subject/V agreement	45/82 (54.9)	18/97 (18.6)	(0)

** Percentages are in parentheses.
* For comparison we have included the performance of an "agrammatic" and a normal subject.

There are several features of the patient's performance that are worth focusing on. First, and most important for our present purposes, it is clear that the patient omits (22.3%) or misselects (19.8%) free-standing grammatical markers and misselects inflectional affixes (20.4%). Especially striking is the large proportion of violations of Subject/Verb agreement (55.9%), but the patient also made a substantial number of Determiner/Noun and Noun/Adjective agreement violations (13.8% and 20%, respectively). These difficulties are reflected directly in two other measures of the grammatical appropriateness of the patient's speech: mean phrase length of syntactically (MPL-S) and morphologically (MPL-M) appropriate speech. The former measure (MPL-S) captures the length of lexically appropriate strings, whether or not there are violations of agreement (e.g., the string 'c'e *la mia studia* ancora aperto' would be scored as length 7 even though the phrase "la mia studia" is morphologically deviant). The other measure (MPL–M) captures the length of grammatically correct strings including agreement. As can be seen in Table 2, F.S. has a reduced MPL–S (6.1) and even shorter MLP–M (3.2) when compared to a matched normal control (10.1 for both measures). However, the reduced MPL is not due to a reduction in availability of syntactic frames--that is, it is not due to an inability to produce subordinate clauses (the ratio of main to subordinate clauses is 2 and 1.7 for F.S. and the normal control, respectively) or prepositional phrases (11.4% and 11.7% of total noun phrases were prepositional phrases for F.S. and the normal control, respectively)--the patient appeared to be quite normal in this regard. The reduced phrase length appears to result from the omission of free-standing grammatical markers or the misselection of both free and bound grammatical markers.

It is instructive to compare F.S.'s performance to that of another patient who would also be clinically classified as "agrammatic." For this purpose we compared his performance to patient C.D.A. The two patients differ on a number of measures as can be seen in Table 2: They differ in the mean phrase length of their speech (both MPL–S and MPL–M), in the proportion of words produced out of grammatical context, in their use of subordinate clauses and prepositional phrases, and in the proportion of agreement violations--whereas F.S. is less impaired than C.D.A. in the first three measures of grammaticality of speech, there is a clear reversal in severity of impairment for the last mentioned measure. It is unlikely that the underlying deficit for these two patients is the same. Thus, the mere classification of these two patients as "agrammatic" would be misleading, at best. In any case, the point here is that F.S.'s spontaneous speech clearly reflects an impairment in morphological processing. What is not clear is whether the disorder arises from damage to the lexical or to the syntactic component of the sentence processing system.

Two hypotheses (at least) may be entertained about the possible locus of functional damage to the sentence production system which would give rise to the pattern of omission and misselection errors produced by F.S. in spontaneous speech. The Lexical Deficit Hypothesis assumes that the locus of damage is to some component of the lexical system. For this hypothesis to be entertained seriously, however, the structure of the lexicon must be articulated in such a fashion that function words and inflectional affixes may be damaged selectively. That is, function words must form an autonomous subcomponent of the lexicon, and the inflectional component of the lexicon must similarly be autonomously represented within the lexicon. (Of course, function words and inflectional affixes could functionally constitute a single processing component.) The other hypothesis, the Syntactic Deficit Hypothesis, assumes that the locus of damage is to a level of sentential processing which distinguishes grammatical features (such as free and bound grammatical markers) from the major lexical items of a sentence--perhaps the Positional Level in Garrett's model of sentence production (Garrett, 1980, 1982; see also Lapointe, 1985). Of course, it is entirely possible that F.S. may have damage to both components of processing.

While it is difficult to provide evidence which would rule out the contribution of damage to the syntactic processing component to the overall pattern of speech production impairment in our patient, it is a relatively simple matter to state the conditions under which we would accept the hypothesis that damage to the lexical system is a major contributor to the patient's impairment. Thus, if it could be demonstrated that F.S. has difficulties in single word processing that are explicable by appeal to the morphological structure of words, we would be inclined to accept the hypothesis that at least part (if not all) of the spontaneous production disorder is due to damage to the lexical system. Of course, this latter inference is only justified if the single word processing impairment can be shown to involve the relevant subcomponent of the lexical system--the inflectional component in this case. To address this issue we assessed F.S.'s ability to process single words with a variety of tasks.

2. Repetition Tests

The patient was asked to repeat, in several sessions, 1832 words and 283 nonwords. The word sample contained several sublists, controlled for form class, frequency, length, morphological complexity, type of suffix (inflectional vs. derivational), and presence of prefix vs. pseudoprefix. The stimuli were presented in random order, at a normal rate of articulation. Some sublists only contained words, whereas others contained both words and nonwords intermixed in random order. The examiner pronounced each stimulus aloud, and the patient was asked to repeat it.

a. Word repetition
F.S.'s ability to repeat single words is severely impaired: He repeated incorrectly 919/1832 (50.2%) stimuli. A breakdown of repetition performance as a function of the form class of the stimulus word (without controlling factors such as word length, frequency, and abstractness/concreteness; but see below) reveals major effects of form class (see Table 3). The patient performed equally poorly on function words and nouns (31.0% and 29.6% errors, respectively) and even worse on adjectives (49.2% errors) and verbs (64.3% errors).

Table 3. Performance obtained by F.S. in word repetition tasks.

Part of speech	Errors	%
Nouns	121/409	29.6
Adjectives	290/589	49.2
Verbs	482/750	64.3
Function words	26/84	31.0
TOTAL	919/1832	50.2

A quantitative analysis of the errors produced by F.S. (a total of 919 errors) is shown in Table 4. Responses were scored as correct or as one of a number of incorrect response types. A description, with examples, of each of the error categories used in this analysis is shown in Appendix I.

F.S. produced 663/919 (72.1%) incorrect word responses. If we restrict the analysis of errors to polymorphemic words in the sample (i.e., words which permit morphologically legal errors--nouns, adjectives, and verbs), 659/893 (73.8%) errors resulted in word responses and, most importantly, they were almost all (636; 96.5% of the word responses or 71.2% of the total corpus of errors) morphologically based. These latter errors consist of the correct repetition of the root of the stimulus word and a substitution of the affixal part of the word (e.g., *settimana* (week) → *settimane* (weeks); *povera* (poor; f.sg.) → *overo* (poor; m.sg.); *vestire* (to wear) → *vestivi* (you were wearing)). A striking feature of these morphologically-based errors is that they are essentially all (615/637 or 96.7%) inflectional errors. Admittedly the sample of words we are considering here is not a random sample of the words in the language--verbs and adjectives are overrepresented--but, the dissociation between inflectional and derivational errors cannot be attributed to this sampling bias (see below for F.S.'s performance on controlled sublists). Of the remaining, nonmorphological errors, very few word responses consisted of semantic paraphasias (4; 0.4%) or unrelated word responses (19; 2.1%; e.g., *reca* (he brings) → *creda* (that he believes)). Clearly, the primary dimension along which we can characterize the word-error responses is a morphological one.

The pattern of nonword responses (186/893; 20.8%) is also informative. A nonnegligible proportion of these errors (55/186; 29.6%) could be considered to be "morphologically-based." This latter type of error involves a substitution of inflectional or derivational affixes. Some of them consist of a correct root plus a suffix not permissible for that root (22/55; 40.0%; e.g., *resisteva* (he was resisting) → *resistire* (nonword)--the affix -*ire* is the infinitival form for verbs of the 3rd conjugation and is

Table 4. Distribution of errors made by F.S. in word repetition tasks.*

	Nouns	Adjectives	Verbs	TOTAL	Function Words	TOTAL
Inflectional	55 (45.5)	201 (69.4)	345 (71.6)	601 (67.3)	----	601 (65.4)
Phonemic subst. on root and inflect. subst.	6 (5.0)	16 (5.5)	23**(4.8)	45 (5.0)	2 (7.7)	47 (5.1)
Illegal inflections	5 (4.1)	1 (0.4)	9 (1.9)	15 (1.7)	3 (11.5)	18 (2.0)
Prefix omission	1 (0.8)	----	1 (0.2)	2 (0.2)	----	2 (0.2)
Derivational	14 (11.6)	3 (1.0)	4 (0.8)	21 (2.4)	----	21 (2.3)
Illegal derivations	4 (3.3)	3 (1.0)	----	7 (0.8)	----	7 (0.8)
Phonemic substitution	27 (22.3)	40 (13.8)	64 (13.3)	131 (14.7)	11 (42.3)	142 (15.5)
Semantic substitution	----	2 (0.7)	2 (0.4)	4 (0.4)	3 (11.5)	7 (0.8)
Other word response (phonologically related)	1 (0.8)	3 (1.0)	15 (3.1)	19 (2.1)	1 (3.9)	20 (2.2)
Fragments	6 (5.0)	12 (4.1)	7 (1.4)	25 (2.8)	2 (7.7)	26 (2.8)
No response	2 (1.6)	9 (3.1)	12 (2.5)	23 (2.6)	4 (15.4)	27 (2.9)

* Percentages are in parentheses.
** Twelve errors are incorrect word responses consisting of the substitution of the verb stem with a phonologically-related stem and of the verb inflection (e.g., RIDARO' (I will give again) → RIDIRA' (he will say again)); eleven errors are nonword responses consisting of the substitution of the verb stem with a phonologically-related pseudo-stem and of the verb inflection (e.g., SUDAVA (he was sweating) → SUGIARE (nonword)).

not appropriate for the root *resist-* which requires the affix \-*ere* for verbs of the 2nd conjugation); the other errors in this category consist of phonologically similar pseudoroots with substituted suffixes (33/55; 60.0%; e.g., *fiatavi* (you were breathing) → *fiafare*--a pseudoroot *fiaf-* + the "appropriate" (for *fiat-*) infinitival affix *-are*). The remaining nonword errors (131/186; 70.4%) are morphologically nondecomposable responses which result from phonemic substitutions of one or more phonemes in the stimulus word.

The error corpus also contained a small proportion of "fragment" responses (29/893; 2.8%; e.g., 'unirono' (they united) → 'uni'...) and omissions (23/893; 2.6%). These errors will not be discussed further.

F.S.'s repetition performance for function words contrasts markedly with that for other word classes. Specifically, the majority of errors for function words consist of phonemic substitutions.[1] This result reflects the fact that the great majority of function words used in the repetition task are uninflected and, therefore, there is no possibility for making morphological errors. We wish to stress, however, that overall performance for this class of words is not worse than for other word classes. In fact, as already indicated, the level of performance for function words was comparable to that for nouns, which is better than that for adjectives and verbs.

The results we have reported thus far are striking in at least two respects. First, the patient's single-word repetition difficulty is characterized by morphological errors; of the total scorable errors produced, 84.5% were morphologically-based and only 15.5% were phonemic paraphasias. This distribution of errors suggests that while the patient does have a phonological processing deficit (at some level of processing), it cannot account (in any simple way) for the massive presence of morphological errors. Second, and perhaps more importantly, the great majority of morphological errors were inflectional (96.7% vs. 3.3% for inflectional and derivational errors, respectively). On the face of it, this latter result rather compellingly suggests a selective deficit to the inflectional component of the lexicon and, therefore, implies functional autonomy for this subcomponent of the lexicon. However, before drawing such a strong conclusion with its associated inferences for the structure of the lexical system, there are several issues that should be addressed: We should investigate the parameters that determine the probability of making an error in repetition and, specifically, a morphological error; we should more carefully evaluate the dissociation between inflectional and derivational errors; we should evaluate possible differences in processing prefixes and suffixes; we should characterize the pattern of morphological errors--that is, the distribution of responses as a function of stimulus characteristics; and, we should attempt to determine whether functional damage is restricted to the output lexicon, the input lexicon, or both. We next turn to these issues through the analysis of various sublists included in the total corpus of words we have just discussed.

The effects of word length, word frequency, and form class on repetition performance. In order to assess the effects of word length, word frequency, and form class on F.S.'s repetition performance, we asked him to repeat a list of 156 words controlled for these factors. The list consisted of 52 nouns, 52 adjectives, and 52 verbs. Half of the total set of stimuli (78) had a mean frequency of 150/million, range 100-300/million; the other half had a mean frequency of 20/million, range 10-30/million (frequencies from Bortolini, Tagliavini & Zampolli, 1971); half of the total set of stimuli ranged from 4 to 6 phonemes; the other half ranged in length from 7 to 9 phonemes. The high and low frequency and the short and long words were distributed evenly among the three classes of words. We also included in the list 52 function words. However, for these words we could not control the factors of length and frequency.

Repetition results for this list of words is shown in Table 5. There are clear effects of length (X^2 = 10.649; p < .01) and frequency (X^2 = 10.649; p < .01). The form class condition did not reach an acceptable level of significance (X^2 = 4.912; p = 4.2) but there is a trend for verbs to be repeated more poorly than adjectives, which in turn are repeated more poorly than nouns. It is worth stressing that the proportion of morphological errors remains roughly invariant as a function of the factors manipulated in the experimental list.

The results in this section confirm conclusions reached earlier in the paper. Specifically, the effect of word length--a nonlexical factor--suggests that a factor contributing to the patient's performance is the phonological "complexity" of the stimulus; that is, the sheer number of phonological segments to be processed affects the probability of a correct response. The effect of word frequency points instead to a deficit in the lexicon. The assumption here is that the availability of the whole-word phonological representation of a lexical entry is a direct function of the frequency of usage of that phonological representation--frequently used words are relatively more accessible than infrequently used words (e.g., Morton, 1979). If we further assume that damage to the lexicon accentuates the relative accessability of phonological representation, then we would expect that words of lower frequency of occurrence in the language would be the ones most difficult to produce. In short, F.S.'s repetition difficulty arises from damage to independent components of the word production system--damage to the lexicon and damage to nonlexical

A. Caramazza

phonological processes, either at the input or the output level. The lexical deficit does not appear to be form-class-specific (there is only a nonsignificant trend in this direction).

Table 5. F.S.'s word repetition performance *

	Total errors	Morphological errors (N.A.V.)
Form class:		
Nouns	15/52 (28.8)	11/52 (21.2)
Adjectives	20/52 (38.5)	16/52 (30.8)
Verbs	26/52 (50.0)	21/52 (40.4)
Function words	21/52 (40.4)	-----
Length:		
Short (4-6 phonemes)	29/104 (27.9)	16/78 (20.5)
Long (7-9 phonemes)	53/104 (51.0)	29/78 (37.2)
Frequency:		
High ($\geq$ 100/million)	29/104 (27.9)	17/78 (21.8)
Low ($\leq$ 10/million)	53/104 (51.0)	28/78 (35.9)

Sublist 2. Root length x Suffix length.

Root:		
Short (2 phonemes)	11/24 (45.8)	5/24 (20.8)
Long (4-6 phonemes)	15/24 (62.5)	10/24 (41.7)
Suffix:		
Short (1 phoneme)	7/16 (63.7)	4/16 (25.0)
Medium (3 phonemes)	9/16 (56.2)	6/16 (37.5)
Long (4-5 phonemes)	10/16 (62.5)	5/16 (31.2)

*Percentages are in parentheses.

Repetition of prefixed words. F.S. was asked to repeat 85 prefixed words, each containing one of 8 different prefixes, interspersed in various sublists. The following prefixes were included in the experimental list: *ri-*, as in *rifare* (to redo); *dis-*, as in *disgrazia* (disgrace); *s-*, as in *scoperto* (uncovered); *in-*, as in *inutili* (useless); *con-*, as in *congiungono* (they conjoin); *re-*, as in *respinto* (pushed); *di-*, as in *distacco* (detachment); and, *pre-*, as in *pregiudizio* (prejudgment). Thirty-nine of these prefixed words, which were part of a large list including items belonging to all word classes, were matched for part of speech, frequency (approximately 20/million), length (mean length: 8.3 letters) and initial letter cluster to 39 pseudoprefixed words (e.g., prefixed word: *rifare* (to re-do); pseudo-prefixed word: *ricevo* (I receive)). The results obtained by F.S. in repeating the entire corpus of prefixed words, and the subsets of matched prefixed and pseudoprefixed words, are shown in Table 6.

Table 6. Repetition of prefixed words.*

	Overall prefixed (n=85)	Matched prefixed (n=39)	Matched pseudo-prefixed (n=39)
1. Correct responses	41 (48.2)	21 (53.8)	21 (53.8)
2. Error distribution			
a. Morphological	27 (61.4)	15 (83.3)	11 (61.1)
Prefix	2 (4.6)	2 (11.1)	-----
Suffix	25 (56.8)	13 (72.2)	11 (61.1)
inflection	20 (45.5)	10 (55.5)	11 (61.1)
derivation	5 (11.3)	3 (16.7)	-----
b. Nonmorphological	17 (38.6)	3 (16.7)	7 (38.9)
Phono.subst.errors	11 (25.0)	3 (16.7)	2 (11.1)
Fragments	5 (11.3)	-----	1 (5.6)
No response	1 (2.3)	-----	4 (22.2)

*Performance obtained by F.S. in repeating the whole sample of prefixed words and matched subsets of prefixed and pseudoprefixed words: Correct responses and error distributions (percentages are in parentheses).

The most relevant aspect of F.S.'s performance is his proficiency in repeating prefixes as opposed to suffixes: Of the 44 errors he made on the prefixed words, only two were prefix errors, both omissions ('stendono' (they stretch) → 'tendono' (they tend, or they stretch); 'slancio' (thrust) → 'lancio' (throw)), but he reproduced incorrectly 25 suffixes, 20 inflectional and 5 derivational errors. It is worth noting that both prefix omissions occurred with consonant clusters (/s/ + consonant) that are both articulatorily complex and relatively infrequent. This consonant cluster proved difficult for F.S. also when it occurred in word–initial position of non-prefixed words (consider the following errors in repetition found in the larger error corpus: 'stivali' (boots) → 'tivali' (nonword); 'strana' (strange) → 'trana' (nonword); 'spina' (thorn) → 'pina').

F.S.'s repetition performance for prefixed words leaves no doubt that he does not have particular difficulties in processing prefixes. Instead, it appears that his morphological processing impairment is restricted to suffixes and, in particular, inflectional suffixes.

Inflectional vs. derivational suffixes. In an earlier section of this paper we reported that for the full corpus of morphological errors there is a striking dissociation between inflectional and derivational errors (96.7% vs. 3.3%, respectively). As we emphasized in that section, however, the stimulus words included in the total corpus were not controlled for potentially relevant factors that may determine the probability of making an inflectional or derivational error. Thus, for example, one of the factors not controlled for in the total stimulus set is the proportion of derived vs. inflected words. Since in Italian all words except a subset of the free-standing grammatical markers are inflected, there is a very large discrepancy between the number of inflected versus derived words in the total stimulus set. If the probability of making a derivational error is a function of whether or not a word is derived, then the paucity of such words in the stimulus set would underestimate the extent of processing difficulties of derivational morphology in our patient. To more accurately assess whether or not inflectional morphology is impaired while derivational morphology is normal in our patient, we analyzed selected subsets of the total stimulus set.

In the first analysis we considered the distribution of errors for suffix-derived words. Our stimulus set contained 305 words which could unambiguously be considered to be derived words. F.S. successfully repeated 135 (44.3%) words from this set. Of the errors 109 (64.1%) were morphologically-based; of these errors 90 (52.9%) were inflectional, 12 (7.0%) were derivational, and 7 (4.1%) could not be unambiguously scored as either derivational or inflectional (e.g., ballavi (you were dancing → 'ballo' (I dance--inflectional--or the dance--derivational).

The second analysis considered the repetition performance for a specially designed list of words. The 106-word list consists of 53 inflected words (all verbs) and 53 derived words (nouns and adjectives). The two subsets of words were exactly matched for length and frequency. Since the frequency of derived words tends to be low, more than two thirds of the stimuli had a frequency of 10/million or less. F.S. repeated correctly 18 (33.4%) inflected and 18 (33.4%) derived words. For the inflected words all the morphological errors were inflectional (25; 71.4%); for the derived words he produced mostly inflectional errors (18; 51.4%), but he also produced a few derivational errors (3; 8.6%).

The results reported in this section confirm the conclusion stated earlier in the paper that the patient has a deficit in processing inflectional morphology. However, there is also some indication that the processing of derivational morphology is not entirely normal in our patient: For the full corpus of morphological errors (136) produced for derived words (either prefixed or suffixed), F.S. made a nonnegligible proportion (10.3%) of derivational errors. We will discuss the discrepancy between the proportion of inflectional and derivational errors in the Discussion section of the paper.

Patterns of inflectional errors. We have argued that F.S.'s repetition impairment results from damage to two independent processing mechanisms: a deficit at some level of phonological processing and a deficit to the morphological processing component of the lexical system. Various arguments may be given in support of this conclusion. The most direct, and the one we will focus on here, is based on the analysis of distributional characteristics of repetition errors. Specifically, we contend that one may plausibly conclude that the functional locus of damage is at some level of phonological processing if the distribution of errors is explicable by appeal to phonological principles. Similarly, one may plausibly conclude that the functional locus of damage is at some level of morphological processing if the distribution of errors is explicable by appeal to morphological principles.

There is already clear evidence for supposing that F.S. has a phonological processing impairment: A substantial proportion of repetition errors consisted of phonemic paraphasias. The issue now is whether or not the putative "morphological" errors might not also merely result from damage to some phonological processing mechanism. This issue was addressed by considering the distribution of inflectional errors made for nouns, adjectives, and verbs. Since the clearest case can be made for adjectives, we will consider this form class first.

F.S. was asked to repeat a set of adjectives which could take one of four alternative inflectional affixes. The four inflectional affixes mark gender and number (e.g., *caro* (dear; m.sg.), *cari* (m.pl.), *cara* (f.sg.), *care* (f.pl.)). This experimental list included 30 m.sg. adjectives, 23 m.pl. adjectives, 30 f.sg. adjectives, and 30 f.pl. adjectives, matched for length (6.9 to 7.2 letters), root frequency (27.4/million to 29.6/million) and surface form frequency (6.4/million to 7/million). F.S. repeated correctly 28 m.sg. adjectives (93.3%), 10 m.pl. adjectives (43.5%), 16 f.sg. adjectives (53.3%), and 8 f.pl. adjectives (26.7%). The patient displayed a marked tendency to produce the m.sg. as the incorrect response: Of the 45 inflectional errors, 36 were substitutions of the m.sg. inflection for other inflectional endings (80.0%).

Since the m.sg. form of the adjective is usually the most frequent, as well as the citation form,[2] F.S. was asked to repeat another list of adjectives to determine whether or not the very high percentage of incorrect m.sg. responses merely reflected a tendency to produce the most frequent form of the adjective. This list included 200 adjectives equally divided among the following four types: (i) adjectives whose m.sg. form is more frequent than non-m.sg. forms, presented in the m.sg. form (root frequency: 40/million; form frequency of the m.sg. form: 20.9/million; form frequency of non-m.sg. forms: 3/million); (ii) a non-m.sg. form of the adjectives in (i); (iii) adjectives whose m.sg. form is very infrequent, presented in the m.sg. form (root frequency: 40/million; form frequency of the m.sg. form: 5/million; form frequency of the non-m.sg. form: 22.5/million; (iv) a non-m.sg. form of the adjectives in (iii). The incidence of the 3 non-m.sg. inflections was balanced across subsets (i) and (iv). Length was balanced across subsets.

Once again, the results are clearcut (see Table 7): F.S. repeated correctly m.sg. adjectives a high proportion of the time (41/50 from subset (i) and 40/50 adjectives from subset (iii)), but non-m.sg. forms were reproduced correctly much less often (5/50 from subset (ii), and 11/50 from subset (iv)). Of the inflectional errors made in this task (71/113; 62.8%), the vast majority (56/71; 78.3%) consisted of the substitution of the m.sg. inflection for a non-m.sg. suffix.

Table 7. Number of correct responses provided by F.S. in repeating a sublist of adjectives with four endings, matched in length and controlled for root frequency and surface form frequency.

		Form administered	
		m.sg.	non-m.sg.
Surface form	m.sg. > non-m.sg.	41/50	5/50
frequency	m.sg. < non-m.sg.	40/50	11/50

If we consider the distribution of correct responses and inflectional errors for the entire set of adjectives that take four inflectional affixes, there is a very strong effect of inflectional form on performance. Table 8a summarizes these data. As is immediately apparent, the m.sg. form is repeated correctly with very high probability (94.9%). The probability of correctly repeating the other inflectional forms is quite low, by contrast, ranging from 25.5% to 34.2% to 39.8% for f.pl., m.pl., and f.sg., respectively. Furthermore, there is an overwhelming tendency to produce the m.sg. form of the adjective independently of the inflectional form of the stimulus. A similar analysis for adjectives that only take two inflectional endings (e.g.,forte (strong, m.sg. and f.sg.), forti (strong, m.pl. and f.pl.) gives comparable results. As is shown in Table 8b, whereas the singular form is very often repeated correctly (81.2%), the plural form is only infrequently repeated correctly (34.5%). And, again here, there is a strong tendency to incorrectly produce the singular form when repeating an adjective marked for plural.

These results leave little doubt that the major determinant of morphological errors in our patient is a deficit to the inflectional processing component of the lexical system. The distribution of repetition errors is explicable by appeal to morphological principles: The most often produced form of an adjective, both correctly and incorrectly, is the citation form. That is, the patient's tendency to produce the m.sg. form for the four-ending adjectives does not merely reflect a frequency effect --the citation form was given both when it is the relatively high and when it is the relatively low frequency form of an adjective--nor, does it reflect a bias to produce the phonological form /o/, which is associated with the m.sg. form of four-ending adjectives (e.g., caro, cara, care, cari) --F.S. also overwhelmingly produced the singular form for two-ending adjectives which take the phonological form /e/, the phonological form associated with f.pl. inflections for four-ending adjectives. In short, F.S.'s pattern of inflectional errors for adjectives cannot be explicated by appealing to the relative frequencies of alternative inflectional forms of adjectives nor by appealing to potential preferences for alternative phonological forms. Instead, there is strong support for the view that the primary determinant of the probability of correctly repeating an adjective is whether or not the stimulus in given in the citation form or in another inflected form--a morphological principle.

Table 8. Confusion matrix for inflectional errors made by F.S. in repeating 4-ending and 2-ending adjectives (percentages are in parentheses).

	M.SG.	M.PL.	F.SG.	F.PL.	TOTAL
a. 4-ending adjectives					
M.SG.	149 (94.9)	8 (5.1)	- - - - -	- - - -	157
M.PL.	40 (52.6)	26 (34.2)	5 (6.6)	5 (6.6)	76
F.SG.	43 (48.9)	1 (1.1)	35 (39.8)	9 (10.2)	88
F.PL.	34 (61.8)	2 (3.6)	5 (9.1)	14 (25.5)	55
TOTAL	266 (70.7)	37 (9.8)	45 (12.0)	28 (7.4)	376
b. 2-ending adjectives					
	SG.	PL.			
SG.	56 (81.2)	13 (18.8)			
PL.	36 (65.5)	19 (34.5)			

Although we don't have nearly as strong a data base for nouns as we have for adjectives and, therefore, we cannot evaluate the effects of such factors as frequency and phonological form on repetition, what little data we have on F.S.'s performance in repeating nouns essentially mirrors that obtained with adjectives. F.S. repeated correctly 300/323 (92.9%) of the nouns when these were given as stimuli in the singular form and only 56/86 (65.1%) when given in the plural form. This result is consistent with the claim that the citation form of a word is relatively spared in comparison to other inflected forms.

The analysis of F.S.'s verb repetition performance provides a further opportunity for evaluating the hypothesis that his deficit is functionally localized in the morphological processing component of the lexicon and, more specifically, in the inflectional processing component. Over a number of sessions, F.S. was asked to repeat 757 verbs. He repeated correctly 268 (35.7%) of these stimuli. Of the 482 errors, the great majority, 345 (71.6%), were inflectional errors. The remaining errors were divided among phonemic substitutions, phonemic substitutions + substitution of the inflection, morphologically illegal substitutions of the inflection, unrelated word responses, fragments and omissions. Only 4 unambiguously derivational errors were produced by F.S. in response to a verb stimulus (0.8% of total errors).

A breakdown of verb stimuli by mood, aspect, and tense reveals that some forms were more difficult to repeat than others (see Table 8). Thus, for example, the imperfect form was more difficult to repeat than the present form in the indicative mood or the past participle form. However, as can be seen in Table 9, inflectional errors always (except for the future and conditional forms) constituted the most frequent type of error.

A stimulus-response matrix for those verb forms with a reasonably large representation in the stimulus set is shown in Table 10. This table shows the probability of producing a response (whether or not correct) of the same form as the stimulus (i.e., given a verb in the present form (e.g., 'Temo' (I fear)) the response is in the present form (e.g., 'temo,' correct, or 'temi' (you fear), 'teme' (he fears), 'temiamo' (we fear), 'temete' (you fear; pl.) or 'temono' (they fear)). The present and past participle are the best preserved, while the imperfect and (simple) past tense are the most impaired verb forms. It is worth noting that there is no indication in the data for preservation of the mood feature of a verb; for example, a verb in the indicative voice, say the imperfect, is not more likely to be repeated as another indicative form, say the (simple) past tense, than a verb form in another mood, say in the infinitival form. It is also worth stressing that unlike nouns and adjectives where the inflectional ending is just a single phoneme (e.g., *mel-a* (apple, f.sg.)), verbal inflections can consist of a single or a series of phonemes (e.g., *am-a* (he loves; present), *am-are* (to love; infinitival), *am-ato* (loved; past participle), *am-assero* (that they loved; subjunctive), *am-erebbero* (they would love; conditional), and so forth). Thus, inflectional errors for verb forms with the longer inflections will necessarily involve multiple-phoneme changes. As can be seen from Table 10, F.S. produced very many such multiple phoneme substitutions. This result is important, because it conclusively demonstrates that inflectional substitutions cannot merely be attributed to chance phoneme-substitution errors (as opposed to inflectional errors). Thus, consider as an example the following error: sping*a* (that he pulls) → sping*ono* (they pull). Here the change involves substituting one phoneme and adding two more. Phonological errors involving multiple phoneme

Table 9. Distribution of the errors made by F.S. in repeating verb forms.*

	Correct	Inflectional	Inflectional Plus[a]	Total Inflectional	Others[c]
Indicative					
Present (n=211)	101 (47.9)	72 (34.1)	10 (4.7)	82 (38.9)	28 (13.2)
Imperfect (n=153)	34 (22.2)	100 (65.4)	6 (3.9)	106 (69.3)	13 (8.5)
Past Tense (n=64)	12 (18.7)	41 (64.1)	3 (4.7)	44 (68.6)	8 (12.5)
Future (n=31)	9 (29.0)	3 (9.7)	2 (6.4)	5 (16.1)	17 (54.9)
Total (n=459)	156 (34.0)	216 (47.0)	21 (4.6)	237 (51.6)	66 (14.4)
Subjunctive (n=29)	2 (6.9)	21 (72.4)	1 (3.4)	22 (75.8)	5 (17.3)
Conditional (n=6)	(0)	2 (33.3)	1 (16.7)	3 (50.0)	3 (50.0)
Participle					
Present (n=2)	(0)	2(100.0)	(0)	2(100.0)	(0)
Past (n=125)	52 (41.6)	54 (43.2)	6 (4.8)	58 (48.0)	13 (10.4)
Gerund (n=12)	9 (75.0)	(0)	(0)	(0)	3 (25.0)
Infinitive (n=83)[b]	40 (48.2)	29 (34.9)	1 (1.2)	30 (36.1)	13 (15.7)
Ambiguous (n=35)[b]	9 (25.7)	23 (65.7)	2 (5.7)	25 (71.4)	1 (2.9)

* Percentages are in parentheses.

[a] incorrect responses that contain an inflection substitution error, resulting in a non-permissible combination of root + inflection (e.g., resistere (to resist) → resistivo (nonword)), and incorrect responses that contain a substituted inflection + a substituted root (e.g., testare (to test) → distate (to be distant, ind.pres.2nd pl., or past participle, f.pl.)), or a substituted inflection + phonologically-related pseudoroot (e.g., fiatavi (you were breathing) → fiafare (nonword))

[b] verb forms that cannot be unambiguously identified (e.g., tirate (to pull), ind.pres.2nd pl., or past part. f.pl.; esclusi (to exclude), ind.past.1st. sg., or part.past., m.pl.

[c] includes all the remaining incorrect (word and nonword) response types listed in Table 3

Table 10. Stimulus-response matrix of the errors made by F.S. in repeating verb forms of some verb tenses.*

	Indicative Present	Indicative Imperfect	Indicative Past Tense	Infinitive	Past Participle	Ambiguous**	Other Verb Forms	Total
Indicative Present	152 (87.9)	1 (0.6)	3 (1.7)	6 (3.4)	9 (5.2)	1 (0.6)	1 (0.6)	173 (100)
Indicative Imperfect	11 (8.2)	50 (37.3)	1 (0.7)	37 (27.6)	20 (14.9)	13 (9.7)	2 (1.5)	134 (100)
Indicative Past Tense	5 (9.4)	2 (3.8)	20 (37.8)	8 (15.1)	9 (17.0)	5 (9.4)	4 (7.5)	53 (100)
Infinitive	6 (8.7)	6 (8.7)	(0)	40 (58.0)	12 (17.4)	5 (7.2)	(0)	69 (100)
Past Participle	5 (4.8)	4 (3.9)	1 (1.0)	10 (9.6)	77 (74.0)	7 (6.7)	(0)	104 (100)
TOTAL	179 (33.6)	63 (11.8)	25 (4.7)	101 (18.9)	127 (23.8)	31 (5.8)	7 (1.3)	533 (100)

* Percentages are in parentheses.

** This category includes incorrect verb responses that cannot be unambiguously assigned to one of the other response categories (e.g., lavavi (you were washing) → lavate (you wash, indicative present, 2nd plural, or washed, past participle, f.pl.)).

substitutions, additions, or deletions which resulted in the production of nonwords (e.g., *tem-o* (I fear) → *tem-elo* or *tem-aro*, where *elo* and *aro* are *not* legal affixes) as opposed to inflectional errors were *not* found in the corpus of errors.

b. Nonword repetition

In order to assess nonlexical processing mechanisms in repetition, we asked F.S. to repeat 283 nonwords, randomly interspersed with words. F.S. performed very poorly in this task. He repeated correctly only 28/283 (9.9%) nonwords. There was no clear effect of stimulus length on performance: 11/101 (10.9%) correct versus 17/182 (9.3%) correct, for short (4 to 6 phonemes) and long (7 to 9 phonemes) nonwords, respectively. The absence of a length effect should not be given undue weight, however, since performance may have been too poor (floor effect) for drawing strong implications from these data. F.S.'s performance in nonword repetition clearly reflects major damage to phonological processes, either at the input or output level, but most likely at both levels.

Interim summary

The results we have reported to this point paint a coherent picture. F.S. presents with morphological processing difficulties both in spontaneous speech and single-word repetition. These difficulties are certainly compounded by a moderate deficit in phonological processing (as is indicated by nonword repetition performance) but are not reducible to a phonological processing disorder. The strongest evidence against such a possibility is the patterned nature of the inflectional errors produced by F.S. in the repetition task. The pattern of inflectional errors is explicable by appeal to morphological and not phonological principles of the language. On these grounds it is reasonable to conclude that the morphological errors produced by F.S. in spontaneous speech and in repetition are properly characterized as resulting from damage to a morphological processing mechanism. Furthermore, since F.S. produced inflectional errors not only in spontaneous speech but also in single-word repetition, we are justified in entertaining the parsimonious hypothesis that damage to the inflectional component of the lexical system is the common source of damage for both forms of impairment.

The preliminary conclusion we have reached here identifies as the most probable locus of functional damage the inflectional component of the output lexicon. However, as already noted, F.S. also presents with phonological processing difficulties. Some of these difficulties clearly involve speech production mechanisms as indicated by his performance in spontaneous speech. We have argued that such a deficit cannot be the basis for the morphological errors in spontaneous speech or repetition. By the same token neither could a deficit in processing the auditory input serve as the basis for the morphological errors in repetition. But, rather than relying just on argument to draw this latter conclusion, we assessed F.S.'s ability to process auditory inputs.

Auditory processing

F.S.'s auditory processing ability was first evaluated through a lexical decision task. The lexical decision test consisted of 560 items, equally divided between words and nonwords. Half of the words (N=140) were verbs, the remaining 140 words belonged to the other grammatical classes (nouns: N=78; adjectives: N=33; functors: N=29). Two sets of nonwords, exactly matched in length to the word stimuli were used for this task. The first set consisted of 140 stimuli. Half of the nonwords in this set (N=70) were "morphologically legal," that is, they could be morphologically decomposed into a real root and a real inflection; the remaining 70 nonword stimuli in this set were exactly matched to the other nonword stimuli in length and in degree of similarity to real words, but could not be morphologically parsed into a verb root and a verb inflection. Nonwords in the second set (N=140) were matched in length to the nonwords in the first set, and were all of the "morphologically non-decomposable" type. An example of the "morphologically decomposable" nonword stimuli is *veneva*, resulting from the root *ven-* ('venire,' to come), with the non-permissible inflection *-eva* (legal for verbs like *volere* (to want)--*voleva*, he was wanting). The corresponding non-decomposable stimulus is *voreda*, which contains neither a verb root nor a verbal inflection.

F.S. performed relatively well on this task: He produced 11/280 (3.9%) false rejections on words, and 7/280 (2.5%) false alarms on nonwords. F.S. incorrectly rejected as nonwords 1/78 (1.3%) nouns, 1/33 (3.0%) adjectives, 0/29 functors and 9/140 (6.4%) verbs, and, he incorrectly accepted as words 2/70 (2.9%) decomposable nonwords, 0/70 matched non-decomposable nonwords, and 5/140 (3.6%) 'other' nonwords.

F.S.'s performance on this test demonstrates that he can reliably (though not flawlessly) distinguish words from nonwords. However, his good performance in a lexical decision test does not say much about the nature of the information that is available to him upon the presentation of a word stimulus. For example, even though he might be able to say that *chiamavo* (I was calling) is a word, he may do so on the basis of incomplete information about the input string (i.e., based on the recognition of the root morpheme and the presence of an unspecified, but permissable suffix). In order to obtain more information on this issue, an auditory, same-different judgment task was administered.

Same-Different auditory judgment task

F.S. was presented with 428 pairs of verbs: Half of the pairs consisted of the same stimulus; the remaining pairs consisted of different verb forms. Two lists of "different" pairs were constructed. In one list (N=107), verbs differed by one phoneme in the root morpheme part of the word; in the other list (N=107) they differed by one phoneme in the suffix part. Different verb pairs were matched across lists, so as to include the same phoneme contrasts. So, for example, the first list included items like spara (he shoots) - spira (he dies), or like compativo (I was pitying) - comparivo (I was appearing). The corresponding stimuli in the second list would be speri (you hope) - spera (he hopes), or spezzare (to break) - spezzate (broken; f.sg.). One of the two verbs used in each different pair was used to construct "same" pairs. The stimuli included in the two sets of "same" and "different" pairs were matched for length and frequency. The 428 pairs were presented in random order. The examiner read aloud the first verb. The patient was then invited to count aloud backwards from 4 to 0 (which usually took F.S. more than 5 seconds). Subsequently, the examiner pronounced the second stimulus and the patient was invited to say whether the two stimuli he had heard were "same" or "different."

F.S. made 12/214 (5.6%) errors on "same" pairs and 14/214 (6.5%) errors on "different" pairs. He made the same number of errors on pairs that differed in the root morpheme and on pairs that differed in the suffix (7/107, 6.5%). Although not perfect, F.S.'s performance on this test is quite good.

Some of the verbs used in the "same-different" auditory judgment task were included in a repetition test (N=200). Compared to his good performance in the former task, the performance obtained by F.S. in repetition was extremely poor: He repeated correctly only 74 (37.0%) verb stimuli. Out of 126 errors, he produced, as usual, a very high number of substitutions of inflections (94/126; 74.6%). The remaining errors were phonologically similar nonword responses (21/126; 16.7%), or substitutions of a phonologically related word for the correct target (e.g., *rimango* (I remain) → *rimando* (I postpone)) (9/126; 7.0%). F.S. also produced 1 semantic substitution (*giurero* (I will swear) → *giudice* (judge)), and failed to produce any response in one case.

Taken together, the results obtained by F.S. in the auditory lexical decision task and in the auditory "same-different" judgment task (especially when considered in light of performance on the repetiton task in which some of the stimuli used in the "same-different" judgment task were included), rule out the possibility that the patient's repetition disorder is merely the consequence of a reduced ability to process morphologically complex input strings under auditory presentation.

DISCUSSION

Although the pattern of language dysfunction in our patient is complex and, therefore, unlikely to be the result of damage to a single processing mechanism, there are aspects of his performance which can sustain conclusions specifically about the structure of the lexical system. Our discussion will focus on this latter issue. But, first, a brief summary of the major features of F.S.'s language and cognitive performance that are relevant to questions about lexical processing.

There are four major features of F.S.'s performance that are relevant to our discussion: First, there is the fact that F.S.'s spontaneous speech is characterized by morphological errors which involve the substitution of inflectional affixes and the substitution or omission of free-standing grammatical markers; second, the patient's spontaneous speech and repetition of sentences and single words contain phonological errors (phonemic paraphasias); third, his markedly impaired single-word repetition performance results most frequently in inflectional errors; and, fourth, even though F.S.'s auditory/perceptual processing ability is not intact, the nature of this particular impairment does not appear to be quantitatively nor qualitatively of the sort that could account for the qualitative and quantitative features of his repetition disorder. The overall pattern of results we have described suggests as the functional locus of damage the morphological processing component of the lexicon. We elaborate on this conclusion below. There are three issues we wish to take up here: We will argue that damage to nonlexical phonological processes cannot account for the pattern of morphological errors produced by our patient; we will consider the possibility that the morphological errors in spontaneous speech and in single-word repetition have a common source; and, we will discuss the pattern of repetition errors in relation to claims about the organization of the lexicon and, in particular, the morphological processing component.

Phonological deficit and morphological errors

There is no doubt that F.S. has damage at some level of phonological processing. His almost total inability to repeat nonwords indicates a deficit in processing segmental phonology. Furthermore, a nonnegligible proportion of repetition errors for word stimuli can confidently be attributed to a phonological impairment since these errors involved phonemic transformations of a to-be-repeated word (e.g., 'pagata' (paid, past part., f.sg.) → 'pagara' (nonword); 'avverte' (he warns) → 'averre' (nonword)). A similar conclusion can be reached for some of the errors in spontaneous production (e.g., 'divertimento' (amusement) → 'diritimento' (nonword)). An important characteristic of these errors is that the locus of phonological transformation was as likely to be the root as the affixal part of a word, as might be expected if the determining factor for these errors were to be non-morphologically-based. One issue that cannot be resolved with the available data on this patient is the extent to which an auditory/perceptual processing deficit contributes to phonological errors. Although it is entirely possible that a proportion of the phonological errors in repetition reflect misperception of the stimuli, it must, nonetheless, be the case that the patient has a phonological disorder at the production level since phonological errors also occurred in spontaneous speech. Thus, the most conservative conclusion we can reach is that F.S. may have a processing deficit for segmental phonology both at the perceptual and production levels.

The critical issue here, however, is whether or not such a deficit could account for the putative morphological errors produced by our patient. In the Results section we argued against this possibility. There are several arguments that can be offered for this position. First, the nature of the perceptual deficit in our patient is not commensurate with the extent and type of morphological errors produced by F.S. in the repetition task. And, in any case such a deficit is irrelevant to the production of morphological errors in spontaneous speech. Second, if we were to adopt the position that it is a phonological production deficit that is responsible for the putative morphological errors, we would be hard pressed to explain the patterned nature of the inflectional errors obtained with nouns and adjectives. Recall that the inflectional errors produced by F.S. were not distributed randomly among the various inflectional endings but appear to follow a specific pattern--the production of the singular form of nouns and the singular masculine form of adjectives (the citation forms for these two word-classes, respectively) were much better preserved than other inflectional forms. And, finally, the great majority of morphological errors were inflectional, even when a stimulus was unambiguously a derived word. It is unclear how a nonlexical deficit hypothesis could account for this pattern of morphological errors. We must conclude, therefore, that the putative morphological errors are, afterall, really morphological errors.

On the Possible Relationship Between Morphological Errors in Spontaneous Speech and Single-Word Repetition

The second issue we would briefly like to consider is the possibility that the morphological errors in F.S.'s spontaneous production and in single-word repetition have a common basis. This issue cannot be resolved unambiguously given the available data, but its consideration is instructive. There are at least three possible accounts we can give for the co-occurrence of morphological errors in spontaneous production and single-word repetition. We briefly discuss these below.

One possibility is that these two types of errors arise from damage to *distinct* functional mechanisms: Damage to a syntactic processing mechanism accounts for the impairment in spontaneous production and damage to the morphological component of the lexicon accounts for the single-word repetition impairment. If we were to adopt this position, we would have to hypothesize a fairly specific form of damage to the syntactic component of the language production system (the S-structure level in current syntactic (transformational) theory (e.g., Chomsky, 1981), or the Positional level in Garrett's (1980) model of sentence production). That is, the hypothesized deficit would have to be restricted to just those morphosyntactic features of S-structure that govern selection of inflectional affixes, determiners, prepositions and auxiliaries which appear to be most severely impaired in our patient. However, subordinating conjunctions, which presumably are also selected at the S-structure level, are relatively unaffected. Indeed, the syntactic complexity of our patient's speech as indexed by the ratio of main to subordinate clauses does not differ from that of a normal control subject (see Table 2). Thus, F.S.'s speech contained constructions such as the following:

```
           la                faccio
Poi io ascolto il televisione o poi fare il pranzo
Then I listen the (m.sg.) TV (f.sg.) or then to make (infin.) the lunch
Then I watch TV or then make lunch
```

vivo
perché, caro dottore, io *vive* solo!
because, dear doctor, I lives alone!
because, dear doctor, I lives alone!

C'era un processo che c'era questo professore
There was a trial that there was this professor
There was a trial where this professor was

interessava
perché [era] una perizia per un omicidio che *interessa* me.
because [it was] a consult for a murder that interests (pres.,1sg.) me
because a consult for a murder that interests me.

Although this Dual Deficit Hypothesis is logically possible, it is unparsimonious and fails to capture an important similarity in the types of morphological errors produced by the patient in spontaneous sentence production and single-word repetition.

Another possibility is that damage to only the morphological component of the lexicon is responsible both for the morphological errors in spontaneous sentence production and for the morphological errors in single-word repetition. This hypothesis can readily account for the presence of inflectional errors in both types of tasks. However, we are forced to make a strong assumption about the kind of information represented in the morphological component of the lexicon in order to account for the substitution and omission of free-standing grammatical markers. Since F.S. omitted or substituted these latter items in spontaneous production, a unitary hypothesis of the locus of functional damage for spontaneous production and single-word repetition would have to assume that free-standing grammatical markers and inflectional affixes are represented in a common subcomponent of the lexicon as proposed by Caramazza, et al. (1985). However, whether or not this assumption can be given independent linguistic motivation is unclear (but see Kean, 1977).[3]

The third possibility is that the morphological errors in spontaneous sentence production result from damage to both a syntactic processing mechanism *and* the morphological component of the lexicon, while the morphological errors in single-word repetition result from damage to the lexicon alone. This hypothesis could easily be the correct one, but it is also the least interesting because it is the most difficult to disconfirm. Unless there is a principled way for distinguishing the relative contribution, both quantitatively and qualitatively, of damage to the syntactic and morphological processing components, this complex hypothesis about the underlying cause of the patient's impairment in spontaneous speech is not especially illuminating.

Despite our inability to decide which of the three hypotheses of the locus (loci) of functional damage best accounts for our patient's morphological errors in spontaneous sentence production and single-word repetition, we can, at least, draw a firm conclusion about one issue--we must postulate a deficit to the lexicon in order to account for the morphological errors produced by the patient in the single-word repetition tasks.

The difficulty we encountered in our effort to provide a general account of all the morphological errors (i.e., both in spontaneous production and repetition) produced by our patient illustrates the futility of certain efforts to provide a motivated explanation of clinically-defined disorders such as agrammatism, paragrammatism, deep dyslexia, and the like. The correct explanation of the basis for a pattern of language dysfunction depends crucially on a reasonable characterization of the structure of the impaired performance (see Badecker & Caramazza, 1985; Caramazza, 1986, for discussion). This task is hard enough for extensively-studied, individual patients (such as the present case, for example); it requires, at the very least, a proper characterization of a patient's relevant performance. When one seeks to provide an explanation of ill-defined categories such as "agrammatism," it is not clear whether such an effort is meaningful: Categories of this latter sort reflect groupings based either on theoretically arbitrary features of language or empirically indefensible abstractions; in either case, the sought for explanation of the clinically-defined disorder contributes neither to the development of a theory of normal language processing nor to an understanding of the nature of language disorders.

The Dissociation of Inflectional and Derivational Morphology

F.S.'s performance in the single-word repetition task is unambiguous in at least two respects: First, the great majority of errors were morphologically -based, and, second, there is a striking dissociation between inflectional and derivational morphology in repetition errors. Of the total corpus of repetition errors (N=893) for which a morphological error was possible, the great majority (637; 71.2%) were morphologically based. Crucially, however, these errors were almost all (96.7%) inflectional.

It is our contention that these results support a model of the lexicon in which lexical items are represented in morphologically decomposed form. However, before discussing this possibility in any detail we wish to discuss several alternative accounts, of varying degrees of plausibility, which may be offered as explanations for the results we have reported.

One rather implausible account, as a full explanation of the reported results, is based on the assumption of a phonological processing deficit--both at the input and output levels. On this account, the patient misperceives the stimulus and produces a phonologically similar response. This explanation will simply not do on several counts. First, it is completely silent on the presence of morphological errors in spontaneous production where an input phonological disorder is irrelevant. Second, it fails to account for the distribution of errors--of the total corpus of repetition errors that resulted in word responses (N=659), the vast majority were morphological errors (N=636; 96.5%). It is difficult to imagine how a strictly perceptual/phonological deficit (or, output phonological deficit, for that matter) could explain this distribution of errors. And, third, a direct test of the patient's ability to perceptually discriminate phonologically similar word stimuli failed to reveal a significant impairment in input phonological processing. This is not to say, of course, that F.S. does not have a phonological processing impairment--*vide* his phonemic paraphasic errors in repetition. However, this deficit fails to account for the patterned nature of the repetition errors where inflectional errors were the most conspicuous. And, within this class of errors there was further structure explicable along morphological and not phonological principles--e.g., the distribution of errors for adjectives. In sum, although F.S. most likely has a deficit in phonological processing, this deficit is in addition to some other deficit that is responsible for the morphological errors (most of them, at least) in repetition and spontaneous production.

A second explanation, not based on the assumption of morphological decomposition, which may be offered as an account of the reported pattern of results assumes an impairment in lexical retrieval from the phonological output lexicon. On this account, the patient computes the correct meaning of the stimulus word, but this semantic representation fails to activate the correct phonological representation in the output lexicon and instead activates a semantically related word. This unadorned explanation is completely inadequate on the face of it--it fails to account for the distribution of inflectional versus derivational errors; and, within the class of inflectional errors, it fails to explain the preference for the citation form of nouns and adjectives. Furthermore, this hypothesis of the nature of the impairment in F.S. would predict the massive presence of semantic paraphasic errors, errors that were virtually nonexistent in the corpus collected.

A more plausible version of this hypothesis may be offered. This hypothesis--the Satellite Hypothesis--will have to assume a richer

A. Caramazza

structure for the phonological output lexicon, although still not assuming morphological decomposition. This hypothesis is based on a related proposal by Lukatela, Gligorijevic', Kostic' and Turvey (1980) for word recognition. The basic proposal is that lexical entries are organized about a central lexical form (the nominative case in Serbo-Croatian). It is not clear what would be the corresponding organization in Italian where nouns are not case-inflected. Nonetheless, we could make one of two assumptions: either that all morphologically (derivationally and inflectionally) related words cluster about a major lexical form (Satellite Hypothesis I) or, alternatively, that there is a family of clusters where each cluster consists of inflectionally related forms (Satellite Hypothesis II). In the former case we would cluster together nouns, adjectives, verbs, and adverbs with the same root form (e.g., blame: *colpa* (N); *colpevole* (Adj.); *colpevolizzare* (V); *colpevolizzazione* (N); *colpevolmente* (Adv.); etc.; and related inflected forms); in the latter case, each syntactic category of a lexical family would be represented independently in a subcluster (e.g., blame: *colpa* (N.sing.) and *colpe* (N.pl.) would be represented separately from *colpevole* (Adj.sing.) and *colpevoli* (Adj.pl.)). Figures 3 and 4 graphically represent these alternative Satellite Hypotheses.

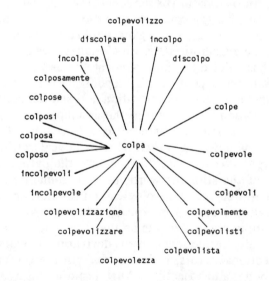

Figure 3. Schematic representation of Satellite Hypothesis I.

It is immediately apparent that Satellite Hypothesis I cannot provide a motivated account for the results we have reported. In this hypothesis no distinction is made among various inflectional and derivational forms of a word and, therefore, errors should not reflect morphological structure, contrary to the results we have obtained.

Satellite Hypothesis II is superficially more interesting. This hypothesis incorporates in the organization of the lexicon the basic distinction between derivational and inflectional morphology: Each subcluster represents inflectional variants of the base and derived forms of a word. To retrieve a specific lexical form (e.g., *colpevoli*) one must enter a lexical cluster through the designated entry point--*colpa* in the example considered here. Even a brief consideration of how this retrieval process might work reveals immediately that this Satellite Hypothesis is forced to make assumptions as strong as those made by the Morphological Decomposition Hypothesis without any of the advantages of this latter hypothesis.

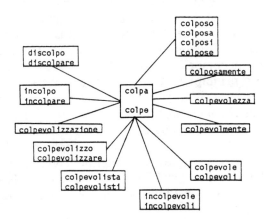

Figure 4. Schematic representation of Satellite Hypotheses II. (Verb paradigms are abbreviated by reporting only the Indicative Present 1st person and the infinitive, e.g., incolpo, incolpare.)

Lexical retrieval within the Satellite Hypothesis II requires that the semantic representation of a word specify three independent sets of semantic values: one for the root morpheme which specifies the entry point for a lexical cluster (ROOT SEMANTICS); one for the derivational affix which specifies the appropriate subcluster within a lexical cluster (DERIVATIONAL AFFIX SEMANTICS); and, one for the inflectional affix which specifies the particular lexical form to be retrieved (INFLECTIONAL AFFIX SEMANTICS). The semantics of a word would, then, have the following structure: [ROOT SEM.; (DER. AFFIX SEM.) INFL. AFFIX SEM.], where the material in parentheses is assumed to be an optional component. Thus, for example, the word colpevoli should have the semantic representation [(COLPA) (ADJ.) (PL.)], where COLPA is the semantic component for the root morpheme (COLP-), ADJ. is the semantic component for the selection of an adjectival affix (EVOL-), and PL. is the semantic component for the selection of the appropriate inflectional affix plural (I). Each component part of the semantic representation serves a specific role in lexical retrieval. The whole representation is needed to select a particular phonological form.

The Satellite Hypothesis II is consistent with the pattern of morphological processing impairment in our patient. To account for the reported results all we need assume is that F.S. has a selective deficit either at the level of the semantic units that specify inflectional forms in a subcluster or at the level of the inflectional forms themselves. Despite the success of this hypothesis in accounting for the reported results we contend that it should not be accorded the status of a serious alternative to the Morphological Decomposition Hypothesis. The reason for taking this position is quite compelling. Note that the Satellite Hypothesis II, in order to provide a principled means for lexical access, *de facto* includes morphological decomposition at the semantic level. However, it does not include provisions for *morphological productivity*. This hypothesis only allows access to stored phonological representations in the phonological output lexicon--it cannot produce novel, morphologically-legal forms. This limitation decisively rules out Satellite Hypothesis II as a viable alternative to the Morphological Decomposition Hypothesis (For related arguments against a morphologically nonproductive lexicon see Stemberger, 1985).

In other papers (Caramazza, Laudanna & Romani, in press; Caramazza, et al., 1985) we have argued for a morphologically decomposed structure of the lexicon on the basis of experimental results we have obtained with normal subjects, the reading performance of a dyslexic patient and various other published results with normal subjects (e.g., Burani, Salmaso & Caramazza, 1984; MacKay, 1979; Taft, 1984) and brain-damaged patients (e.g., Job & Sartori, 1984; Patterson, 1980; but see Badecker & Caramazza, 1986). F.S.'s highly selective disorder of morphological processing reported here provides one of the clearest experimental results yet in favor of the Morphological Decomposition Hypothesis for the organization of the lexicon.

An even more important implication of the reported results concerns whether or not inflectional and derivational morphology constitute independent subcomponents of the morphological processing system. The answer from F.S.'s performance would appear to be clearly affirmative-- F.S. is severely impaired in processing inflectional morphology and only mildly (if at all) impaired in processing derivational morphology. Furthermore, the patient almost never made derivational errors on words that did not contain a derivational affix, despite the fact that he made many inflectional and other errors on these words. That is, there is literally a categorical dissociation of error types: F.S. made inflectional errors on inflected words (both derived and nonderived) and occasionally derivational errors on derived words. This categorical dissociation could only occur if the two classes of affixes, inflectional and derivational, were functionally distinct. The basis for this conclusion is as follows. Let us suppose that inflectional and derivational affixes are not organized into functionally distinct subcomponents of the lexicon but, instead, constitute a single morphological component that stores together both types of affixes. If this component were to be damaged, the retrieval of morphological affixes, both inflectional and derivational, would be affected. In such a case there is no reason to expect different levels of performance for inflectional and derivational affixes. However, we found a large discrepancy in performance for inflectional and derivational affixes. Furthermore, since, on this account, the two types of affixes are "stored" in the same damaged component of the lexicon we would expect affix misselections *not* to honor the distinction between inflectional and derivational affixes. In other words, if affix x were, for whatever reason, not accessible, then some other affix, y, might be selected, independently of the morphological status of x and y. Thus, if F.S. were to be asked to repeat the adjective 'bella' (beautiful, f.sg.) we would expect him to produce errors not only like 'bello' (beautiful, m.sg.; an inflectional error) but also like 'bellezza (beauty; a derivational error). However, cross-category errors almost never occurred--affix misselections respected morphological distinctions. This means that the mechanism for selecting affix type, inflectional or derivational, must be intact in our patient and that damage is restricted to those processes that select specific affixes *within* the inflectional subcomponent of the lexicon.

The view of lexical organization that emerges from these considerations is the following. A lexical semantic representation which may take the form already discussed for the Satellite Hypothesis serves as input to the phonological output lexicon. The semantic representation is articulated into distinct parts, each part specifying different aspects of the lexical form. That is, the semantic representation includes what we have called root semantic features, derivational semantic features (where present) and inflectional semantic features. The root plus derivation semantic features jointly specify a stem plus default inflectional affix in the phonological lexicon. The default inflectional affix is the citation form of a word which we take to be the singular form for nouns, the masculine singular form for adjectives, and the infinitive form for verbs (and possibly the past participle form for verbs since this lexical form behaves differently from other verbal inflections).

The critical assumption we have made here is that although the lexicon is derivationally productive, those derived forms that have been experienced are stored in the phonological lexicon and are accessed by the root and derived semantic features directly. Novel derived forms must be computed by the application of the Derivational Processes Component. The other important assumption we have made is that the phonological form of a lexical item stored in the lexicon is the citation form. This form is transformed by the application of appropriate inflectional processes driven by the inflectional semantic features.[4] It is important to note that we assume that the phonological lexicon may store well-learned inflected forms, and certainly irregularly inflected forms.

In conclusion, we have provided the strongest yet experimental evidence for a dissociation of inflectional and derivational processes in the lexicon. These results are consistent with the model of morphological processing discussed in the *Introduction*. Specifically, our results are consistent with the view that both derivational and inflectional morphology are located in the lexicon--the Strong Lexicalist Hypothesis (e.g., Lapointe, 1979). However, our results also suggest that inflectional and derivational affixation constitute different processes (e.g., Anderson, 1982; Aronoff, 1976). The view of lexical organization that emerges from our results is well captured by the model presented in Figure 1, where we distinguish among three subcomponents of the lexicon: the Root Morpheme Component, the Derivational Processes Component, and the Inflectional Processes Component.

ACKNOWLEDGEMENTS

The research reported here was supported by NIH Grant NS23836 and a grant from the Consiglio Nazionale delle Ricerche, Italy. We thank Bill Badecker and Cristina Burani for their comments on an earlier version of this paper and Kathy Yantis for her assistance in the preparation of this manuscript. We are especially grateful to F.S. for his unfailing patience and cooperation throughout all phases of this research.

REFERENCES

Anderson, S. (1982). Where's morphology? Linguistic Inquiry, 13, 571-612.

Aronoff, S. (1976). Word formation in generative grammar. Cambridge, MA: MIT Press.

Badecker, W. & Caramazza, A. (1985). On considerations of method and theory governing the use of clinical categories in neurolinguistics and cognitive neuropsychology: The case against agrammatism. Cognition 20, 97-125.

Badecker, W. & Caramazza, A. (1986). The analysis of morphological errors in a case of acquired dyslexia. Reports of the Cognitive Neuropsychology Laboratory. The Johns Hopkins University, Baltimore, MD.

Bortolini, V., Tagliavini, C. & Zampolli, A. (1971). Lessico di frequenze della lingua italiana contemporanes. Milano: Garzanti.

Burani, C., Salmaso, D. & Caramazza, A. (1984). Morphological structure and lexical access. Visible Language, 18, 342-352.

Butterworth, B. (1983). Lexical representation. In B. Butterworth (Ed.), Language production (Vol. 2). New York, NY: Academic Press.

Caplan, D., Keller, L. & Locke, S. (1972). Inflection of neologisms in aphasia. Brain, 95, 169-172.

Caramazza, A. (1986). On drawing inferences about the structure of normal cognitive systems from the analysis of patterns of impaired performance: The case for single-patient studies. Brain and Cognition, 5, 41-66.

Caramazza, A. & Berndt, R. S. (1985). A multicomponent deficit view of agrammatic Broca's aphasia. In M.-L. Kean (Ed.), Agrammatism, pp 21-63. Orlando, FL: Academic Press.

Caramazza, A., Laudanna, A. & Romani, C. (in press). Lexical access and inflectional morphology. Cognition.

Caramazza, A., Miceli, G., Silveri, M. C. & Laudanna, A. (1985). Reading mechanisms and the organization of the lexicon: Evidence from acquired dyslexia. Cognitive Neuropsychology, 2, 81-114.

Chomsky, N. (1981). Lectures on government and binding. Dordrecht, Netherlands: Foris Publications.

Coltheart, M. (1985). Cognitive neuropsychology and the study of reading. Attention and Performance, XI. Hillsdale, NJ: LEA.

Cutler, A. (1983). Lexical complexity and sentence processing. In G. B. Flores d'Arcais & R. J. Jarvella (Eds.), The processes of language understanding. London: John Wiley & Sons.

Dell, G. (1986). A spreading-activation theory of retrieval in sentence production. Psychological Review, 93(3), 283-321.

De Villiers, J. G. (1978). Fourteen grammatical morphemes in acquisition and aphasia. In A. Caramazza & E. B. Zurif (Eds.), Language acquisition and language breakdown: Parallels and divergences, pp 121-144. Baltimore, MD: The Johns Hopkins University Press.

Garrett, M. (1980). Levels of processing in sentence production. In B. Butterworth (Ed.), Language production (Vol.1). New York, NY: Academic Press.

Garrett, M. (1982). Production of speech: Observations from normal and pathological language use. In A. Ellis (Ed.), Normality and pathology in cognitive functions. London: Academic Press.

Gleason, J. B. (1978). The acquisition and dissolution of the English Inflectional System. In A. Caramazza & E. B. Zurif (Eds.), Language acquisition and language breakdown: Parallels and divergences, pp 109-120. Baltimore, MD: The Johns Hopkins University Press.

Goodglass, H. (1976). Agrammatism. In H. Whitaker & H. A. Whitaker (Eds.), Studies in neurolinguistics (Vol.1). New York, NY: Academic Press.

Goodglass, H. & Berko, J. (1960). Agrammatism and inflectional morphology in English. Journal of Speech and Hearing Research, 3, 257-267.

Goodglass, H., Gleason, J., Ackerman-Bernholtz, N. & Hyde, M. (1972). Some linguistic structures in the speech of a Broca's aphasic. Cortex, 8, 191-212.

Goodglass, H. & Kaplan, E. (1972). The Assessment of aphasia and related disorders. Philadelphia, PA: Lea and Febiger.

Henderson, L. (1985). Towards a psychology of morphemes. In A. W. Ellis (Ed), Progress in the psychology of language, pp 15-68 (Vol.1). London: LEA Limited.

Jackendoff, R. (1975). Morphological and semantic regularities in the lexicon. Language, 51, 639-671.

Job, R. & Sartori, G. (1984). Morphological decomposition: Evidence from crossed phonological dyslexia. The Quarterly Journal of Experimental Psychology, 36A, 435-458.

Kean, M.-L. (1977). The linguistic interpretation of aphasia syndromes: Agrammatism in Broca's aphasia, an example. Cognition, 5, 9-46.

Lapointe, S. (1979). A theory of grammatical agreement. Unpublished doctoral dissertation, University of Massachussetts, Amherst, MA.

Lapointe, S. (1985). A theory of verb from use in the speech of agrammatic aphasics. Brain and Language, 24, 100-155.

Lieber, R. (1980). On the organization of the lexicon. Unpublished MIT PhD thesis.

Lukatela, G., Gligorijevic', B., Kostic', A. & Turvey, M. T. (1980). Representation of inflected nouns in the internal lexicon. Memory and Cognition, 8, 415-423.

MacKay, D. (1979). Lexical insertion, inflection, and derivation. Journal of Psycholinguistic Research, 8, 477-498.

Matthews, P. (1974). Morphology. London: Cambridge University Press.

Morton, J. (1979). Word recognition. In J. Morton & J. Marshall (Eds.), Psycholinguistics 2: Structures and Processes. Cambridge, MA: MIT Press.

Parisi, D. & Pizzamiglio, L. (1970). Syntactic comprehension in aphasia. Cortex, 6, 204-215.

Patterson, K. (1980). Derivational Errors. In M. Coltheart, K. Patterson & J. Marshall (Eds.), Deep dyslexia. London: Routledge, Kegan and Paul.

Patterson, K. E. (1982). The relation between reading and phonological coding: Further neuropsychological observation. In A. W. Ellis (Ed.), Normality and pathology in cognitive functions. London: Academic Press.

Scalise, S. (1980). Towards an "extended" Italian morphology. Journal of Italian Linguistics, 1/2, 197-244.

Scalise, S. (1984). Generative morphology. Dordrecht, Netherlands: Foris Publications.

Selkirk, L. (1982). The syntax of words. Cambridge, MA: MIT Press.

Siegel, D. (1974). Topics in English morphology. Unpublished manuscript, MIT, Cambridge, MA.

Stemberger, J. P. (1985). An interactive activation model of language production. In A. W. Ellis (Ed.), Progress in the psychology of language, pp 143-183 (Vol. 1). London: LEA Limited.

Taft, M. (1984). Evidence for an abstract representation of word structure. Memory and Cognition, 12, 264-269.

Taft, M. (1985). The decoding of words in lexical access: A review of the morphographic approach. In D. Besner, T. Waller & G. Mackinnon (Eds.), Reading research: Advances in theory and practice (Vol.5). NY: Academic Press.

Williams, E. (1981). X features. In S. Tavakolian (Ed.), Language acquisition and linguistic theory. Cambridge, MA: MIT Press.

Appendix I: LEGEND FOR TABLES

Inflectional error: incorrect word response, consisting of the production of the correct stem + incorrect inflection.

Examples: finestr*e* (windows, f.pl.)   → finestr*a* (window, f.sg.)
                 gross*a* (big, f.sg.)   → gross*o* (big, m.sg.)
                 legg*eva* (he was reading)   → legg*ere* (to read)

Derivational error: incorrect word response, consisting of the production of the correct stem + incorrect derivational suffix, substituting for the correct inflection.

Examples: pitt*ura* (painting, noun)   → pitt*ore* (painter)
                 illus*orie* (illusory, f.pl.)   → illus*ione* (illusion)
                 pass*ando* (passing, gerund)   → pass*aggio* (passage)

Prefix omission: incorrect word response, consisting of the production of the correct stem and of the correct suffix, with omission of the prefix.

Example: *s*cambio (exchange)   → cambio (change)

Semantic substitution: incorrect word response, consisting of the production of an item semantically (but not phonologically) related to the target.

Examples: geniale (brilliant)   → un tipo originale (a character)
                 giurero' (I will swear)   → giudice (judge, noun)

Other word response: production of a word phonologically (but not semantically) related to the stimulus.

Examples: rimango (I remain)   → rimando (I postpone)
                 vieta (he prohibits)   → dieta (diet, noun)

Illegal inflection: incorrect nonword response, consisting of the production of the correct stem + incorrect inflection, present in the language, but not permissible for that particular stem.

Examples:
Stimulus   aspett*are* (you are waiting)   riemp*ito* (filled, m.sg.)
Error   aspett*iva* *   riemp*iere* *

Permissible, incorrect	aspett*ava* (he was waiting)	riemp*ire* (to fill)

Correct use of inflection	sent*iva* (he was hearing)	cogl*iere (to pick)*

Illegal derivation: incorrect nonword response, consisting of the production of the correct stem + substituted derivation, present in the language but not permissible for that stem.

Stimulus	Error	Correct instance of deriv.
autunn*ale* (autumnal) →	autunn*aio*	fior*aio* (florist)
pront*ezza* (readiness) →	pront*enza*	pot*enza* (power)

Phonological error: incorrect nonword response, phonologically related to the stimulus. It can contain the target stem only, the target inflection only, or neither (see Note).

Examples:

càdono (they fall)	→ càdote
misi (I put, past)	→ mensi
sopravvìvere (to survive)	→ sopravìsimo

Phonological error on root + substituted inflection: incorrect nonword response, consisting of the production of a pseudoroot, phonologically related to the target + an incorrect inflection.

Examples:

fiat*avi* (you were breathing)	→ fiaf*are*
cont*ato* (counted, m.sg.)	→ colt*are*

Appendix II

We briefly present some general principles of Italian inflectional morphology.

Nouns usually carry number inflection; gender is lexically determined. The most frequent ending of the masculine singular (m.sg.) is -*o*, and the corresponding plural form (m.pl.) is -*i* (e.g., cappott*o* (coat), cappott*i* (coats)); the most frequent form of the feminine singular (f.sg.) is -*a*, and the corresponding plural form (f.sg.) is -*e* (e.g., piant*a* (plant), piant*e* (plants)). Since noun gender is lexically determined, however, there are many exceptions to this general case, and the morphology of a noun is not an indicator of its gender (e.g., elefant*e* (elephant, m.sg.), elefant*i* (elephants, m.pl.); poet*a* (poet, m.sg.), poet*i* (poets, m.pl.); artist*a* (artist, m.sg. and f.sg.), artist*i* (artists, m.pl.), artist*e* (artists, f.pl.); pell*e* (skin, f.sg.); pell*i* (skins, f.pl.), etc.). Some nouns are invariable (e.g., citta' (city, f.sg., and cities, f.pl.).

Adjectives can be broadly divided in two categories. Some carry 4 different endings, corresponding to m.sg. (*-o*), m.pl. (*-i*), f.sg. (*-a*), f.pl. (*-e*)--see for example buon*o*, buon*i*, buon*a*, buon*e* (good). Other adjectives only carry 2 inflections, that mark number (sg.: *-e*; pl.: *-i*) and are ambiguous with respect to gender--see for example, fort*e* (m.sg. and f.sg.), fort*i* (m.pl. and f.pl.) (strong).

In connected speech, adjectives always agree with the name that they modify, in gender and number. The gender of the noun also determines the choice of the article (e.g., in the most typical cases, il cappott*o* ner*o* (the black coat, m.sg.), *i* cappott*i* ner*i* (the black coats, m.pl.), *la* piant*a* san*a* (the healthy plant, f.sg.), *le* piant*e* san*e* (the healthy plants, f.pl.).

Verbs have an inflectional paradigm that is much more complicated than the paradigm of either nouns or adjectives. Italian verbs belong to one of 3 conjugations. For each verb in each conjugation, Italian has 4 finite modes (indicative, subjunctive, conditional, imperative) and 3 non-finite modes (gerund, participle and infinitive). Some of the verb forms are generated by adding an inflection to the verb root; others are generated starting from a *aux + V root + past participle* structure, where *aux* can be either 'essere' (to be) or 'avere' (to have).

For forms of the first type (*V root + inflection*), within the finite modes, indicative has 4 tenses (present, imperfect, past and future), subjunctive has 2 tenses (present and imperfect), conditional and imperative each have 1 tense (present); each finite mode has 6 voices, corresponding to the 1st, 2nd and 3rd singular, and to the 1st, 2nd and 3rd plural. Within the non-finite modes, the gerund and the infinitive have one tense (present), and the participle has two (present and past). These forms are invariable, except for the past participle, which under certain conditions behaves like an adjective with four endings (e.g., "I bambini sono baciati dalla mamma" (The boys are kissed (m.pl.) by their mother; "La mamma li ha baciati" (The mother them has kissed (m.pl.)).

The forms of the second type (*aux + V root + past participle inflection*) are much less frequent in the language, but are just as numerous as the forms of the type *V root + inflection* (4 indicative tenses, 2 subjunctive and participle tenses, 1 conditional, imperative, gerund and infinitive tense).

The paradigm of the *V root + inflection* forms of the verb 'amare' (to love), a regular verb of the 1st conjugation, is reported below.

INDICATIVE

Present	Imperfect	Past	Future
am-o	am-avo	am-ai	am-ero'
(I love)	(I was loving)	(I loved)	(I will love)
-i	-avi	-asti	-erai
-a	-ava	-o'	-era'
-iamo	-avamo	-ammo	-eremo
-ate	-avate	-aste	-erete
-ano	-avano	-arono	-eranno

SUBJUNCTIVE

Present	Imperfect
am-i	am-assi
(that I love)	(that I loved)
-i	-assi
-i	-asse
-iamo	-assimo
-iate	-aste
-imo	-assero

CONDITIONAL

Present
am-erei (I would love)
-eresti
-erebbe
-eremmo
-ereste
-erebbero

IMPERATIVE

Present
am-a   (2nd sg.)
-ate (2nd pl.)
The remaining forms are borrowed
from the Subjunctive

PARTICIPLE

GERUND			INFINITIVE
Present	Present	Past	Present
am-ando	am-ante	am-ato	am-are
(loving)	(loving)	(loved,m.sg.)	(to love)

NOTES

[1] This result is somewhat surprising given the commonly accepted position that errors on this word class tend not to be phonemic substitutions. However, it must be noted that the particular sample of words used in our task consisted of bi- and polysyllabic words, unlike most of the high

frequency function words for which the claim on non-occurrence of phonemic substitutions is made.

[2] By citation form of a word, we mean that form which is considered to be basic in respect to other inflected forms. It is the form which is listed in dictionary entries and is usually given in response to questions such as "How do we say x in such and such a language?".

[3] Alternatively, we could assume that function words and inflectional affixes form distinct subcomponents of the lexicon and that both are damaged in our patient.

[4] It should be noted that, although we have emphasized how inflectional affixes are activated from the semantic component of the lexicon, these phonological forms may also be accessed directly from information specified in a syntactic frame in sentence production. That is, we assume that inflectional affixes may be accessed either through semantic or syntactically specified information depending on whether single-word or sentence production is being considered.

CHAPTER ELEVEN

THE DISRUPTION OF SENTENCE PRODUCTION:
A CASE OF SELECTIVE DEFICIT TO POSITIONAL
LEVEL PROCESSING

INTRODUCTION

Sentence production is an extremely complex process involving the construction of several types of linguistic representations by a number of independent processing mechanisms. Damage to this system will undoubtedly result in varied forms of sentence production deficits depending on the "locus" and type of damage to the system. Thus, we expect one pattern of impairment in the case where brain damage were to affect lexical processing mechanisms, another pattern were the damage to affect sentence planning mechanisms, yet another were the damage to affect working memory mechanisms, and so forth. The variety of expected patterns of sentence production impairment is, then, a function of the complexity of the normal processing system and the possible forms of damage to that system. On this uncontroversial view, and assuming 1) that the structure of the sentence production system is at least as complex as the model proposed by Garrett (1980; 1982) and 2) that the components comprising the system may be damaged differentially, we expect sentence production impairments to be of many different forms. And, yet, until very recently the only forms of sentence production impairment discussed in the aphasia literature were the classical clinical syndromes of agrammatism and paragrammatism; that is, impairments of sentence production were studied within the narrow confines of these latter clinical syndromes.

In a recent discussion of the cognitive and linguistic mechanisms that may be implicated in the complex clinical disorder of agrammatism, Caramazza and Berndt (1985; see also Goodglass & Menn, 1985; Berndt, 1987) argued that the syndrome is multiply dissociable and that, therefore, we must assume that the observed clinical picture results from damage to several autonomous processing components. This proposal contrasts with various unitary deficit accounts of the clinical syndrome--accounts that place the locus of functional deficit either at the level of a general syntactic processing component (Berndt & Caramazza, 1980; Saffran, Schwartz, & Marin, 1980), the phonological processing component (Kean,

1977), the lexical component (Bradley, Garrett, & Zurif, 1980), or a general cognitive mechanism involved in temporal control (Kolk, van Grunsven, & Keyser, 1985). Caramazza and Berndt (1985) cite in support of their proposal various patterns of language processing impairment which they interpret as reflecting the differential dysfunction of autonomous components of the sentence production system. However, an even stronger conclusion than that reached by Caramazza and Berndt is possible: There are compelling theoretical and methodological arguments (Badecker & Caramazza, 1986) and empirical observations (Miceli, Silveri, Romani, & Caramazza, in press) which undermine plausible considerations of the clinical syndrome of agrammatism as a theoretically coherent functional category. On this view there is nothing to be gained by attempting to formulate an explanatory account of the intrinsically heterogeneous clinical disorder of agrammatism. Instead, individual patterns of language production impairment--whether clinically identifiable as agrammatism, paragrammatism, or some other clinical type --may be used to constrain models of sentence production. In this paper we report an analysis of the language production impairment in a patient who may be clinically classified as an agrammatic aphasic. Her pattern of performance is interpretable as reflecting a deficit at the level at which the phrasal geometry of a sentence frame is specified (positional level in Garrett's model of sentence production).

In a series of papers Garrett (1975; 1980; 1982) has developed a highly detailed model of the sentence production process. This model, in addition to the high degree of explicitness by comparison to other psycholinguistic models, has the virtue of providing a reasonable account for the principal source of data in this domain of investigation--speech errors. Other models of sentence production (Dell, 1986; Bock, 1982) differ from Garrett's in a number of details, but they all share an important characteristic that is the focus of the present investigation. All extant models assume that there is a level of representation that specifies the surface structure of the to-be-produced sentence. This representation together with other information about the semantic content of the sentence jointly determine the selection of phonological representations from the lexical system. Thus, a distinction is made between an abstract level of representation that specifies a sentence frame with lexical slots and the phonological shapes that are selected from a phonological (or orthographic) lexicon for insertion in the appropriate slots in the sentence frame. In Garrett's model the phonologically specified sentence frame representation is referred to as the "positional level representation."

Garrett's model makes another important distinction, that between two classes of vocabularies: closed-class and open-class vocabularies. The former--closed-class vocabulary--refers to the set of free-standing and bound grammatical morphemes of the language, such as articles, auxiliaries, inflections and so forth. The other vocabulary--the open-class vocabulary--refers to the content words of the language; i.e., nouns, verbs, adjectives, and some types of adverbs.

The distinction between the two types of vocabularies corresponds to a computational distinction in the model. The selection of open-class items is made on the basis of semantic information (message level representation in Garrett's words). More specifically, meaning relations at the message representation level serve as the basis for lexical selection and the determination of functional structures which specify the relations that obtain among lexical representations. The functional level representation thus constructed serves, in turn, as the basis for the retrieval of word forms (for open-class words) and the selection of sentence planning frames. The sentence planning frames contain the necessary information for the selection of closed-class items. At this point in the process of sentence production the representation that has been constructed consists of a string of phonologically specified items--the positional level representation. For present purposes the important point to note is that there is a computational distinction between the selection of open- and closed-class items: The former are selected on the basis of semantic information, and the latter are selected on the basis of information specified in sentence planning frames; furthermore, the two classes of items are specified at distinct levels of representation.

The model of sentence production we have adopted allows (relatively) precise predictions about the possible forms of impairment in sentence production under conditions of brain damage. On the assumption that each of the components of the proposed model may be damaged selectively, there are various forms of impairment that should be observed. We expect different forms of sentence production impairment depending on whether the damage is localized to the processes that determine the construction of functional level representations, or the processes that determine the construction of positional level representations, or the lexical system, and so forth. Thus, for example, if a patient were to have selective damage localized to the mechanisms involved in processing positional level representations, we would expect the following pattern of performance: normal sentence comprehension, normal production of single words, and impaired sentence production characterized by difficulties in the selection of grammatical morphemes[1] (independently of modality of output, written or spoken)--those elements that are selected by information specified at the positional level representation in sentence production. In this paper we describe a patient whose pattern of language processing performance takes this latter form--a pattern that is explicable by assuming that she has damage localized to the positional level representation.

CASE HISTORY

M.L. is a 55 year-old, left-handed female with a 12th grade education. She previously held a clerical position with the Census Bureau. She suffered a small, right hemisphere stroke in June of 1986, resulting in mild paresis of both left extremities and mild dysarthria, but without aphasia. A CT scan at that time was normal. One month later, she suffered a new thromboembolic stroke, resulting in dense left hemiplegia, left neglect, and aphasia. A CT scan in August of the same year revealed a large infarct in the right parietal and frontal regions and right basal ganglia. Neurologic examination indicated left facial palsy, a slight decrease in the left visual field, trace to poor movement and increased tone in the left extremities, with intact tactile sensation and proprioception. It was noted that her comprehension appeared to be intact, although her speech was limited to occasional single words.

A clinical speech-language pathology evaluation in December 1986 indicated unilateral upper motor neuron involvement of cranial nerves VII, IX, and X, manifested in harsh phonation and slightly reduced range of volitional (but not reflexive) movements of the face and velum on the left side. Single word repetition showed normal articulation. M.L. responded with 100% accuracy on the auditory comprehension and naming subtests of the Boston Diagnostic Aphasia Examination (BDAE, Goodglass and Kaplan, 1972) and received a score of 35.5/36 on the Modified Token Test (DeRenzi and Faglioni, 1978). M.L. was able to recall a maximum of 6 digits forward and 3 digits backward, 6 semantically unrelated words and 6 semantically related words. She received a score of 59/60 on the Revised Boston Naming Test (Goodglass, Kaplan, & Weintraub, 1983). Spontaneous speech and repetition are described below. Persisting left neglect was evidenced in visual reproduction and direct copying of abstract designs, although direct copying of drawn objects and line cancellation tasks were within normal limits. She also showed extinction of left-sided tactile and visual stimuli with bilateral stimulation.

EXPERIMENTAL TASKS

General Methods

A variety of tasks were used to elicit verbal and written sentence production. Stimuli and instructions for each task are described in greater detail in the sections that follow. All reading stimuli were printed in large, capital, bold-face letters. Picture stimuli were black and white line drawings. Each verbal response was recorded for later transcription. The tapes were transcribed by two clinicians who were familiar with the subject for interjudge reliability measures. Written sentences were also scored independently by the two clinicians. Percent agreement between judges (number of words agreed upon/total number of words x 100) on transcription of verbal responses and written responses was 98.8% and 98.6%, respectively. Point-to-point percent agreement on grammatical accuracy was 93.8% for verbal sentences and 97.6% for written sentences.

M.L.'s oral and written sentence production ability and her ability to perform sentence anagram tasks were contrasted to her performance on grammaticality judgment, word insertion in sentence frames, and sentence comprehension tasks. Comprehension of auditory and printed sentences was assessed through sentence-picture matching tasks. Responses in testing comprehension and grammaticality judgment required pointing to printed yes/no cards. All sentences were presented face-to-face by the examiner.

"Unconstrained" Production Tasks

Oral production. The connected speech samples used for analysis included story telling (Little Red Riding Hood, Goldilocks and the Three Bears), story re-telling (free recall of the passages in the Weschler Memory Scale form I; Weschler, 1972), and picture description (the "Cookie Theft" picture from the BDAE (Goodglass & Kaplan, 1972) and the picnic picture from the Western Aphasia Battery (WAB; Kertesz, 1982)). M.L. was instructed to tell each of the stories as completely as she could remember them. For picture description tasks, she was instructed to describe "everything happening in the picture." M.L. was encouraged to speak in complete sentences. Additionally, she was cued to look at the whole picture by drawing her attention to the left side, the side of mild neglect. A transcription of each of these connected speech samples is contained in Appendix A.

The striking characteristics of M.L.'s speech are reduced phrase length and the paucity of both bound and free grammatical morphemes. The mean length of utterance (MLU) for the speech samples collected was 2.48 words (range = 1 to 4 words; S.D. = 1.13). The median phrase length was two words. Phrases were identified as utterances separated by pauses longer than 2 seconds.[2] It was not possible to analyze in detail M.L.'s speech in terms of intended morphemes, since in most instances the surface structure of her intended utterance could not be surmised from the words produced. However, several types of specific errors were evident in the transcriptions. M.L.'s omission of articles and auxiliaries was clearly evident in phrases such as, "[A] couple [is] having [a] picnic...A boy [is] flying [a] kite." (The material in square brackets was omitted by the patient.) The omission of prepositions is exemplified in the following sentence produced by M.L.: "Water [is] flowing [to/onto the] floor." Sometimes these errors were self-corrected, as in "[They] made up [a] purse her...for her." An example of her omissions of bound morphemes is found in the phrase, "[...] touch[ed] by the story." Bound morpheme errors always involved inflectional, never derivational, errors. While errors on obligatory free-standing morphemes were noted in virtually every phrase, only two errors on obligatory bound morphemes were noted in 58 utterances. M.L. also made many omission errors involving multiple word sequences, making it impossible to score a response in terms of lexical omissions. Some examples of these latter utterances are: "[...] [...] too soft," "[...] [...] just right," and "[...] [...] tired."

M.L.'s narrative speech contained a number of possible word-order errors. For example, she produced the utterances "...little girl blond" and "What are you in...grade?". Unfortunately, it could not be determined from the context whether the observed errors were truly word-order errors or the consequence of efforts to 'repair' omission errors. That is, the patient could have produced a word-order error when, as a consequence of realizing that she had omitted a word(s), she attempted to correct the error by producing the previously omitted word(s) at the point where she noted the omission. As we will see below, however, there are a few cases in other tasks where the attribution of word-order error could be made with somewhat greater confidence.

To further assess M.L.'s sentence production ability, she was asked to produce sentences incorporating specific target words. M.L. was asked to produce 60 sentences in response to 20 nouns, 20 verbs, and 20 adjectives. Her sentence production in these structured, sentence formulation tasks resembled her production in open-ended tasks. She produced only 3 (5%) complete sentences. Each of these contained four or fewer words, and was a simple, active-voice sentence (e.g., "He won his case."). Of the other 57 utterances, only 15 contained a single error; the remaining 42 utterances contained multiple errors. The types of errors she produced in this task were the same as those she produced in the story-telling and picture description tasks. Examples of each type of error produced by M.L. in utterances with a single and multiple errors follow below:

a) Omission of pronoun: "Will [...] marry me?"
b) Omission of preposition: "I went [...] school."
c) Omission of article: "I played in [...] band."

d) Inflectional error: "I've got[ten] plump."
e) Inflection & (possible) word-order errors: "Ducks...flat bill[s] have."
f) Pronoun & article omissions: "Are [...] going to [...] fair?"
g) Pronoun & preposition omissions: "Did [...] put money [...] the bank?"
h) Article & preposition omissions + (possible) word-order error: "Who is [...] girl [...] nose...big?"

M.L.'s self-initiated speech was also recorded during a one hour speech therapy session. The MLU for this sample of conversational speech was 1.48 words (range = 1 to 3 words; S.D. = O.75). The median utterance length was one word. Her self-initiated speech shows the same types of errors as described above (e.g., Pronoun & article omissions: "[...] heard on [...] radio...[...] more [...]...[...] coming tonight...more snow."; inflection, pronoun & article omissions: "[...] ask[ed] [...] question..."

A quantitative analysis of the speech errors produced by M.L. in the various sentence and narrative production tasks described thus far shows that she omitted free-standing grammatical morphemes in about 60% of scorable obligatory contexts (Table 1). Omission errors for articles, pronouns, conjunctions, and auxiliaries occurred with similar high frequency--about 63-82%. Prepositions and inflectional suffixes were omitted less frequently than other grammatical morphemes. Overall, it is clear that M.L. has extremely severe difficulties in producing the grammatical morphemes and other closed-class words needed for the normal construction of a sentence.

Written production. M.L. made frequent substitutions, deletions, insertions and transpositions of letters in writing all classes of words and nonwords in all spelling tasks (oral and written to dictation, written naming, and delayed copying). Her pattern of spelling errors, explicable by proposing selective damage to the graphemic buffer, has been described in detail elsewhere (Hillis & Caramazza, in press). However, since her misspelled words were always recognizable, it was possible to analyze her sentence construction in connected writing samples.

M.L. was presented with the "Cookie Theft" picture from the BDAE and the picnic picture from the WAB, one at a time. She was instructed to write a complete description of "everything happening in the picture," using complete sentences. There were no time constraints. Transcription of her written picture descriptions are reported in Appendix B. M.L.'s written output shows the same pattern of errors as her verbal output, including shortened phrase length and a reduction of both bound and free grammatical morphemes. As may be seen from the sample of errors shown in Appendix B, errors included clear omissions of articles, inflections, and auxiliaries (e.g.,'[...] dog [...] watch[...] [the] boy'; '[...] couple [...] having [...] picnic'). The mean length of written "phrases" in this task was 3.17 words (range = 2 to 5 words; S.D. = 0.94) The median phrase length was 3 words. Bound morpheme errors again appeared to be less frequent than obligatory free morpheme errors, and were again restricted to inflectional errors. Sixteen omissions of obligatory functors, one functor substitution, and two inflectional errors were counted. Word-order errors were also present ('The drying dishes mother is'; 'The fall stool'; 'Boy kite flying'). For these errors, unlike those recorded for the oral production task, we may rule out the hypothesis that they represent 'repairs' of omission errors, since a repair in a writing task would allow the correct spatial placement of the putatively omitted word. Thus, we may confidently state that M.L. does produce some word-order errors. As in the oral production tasks reported above, most (10/13; 76.9%) of M.L.'s phrases in written narratives contained an appropriate main verb.

Table 1. Number (and % in obligatory contexts) of M.L.'s errors in spontaneous speech.

Omissions in Obligatory Contexts		
Closed-class	108/173	(62.4)
Articles	32/51	(62.7)
Pronouns	26/36	(72.2)
Conjunctions	5/7	(71.4)
Auxiliary Verbs	14/17	(82.4)
Prepositions	13/34	(38.2)
Have/be verbs	14/24	(58.3)
Here/there adverbs	4/4	(100.0)
Open-class	3/79	(3.8)
Adjectives	1/30	(3.3)
Verbs	2/49	(4.1)
Suffixes		
Inflectional	5/27	(18.5)
Derivational	0/6	(0)
Word Substitutions		
Closed-class	4/173	(2.3)
Open-class	0/207	(0)
Total errors/total obligatory contexts	116/380	(30.5)
Possible word order errors:	2	

"Constrained" Production Tasks

The production tasks we have considered thus far pose some difficulties in scoring errors because often it is not possible to reconstruct from the fragmented utterances produced by M.L. the intended target construction.

To (partially) overcome this difficulty and to have a more direct comparison of her spoken and written production we asked M.L. to read, repeat, and write sets of sentences. Stimuli for reading and repetition tasks were drawn from a set compiled for other purposes (The Assessment of Intelligibility of Dysarthric Speech; Yorkston and Beukelman, 1981), which contains sentences selected from adult level reading materials with the following characteristics: 1) all words from among the 30,000 most frequently occurring (Thorndike & Lorge, 1944) and 2) no quotations, parentheses, proper names, quotations, hyphenated words, or numbers >10. While there was no attempt to control for sentence type, sentences varied widely in syntactic structure. Twenty 10-word sentences served as stimuli in both reading and repetition tasks. Stimuli for dictation tasks were selected from among stimuli for the reading and repetition tasks, or constructed from these sentences by deleting or replacing words longer than 6 letters with shorter words (e.g., "I had three tiny, screaming babies in my arms" was dictated as, "I had three tiny babies in my arms."). This modification was undertaken to minimize spelling errors, since we had previously documented that M.L.'s spelling performance was influenced primarily by word length.

Sentence reading. M.L. was asked to read aloud 60 sentences, 9-10 words in length. She made 65 errors (11.6% of the total set of words in the sentences), of which 47 (72.3%) were omissions of closed-class words. These errors are striking in comparison with her consistently accurate reading of closed-class words presented in isolation (see below). The distribution of her reading errors is shown in Table 2. She omitted 23.7% of the closed-class words. Substitution errors accounted for 7.6% of her total responses on closed-class words. Article omissions were the most frequent errors (26.2% of total errors). M.L.'s prosody in oral reading was identical to her prosody in spontaneous speech; she read aloud in halting, 2-3 word "phrases. A typical reading attempt follows:
Stimulus: I have to hide it, because I have young children.
Response: "I have it...hid it...you have...my...young children."
    M.L.'s ability to read connected prose was similarly impaired both in prosody and pattern of errors. M.L. read aloud a 129 word passage, "My Grandfather" (author unknown), in order to compare her reading rate to norms for non-brain damaged adults. M.L. read the passage at a rate of 33.5 syllables per minute (normal = 200-300). Oral reading yielded 22 errors: omission of 18/63 (28.6%) of the functors (81.82% of errors), 2 functor substitutions (9.09% of the errors), and 2 inflectional errors (9.09% of the errors).

Table 2. Number (and %) of M.L.'s errors in 3 production tasks.

	Oral Reading of Sentences		Repetition of Sentences		Writing of Sentences	
Word omissions						
Closed class	47/198	(23.7)	38/139	(27.3)	20/49	(40.8)
articles	17/41	(41.5)	14/29	(48.3)	6/11	(54.5)
pronouns	11/40	(27.5)	6/31	(19.4)	4/13	(30.8)
conjunctions	5/19	(26.3)	6/15	(40.0)	1/2	(50.0)
auxiliary verbs	7/32	(21.9)	5/21	(23.8)	1/5	(20.0)
prepositions	5/30	(16.7)	4/19	(21.1)	6/9	(66.7)
have/be verbs	2/30	(6.7)	3/21	(14.2)	2/7	(28.6)
Open class	1/362	(0.3)	2/191	(1.0)	0/44	(0)
adjectives	1/63	(1.6)	2/41	(4.9)	0/9	(0)
Suffix errors						
inflectional	2/82	(2.4)	1/58	(1.7)	1/7	(14.3)
derivational	0/45	(0)	0/24	(0)	0/0	(0)
Word substitutions						
closed class	15/198	(7.6)	10/139	(7.2)	2/49	(4.1)
open class	0/362	(0)	2/191	(1.0)	0/44	(0)
Total word errors	65/560	(11.6)	53/330	(16.1)	23/93	(24.7)
Possible word- order errors:	2		2		2	
Total errors	67		55		26	

M.L. was also presented with 100 printed sentences, and asked to select "the word or words that would best complete the sentence." Responses required article distinctions, pronoun-number distinctions, inflectional distinctions, or pronoun-gender distinctions. Examples follow:
   a) The man chopped down (the, a) trees.
   b) The horse will (jump, jumps) the fence.
   c) Joe has (skipped, skips) his breakfast.
Although her responses were often quite slow (>60"), she produced only one error in 100 responses in this task. Her spontaneous oral reading revealed that the one error she produced could be attributed to her left neglect--it is possible that she failed to process the initial words, "the boys," making "his" an appropriate response in the remaining context (Stimulus: The boys packed (their, his) lunch for school; Response: Selected the word "his," then read aloud, "Packed his lunch...school.")
Sentence repetition. M.L. was asked to repeat ten 5-word, ten 8-word, and twenty 10-word sentences. M.L.'s repetition of sentences showed the same types and general distribution of errors as in her spontaneous speech and sentence reading. The distribution of M.L.'s errors in repeating sentences is shown in Table 2. Only 3 (15%) of the 10-word sentences, 2 (20%) of the 8-word sentences, and 4 (40%) of the 5-word sentences were repeated without error. She made errors on 16.1% (55/330) of the words. Her sentence repetition attempts were slow and halting. As in her reading

performance, functor omissions predominated (69.1%, or 38/55 of her total errors), but 12 word substitutions (21.8% of her errors, of which 10 were functor substitutions) and 2 (possible) word-order errors (3.6% of errors) were also present, as shown in the following example:

Stimulus: The journeys we took were often long and very strenuous.
Response: [ ] journeys we took...[ ] often ....often strenuous ...[ ] long.

Occasional inflectional errors, but no derivational errors, were observed.

Sentence writing. Because of her discomfort in writing with her right, non-dominant hand, M.L. wrote to dictation only fifteen sentences, 6 to 8 words in length. No sentence was produced fully accurately. As in repetition and oral reading of sentences, the most common errors were omission of closed-class words (76.9%, or 20/26 of her total errors), and of articles (one-third of functor omissions), in particular. She omitted 40.8% (20/49) of the function words, including 54.5% (6/11) of the articles, and 30.8% (4/13) of the pronouns in dictated sentences (Table 2). Functor substitutions and inflectional errors accounted for 2 (7.7%) and 1 (3.8%) of her 26 errors, respectively. M.L. also produced some word-order errors (11.5%, or 3 of her 26 errors). Two examples of these errors are the following:

Stimulus: Fill the big dish with apples.
Response: Fill dish big apples.
Stimulus: The girl was hit by the boy.
Response: The was girl was hit boy by the.

M.L. was also given 30 incomplete printed sentences and instructed to write a word or words to form a complete sentence. In this task she produced similar errors to those described above when the responses required production of functors. When responses required closed-class word responses, her performance was 66.7% (10/15) accurate. For instance, the stimulus "The butcher put the knife ---" elicited "table." When the sentence completion tasks required single open-class word responses, M.L.'s performance was 100% (15/15) accurate.

Single word production tasks

Reading. On The Johns Hopkins University Dyslexia Battery, M.L. made 6 errors in reading aloud 326 single words. All incorrect responses were visual errors at the beginning of words (e.g., germ → term; glove → love), consistent with mild left neglect (Kinsbourne & Warrington, 1962). It is important to note that M.L. read correctly all isolated functors (N=40) on this test and on an additional list of 140 words counterbalanced for grammatical word class, frequency, and letter length.

Repetition. M.L. was asked to repeat 170 prefixed, suffixed, and unaffixed words (including 40 functors) and 100 nonwords. Her performance in this single-item repetition task was flawless. She was also able to repeat accurately series of up to six unrelated words.

Writing. M.L.'s writing performance on single words was the focus of detailed analysis in a different context (see Hillis & Caramazza, in press). For the purpose of this study, it is important to note that she spelled closed-class words at least as well as open-class words (and relatively better than most closed-class words, since functors tend to be short). On a list controlled for length and word frequency, she spelled correctly to dictation 21.4% (6/28) of the nouns, 28.6% (8/28) of the verbs, and 25.0% (7/28) of the adjectives. Similarly, she spelled 35.0% (7/20) of the dictated functors accurately. Nearly all of her responses were phonologically implausible nonwords, with 1 or a few grapheme errors (mostly at the beginnings of words--on the left side). There were no functor substitutions or morphological errors. On all functors, and open-class words, written spelling errors consisted of deletions (e.g., only → nly; before → efore; shall → sall; happen → hppen; absent → bsent), substitutions (e.g., happy → fappy), transpositions (e.g., about → aoubt; circle → cricle), insertions (could → clould; greet → gereet), or combinations of these (e.g., since → scnnce; threat → hreat). Comparable error rates and types of errors were produced for nonwords (e.g., murnee → rmnee; doncept → dncept). M.L.'s spelling performance was not affected by type of task: types and rates of errors were comparable across writing to dictation, oral spelling (e.g., faith → aith), and delayed copying (e.g., through → trogh). We have interpreted these errors as resulting from degradation of the graphemic representation of the word in the graphemic buffer, with a possible contribution of her left neglect reflected in the distribution of errors as a function of letter position within words.

Interim summary

M.L.'s performance in the various production tasks reveals that she has major difficulties in producing grammatically complete sentences. This difficulty is not restricted to a single modality of output, spoken or written, nor to a single modality of input for production--M.L. presented with severe difficulties whether the task involved spontaneous production, reading, repeating, or writing to dictation. By contrast to this severe difficulty in sentence production, involving primarily the production of closed-class words (but also some difficulties with word-order), M.L. appears to have no particular differential difficulty in processing single functors or inflected words, nor does she appear to present with comprehension difficulties when assessed with clinical instruments (BDAE and the Modified Token Test). These results suggest the conclusion that M.L. has selective damage at some level of sentence planning. To further document the observed dissociation we administered to M.L. a set of more demanding comprehension tasks as well as a sentence anagram task.

Sentence anagram and comprehension tasks

Sentence anagram. M.L. was presented with a scrambled set of printed words on separate cards. She was instructed to form a complete sentence using all of the cards. No time limit was set for each anagram. The target responses were ten sentences, four to seven words in length, of varied syntactic structure. She correctly sequenced only one sentence. She succeeded in producing this five-word sentence in 2'55", by attempting numerous possible combinations of the words in the anagram. On eight of the nine remaining trials, she was aware that her final response was inaccurate, but presented the sequences in Table 3 as her "best effort" after 2'2" to 4'41" (mean = 2'33"; S.D. = 38.9"; median = 2'26"). Several of these "best" responses revealed an apparent attempt to structure agent-action-object forms, along with severe difficulties in properly ordering function words. The tenth trial was ended when the patient stated that she was unable to form a reasonable response.

Table 3. M.L.'s responses in anagram task.

```
I AROUND WALKED TRACK THE A MILE
NEW THE ROBBER TURNED A LEAF
YOUR SHE IS FRIEND
DAUGHTER HER WERE WASHED BY THE DISHES.
THE MAN DRINKING IS COFFEE.
WAITER POURED WINE WAS BY THE
THE DOG BROWN MEAN THE CAT CHASED
THE TEENAGER WAS SKIPPED THE CLASS BY
YOU EAT WHEN DO YOU WATCH TELEVISION
```

Auditory sentence comprehension. M.L.'s normal performance on standardized tests (BDAE and The Modified Token Test) of auditory comprehension has been reported above. Auditory comprehension was also assessed through sentence-picture matching tasks. M.L. was presented with a sentence followed by an picture, and asked to state whether or not the meaning of the sentence matched the scene depicted in the picture. Two sets of sentence stimuli were presented. The first set included the following sentence types: 1) 60 active-voice, semantically reversible sentences, 30 with corresponding pictures, 15 with "syntactic" foils (subject-object reversals), 15 with lexical foils (8 noun and 7 verb substitutions); 2) 60 passive-voice, reversible sentences, with the same types and numbers of foils; 3) 60 active, non-reversible sentences, 30 with corresponding pictures, 30 with lexical foils (15 noun and 15 verb foils); and 4) 60 passive, non-reversible sentences, with the same types and numbers of foils. Among the stimuli were sentences that represented every possible combination of animate and inanimate subject and object relationship (e.g., The ball is hit by the boy; The boy is hit by the ball; The boy is hit by the girl; and The ball is hit by the car). The second set consisted of 60 sentences with complex relative clause constructions: 17 sentences (9 active, 8 passive) with embedded relative clauses (e.g., The giraffe that has the bow is watching the monkey); 18 sentences (9 active, 9 passive) with right branching relative clauses (e.g., The giraffe is watching the monkey that has the bow); 16 sentences (8 active, 8 passive) with subject relative clauses (e.g., The giraffe that is watching the monkey has the bow); and 9 sentences (all active) with object relative clauses (e.g., The giraffe that the monkey is watching has the bow). Foils depicted the reversal of the subject and object (15 of 30 sentence/picture mismatches) or a shift of the attribute between the subject and object (15 of 30 sentence/picture mismatches).

A total of 294/300 (98%) of M.L.'s responses were correct. All three of her errors on the first set, and one of her errors on the second set, were rejections of correct sentence-picture matches. (These errors may only reflect M.L.'s difficulty in processing the line drawings to match with the sentences; for example, by self-report she rejected the matching picture of the sentence "The dog is biting the horse" because "...it didn't look like the dog was *biting*" (gloss for "...didn't look like...[the] dog [was] *biting*"). Indeed, her three errors on the relative clause sentences were produced in response to sentences with embedded clauses, and all required distinguishing a bus from a visually similar truck (e.g., "The truck that has the stripes is hit by the bus"). Her performance (57/60; 95% correct) on the relative clause sentences is comparable to performance by non-brain damaged control subjects on these stimuli (Romani, unpublished data). Given M.L.'s visual-spatial deficits and the complexity of the picture stimuli required for this task, her performance was excellent. Thus, her auditory comprehension of sentences was judged to be "intact."

Written sentence comprehension. The above sentence-picture matching tasks were also presented with printed sentence stimuli. M.L.'s performance was again excellent (296/300; 98.7% correct). She made only one error with the printed sentences containing relative clauses (again, possibly confusing the bus and the truck), compared to three errors in the auditory presentation condition. Her remaining three errors (errors on set 1) were rejections of correct matches.

Grammaticality judgments. A total of fifty word strings, 8-10 words in length, were read aloud to M.L. Stimuli were constructed by changing one or two words of sentences presented in the reading, repetition, and dictation tasks. She was asked to state whether or not the words formed an accurate English sentence. Each of 25 sentences contained one word-order error (e.g., I had tiny three kittens in my arms), one inflectional error (e.g., The woman will washes herself at the sink), or functor error (e.g., I think we will happy with this one). M.L.'s responses were 100% accurate.

DISCUSSION

The case we have described presents with a clear dissociation between comprehension and production of sentences--a pattern of performance similar to recently reported cases by Miceli, Mazzucchi, Menn, and Goodglass (1983), Kolk, van Grunsven, and Keyser (1985), and Nespoulous, Dordain, Perron, Ska, Bub, Caplan, Mehler, and Lecours (in press). Our patient's performance in sentence comprehension tasks with both visually and aurally presented sentences was within normal limits, as was her performance in a grammaticality judgment task. M.L.'s comprehension performance contrasted markedly with her sentence production performance, which was severely impaired. Her sentence production was characterized by reduced phrase length, frequent omission of free-standing grammatical morphemes, omission of bound grammatical morphemes, and occasional word substitution and word-order errors. (Unfortunately, it could not be established with any confidence in all cases that these latter errors represent true errors of word-order, instead of efforts by the patient to 'repair' earlier omissions that resulted in the production of words out of grammatical order. In some cases we can be quite confident, however. The word-order errors produced by M.L. in the written production tasks are unlikely merely to reflect 'repair' errors resulting in a misordering of words.) A striking feature of M.L.'s sentence production impairment is that it manifests itself in all types of production tasks--oral and written narrative, sentence reading, sentence repetition, and writing sentences to dictation. In all of these tasks, M.L. produced grammatical morpheme errors characterized primarily by the omission of both free-standing and bound forms, but also by occasional substitution errors. However, as in the case of Mr. Clermont described by Nespoulous et al. (in press), M.L. did not present with problems in single word production--neither with free-standing nor with bound grammatical morphemes.

The pattern of performance reported for M.L. is consistent with theoretical expectations of a functional lesion to the positional level (or some aspect of the processes that generate this level of representation) in Garrett's model of sentence production. The positional level representation specifies two types of information crucially needed for the normal production of sentences: 1) the phrasal geometry of the to-be-produced sentence and 2) the specification of the grammatical morphemes to be inserted in specific sites of the sentence frame. If this representation were to be damaged, the most vulnerable elements would be the closed-class words of the sentence, since these elements are specified *only* at the positional level of sentence production. That is, whereas open-class words and other major syntactic features of a sentence are already specified at the functional level of representation, only closed-class words depend entirely on the positional level of representation for their selection from the phonological (output) lexicon. Thus, damage to the mechanisms that generate or control positional level representations should result in impaired production of both free-standing and bound grammatical morphemes in all sentence production tasks, independently of modality of output--the pattern of performance we have described for M.L.

Although it is possible to plausibly argue that M.L.'s pattern of impairment is consistent with the hypothesis that she has a functional lesion to the positional level of representation, it must be pointed out that this claim fails to account for some important features of our patient's performance. Furthermore, the theoretical framework we have adopted as a basis for M.L.'s performance is unsatisfactory in a number of respects. We discuss these two issues in turn.

We have reported that M.L. makes considerably more omission errors for free-standing than for bound grammatical morphemes (see Tables 1 & 2). This discrepancy in error performance between free-standing and bound grammatical morphemes may or may not be theoretically important, but it remains unexplained by the general hypothesis of a functional deficit to the positional level of sentence production. The hypothesis thus far articulated fails to draw a principled distinction between the omission of free-standing and bound grammatical morphemes. The observed difference in performance for the two classes of grammatical morphemes (see also Miceli, Silveri, Romani, & Caramazza, in press) could signal that our hypothesis about the nature of the deficit in M.L. is wrong. That is, contrary to the hypothesis entertained here, the processing mechanisms involved in the retrieval and placement of free-standing and bound grammatical morphemes could be quite distinct. Hopefully, however, the observed discrepancy only signals that our hypothesis is still too general. In this latter case, further theoretical refinements of the hypothesis, articulating in more detail the processing structure of the positional level, could lead to a motivated explication of the observed variability in performance for the two subclasses of grammatical morphemes in question.

Another aspect of M.L.'s performance that does not find a ready explanation within the hypothesis of a functional lesion to the positional level of the sentence production system concerns the observed contrast between omission and substitution errors of grammatical morphemes. The hypothesis entertained in this paper assumes that damage to the positional level representation (or the mechanisms that generate this representation) should adversely affect the processing of grammatical morphemes (see also Garrett, 1982). However, this hypothesis is silent with respect to whether the impairment should manifest itself as omission or substitution errors for the relevant class of morphemes. The mere claim of "damage to the positional level representation" does not imply anything about the specific form that the behavioral impairment will take. And, yet, it is clear that our patient's errors on grammatical morphemes were primarily omissions. Once again we are confronted with the problem of a hypothesis that is not sufficiently developed to account for relevant details of our patient's performance.

That this latter problem is not restricted to our hypothesis of M.L.'s pattern of sentence production impairment, but applies equally to other recent efforts to explicate the basis for the complex clinical disorder of "agrammatism," is small consolation indeed (see Badecker & Caramazza, 1985, for further discussion of this problem). In recent years there has been much discussion on whether a meaningful distinction can be drawn between those disorders of production principally characterized by the omission of grammatical morphemes and those disorders principally characterized by the substitution of these morphemes (e.g., Goodglass & Menn, 1985; Heeschen, 1985; Kolk et al., 1985). No clear resolution has emerged from this discussion (and, on our view, none is likely to be forthcoming either; see Badecker & Caramazza, 1985, for detailed discussion of the basis for this pessimism). What is clear is that the empirical basis for the putative distinction between omission- and substitution-based disorders of grammatical morphemes in sentence production is not as compelling as might be expected from general discussions of this distinction. In an analysis of a large series (N=20) of clinically classified agrammatic patients we (Miceli et al., in press) found that the relationship between omission and substitution of grammatical morphemes is extremely variable. However, in no case did we find that substitution errors were totally absent in the presence of omission errors. We do not intend by the foregoing to imply that omission and substitution errors must necessarily be treated as reflecting the same kind of functional deficit to the sentence production system. The point here is simply that not only are we without a motivated theoretical basis for the putative distinction, but we also lack a clear analysis of the empirical facts on this issue (but see Miceli et al. (in press) for an extensive set of observations on which to base a profitable discussion of this issue).

Yet another aspect of M.L.'s performance that must be considered is the presence, even if not always of clear status, of word-order errors in the oral and written production of our patient. Saffran, Schwartz, and Marin (1980) were the first to forcefully draw attention to the presence of such errors in the speech of (some) clinically agrammatic patients. The cooccurrence of word-order errors with errors in the production of closed-class words need not be problematic for the hypothesis that M.L.'s performance reflects damage to processing mechanisms involved in computing positional level representations (see below for further discussion of this issue). However, the co-occurrence is not a necessary one, as we have clearly documented in an analysis of a relatively large group of patients with attested difficulties in the production of grammatical morphemes (Miceli et al., in press; see also Nespoulous et al., in press). In that analysis we found that the presence of function word omissions is not always, and in our sample not even frequently, accompanied by word-order errors. We are forced, then, to conclude that production difficulties for function words may have different bases; or if they have the same basis, then we must ascribe the source of word-order errors to a deficit to a distinct mechanism from the one that is responsible for function word errors. With respect to M.L. the best we can do is to note that her word-order errors reflect damage to some aspect of the processes involved in computing positional level representations without commitment to the claim that the damaged processes in question are co-extensive with those that are presumably responsible for the function word errors.

We noted earlier that the theoretical framework we have adopted to explain M.L.'s performance is not entirely satisfactory. Two sorts of problems vitiate the possibility for strong conclusions about the nature of the deficit responsible for our patient's performance and, therefore, undermine the possibility for strong claims about the processing structure of the language production system. One problem concerns the relatively undeveloped nature of the theoretical model guiding our interpretation of the data. The other problem concerns our failure to articulate in sufficient detail the specific form of functional lesion assumed to be the source of M.L.'s sentence production deficit. Thus, suppose that we were correct in concluding that M.L.'s sentence production impairment is the result of damage to the positional level of representation. What precisely are the mechanisms involved in generating this level of representation? What aspect of this complex process is damaged in M.L.? And, What does it mean to say that a component of processing is damaged? Unfortunately we cannot give clear answers to these questions.

Although Garrett's model of sentence production draws a number of important distinctions among the levels of representation presumably involved in the sentence production process, the processing structure of the mechanisms that compute these representations is left mostly unspecified.[3] To be sure, Garrett offers some suggestions about the nature of the problem that must be solved and the processes that may be involved in generating positional level representations. He summarizes the steps involved in generating positional level representations thus: "Procedures applied to Functional level representations construct a representation which reflects utterance order directly. Four aspects of the process are distinguished: (a) determination of positional level phrasal frames specifying phrasal stress and closed-class vocabulary, both bound and free, (b) retrieval of lexical forms, (c) assignment to phrasal sites, and (d) assignment of frame elements to positions in the terminal string of lexically interpreted phrasal frames; representation is phonological." (Garrett, 1982; pg. 67). Unfortunately, the recipe offered by Garrett leaves many of the ingredients and the steps for combining them underspecified.[4] An example may help clarify the basis for this concern.

Consider that aspect of the process involved in generating positional level representations that Garrett has identified as: "determination of positional level phrasal frames specifying phrasal stress and closed-class vocabulary, both bound and free." This is most surely an extremely complex process which may very well consist of a number of distinct subprocesses. Thus, for example, the selection of a phrasal frame does not on its own fully determine the specific form of closed-class items to be inserted in the phrasal-frame-determined sites. To constrain this latter selection process much more specific information than that which determines phrasal frames is needed; for example, the specification that a particular Noun Phrase is located at some point in a phrasal frame leaves indeterminate the form of article (if any) that may be inserted in the Noun Phrase. This distinction suggests that there are different "levels" of information specified at the functional level which interact with various subprocesses in the full determination of positional level representations. These subprocesses may be damaged selectively, resulting in different patterns of sentence production disorders. Specifically, word-order and function word errors may dissociate in some brain-damaged patients because of differential damage to these subprocesses of the complex process that determines "...positional level phrasal frames specifying phrasal stress and closed-class vocabulary..."[5] Or, to state this point differently, whether or not word-order and closed-class vocabulary errors dissociate in a particular patient does not significantly help to constrain the kinds of claims we can make about the structure of the sentence production system or the type of functional lesion responsible for the observed impairment.[6]

The other reason for considering not entirely satisfactory the explanation given for M.L.'s performance concerns our failure to provide an articulated claim about the nature of the deficit hypothesized to be responsible for the observed impairment. That is, the notion "damage (functional lesion) at the level of positional level representation" is insufficiently specific, not only in terms of the mechanisms involved in generating the hypothesized level of representation presumably involved in sentence production, but also in terms of how precisely these mechanisms may be damaged. The fact that the problem of insufficient content to the notion "functional lesion" is not specific to the present effort but afflicts cognitive neuropsychology more generally is, once again, small consolation. Without a more precise articulation of what is intended by "damage," putative explanations of patterns of impaired performance are much too general--there are simply too many possible interpretations of what might be meant by saying that a particular process is damaged. Unfortunately, for now, as much as we would wish it to be otherwise, we must admit to our inability to go beyond the mere identification of a general functional locus of deficit to account for M.L.'s performance.

The final issue we would like to consider in this paper concerns the relationship between our case and recently reported similar cases. Although M.L.'s performance is similar in important respects to that of the cases reported by Miceli et al. (1983) and by Kolk et al. (1985), it is most similar to Mr. Clermont's (Nespoulous et al., in press) and, therefore, our discussion will principally focus on a comparison between our patient and this latter patient.[7] There are two major differences between M.L.'s and Mr. Clermont's performance: 1) the two patients differ dramatically in MLU (about 2 and 6 words, respectively); and, 2) M.L. was severely impaired in a sentence anagram task; whereas Mr. Clermont performed well on this task, albeit with considerable effort. The issue to be addressed is whether or not the same type of functional lesion may be assumed to underlie the two patients' performance.

The principal empirical fact militating against assuming that the two patients may be considered to have a common underlying deficit is their contrasting performance on the anagram task. Mr. Clermont's good performance on this task (together with his good performance on single-word processing tasks) led Nespoulous et al. to exclude a deficit to the positional level of sentence production as an explanation of their patient's performance. Instead, these authors propose that his deficit may be characterized in terms of "reduced processing capacity"--the patient can process grammatical morphemes when the task demand is relatively light (e.g., single word processing) but cannot process these same elements when the task demand is high, as in sentence processing.

In contrast, we have proposed that our patient's performance is best explained by assuming that she has a deficit in processing positional level information. The two hypotheses may not be as different as they at first appear.

Granting the plausibility of Nespoulous et al.'s proposal, there remains the crucial issue of why the "reduced processing" account offered by these authors should affect grammatical morphemes and not open-class items. The mere claim of "reduced processing capacity" does not explain the empirical fact that their patient's difficulties were restricted to processing closed-class items; that is, the specificity of their patient's deficit-- restricted as it is to the processing of closed-class items--does not follow in any obvious way from the simple assumption of "reduced processing capacity." In order to account for this empirical fact the authors must make one of two further assumptions: either motivate a theoretical claim which postulates a hierarchy of processing difficulty with closed-class items being more difficult to process than open-class items or, more parsimoniously if we are also to account for our patient's performance, assume that their patient has an additional (or perhaps only) deficit to the positional level of representation. In the absence of motivated theoretical arguments to support the assumption of a hierarchy of processing difficulty for closed- and open-class items, we prefer the latter of the two accounts for Mr. Clermont's impaired performance.

How, then, do we account for the observed discrepancy between the two patients in their performance on the anagram task? One possibility is to assume that the two patients differ in the "severity" of deficit to positional level representations.[8] Recall that our patient's MLU was about 2, whereas Mr. Clermont's was about 6. This difference could be taken as an index of the "extent" of damage to positional level representations--our patient's positional level representations are severely damaged, whereas Mr. Clermont's are only mildly affected. On this account Mr. Clermont's better (but not normal) performance on the anagram task could reflect the more efficient use of spared information at the positional level to guide the selection of words in local contexts. That is, it is possible that in an anagram task, but not other production tasks, processing may be sequentially focused more efficiently to local contexts, permitting the patient to "reason" through the correct choice at a particular point in a sentence. In contrast, M.L.'s deficit to the positional level is so extensive that she cannot exploit the possibility of using local context processing to guide her performance in this task. However, when context is further constrained, as in the lexical insertion task where only one word has to be inserted locally in a sentence, her performance, while not normal, is appropriately much better.

To conclude, with the caveats raised earlier in this paper, we are able to propose that M.L. has a selective functional lesion to the positional level of sentence production. The caveats concern our present inability to account in a motivated way for some features of our patient's performance. These limitations, while not insignificant, do not undermine our proposal. Clearly, however, further theoretical developments are needed if we are to make efficient use of patients' data to inform and constrain theories of sentence production. For the present, the reported case may be interpreted as empirical support for a theory of sentence production which postulates an autonomous level of representation where the grammatical morphemes of a sentence are specified--the positional level in Garrett's theory of sentence production. Furthermore, this case provides additional support for the dissociation between sentence comprehension and sentence production impairments and, therefore, for theories of sentence processing that distinguish between autonomous systems for sentence comprehension and sentence production.[9]

ACKNOWLEDGEMENTS

The research reported in this paper was supported in part by NIH Grant NS23836. We thank Chris Barry for very helpful comments on an earlier version of this paper. We also thank Kathy Yantis for her help in the preparation of the manuscript and Jessica Richmond for assistance in obtaining interjudge reliability measures. We are especially grateful to M.L. for participating in the study.

REFERENCES

Badecker, W. & Caramazza, A. (1985). On considerations of method and theory governing the use of clinical categories in Neurolinguistics and

Cognitive Neuropsychology: The case against Agrammatism. Cognition, 20, 97-125.

Badecker, W. & Caramazza, A. (1986). A final brief in the case against agrammatism: The role of theory in the selection of data. Cognition, 24, 277-282.

Berndt, R. S. (1987). Symptom co-occurrence and dissociation in the interpretation of agrammatism. In M. Coltheart, G. Sartori & R. Job (Eds.), The cognitive neuropsychology of language, (pp. 221-233). London: Lawrence Erlbaum Associates.

Berndt, R. S. & Caramazza, A. (1980). A redefinition of the syndrome of Broca's aphasia: Implications for a neuropsychological model of language. Applied Psycholinguistics, 1, 225-278.

Bock, J. K. (1982). Towards a cognitive psychology of syntax: Information processing contributions to sentence formulation. Psychological Review, 89, 1-47.

Bradley, D., Garrett, M. & Zurif, E. (1980). Syntactic deficits in Broca's aphasia. In D. Caplan (Ed.), Biological studies of mental processes. Cambridge, MA: MIT Press.

Caramazza, A. & Berndt, R. S. (1985). A multicomponent deficit view of agrammatic Broca's aphasia. In M.-L. Kean (Ed.), Agrammatism, 21-63. Orlando, FL: Academic Press.

Dell, G. (1986). A spreading-activation theory of retrieval in sentence production. Psychological Review, 93, 283-321.

DeRenzi, E. & Faglioni, P. (1978). Normative data and screening power of a shortened version of the Token Test. Cortex, 14, 41-49.

Garrett, M. F. (1975). The analysis of sentence production. In G. Bower (Ed.), The psychology of learning and motivation advance in research and theory. New York, NY: Academic Press.

Garrett, M. F. (1980). Levels of processing in sentence production. In B. Butterworth (Ed.), Language Production (Vol.1). New York, NY: Academic Press.

Garrett, M. F. (1982). Production of speech: Observations from normal and pathological language use. In A. Ellis (Ed.), Normality and pathology in cognitive functions. London: Academic Press.

Goodglass, H. & Kaplan, E. (1972). The assessment of aphasia and related disorders. Philadelphia, PA: Lea and Febiger.

Goodglass, H., Kaplan, E. & Weintraub, S. (1983). The revised boston naming test. Philadelphia, PA: Lea and Febiger.

Goodglass, H., Quadfassel, F. A. & Timberlake, W. H. (1964). Phrase length and the type and severity of aphasia. Cortex, 1, 133-153.

Goodglass, H. & Menn, L. (1985). Is agrammatism a unitary phenomenon? In M.-L. Kean (Ed.), Agrammatism. Orlando, FL: Academic Press.

Heeschen, C. (1985). Agrammatism versus paragrammatism: A fictitious opposition. In M.-L. Kean (Ed.), Agrammatism. Orlando, FL: Academic Press, Inc.

Hillis, A. & Caramazza, A. (in press). The Graphemic Buffer and attentional mechanisms Brain & Language.

Kean, M.-L. (1977). The linguistic interpretation of aphasia syndromes: Agrammatism in Broca's aphasia, an example. Cognition, 5, 9-46.

Kean, M.-L. (1980). Grammatical representations and the description of language processes. In D. Caplan (Ed.), Biological studies of mental processes. Cambridge, MA: MIT Press.

Kertesz, A. (1982). Western aphasia battery. NY: Grune & Stratton.

Kinsbourne, M. & Warrington, E. (1962). A variety of reading disability associated with right hemisphere lesions. Journal of Neurology, Neurosurgery and Psychiatry, 25, 339-344.

Kolk, H. H. J., van Grunsven, M. J. F. & Keyser, A. (1985). On parallelism between production and comprehension in agrammatism. In M.-L. Kean (Ed.), Agrammatism. Orlando, FL: Academic Press, Inc.

Miceli, G., Mazzucchi, A., Menn, L. & Goodglass, H. (1983). Contrasting cases of Italian agrammatic aphasia without comprehension disorder. Brain and Language, 19, 65-97.

Miceli, G., Silveri, M. C., Romani, C. & Caramazza, A. (in press). Variation in the pattern of omissions and substitutions of grammatical morphemes in the spontaneous speech of so-called agrammatic patients. Brain & Language.

Nespoulous, J.-L., Dordain, M., Perron, C., Ska, B., Bub, D., Caplan, D., Mehler, J. & Lecours, A. R. (in press). Agrammatism in sentence production without comprehension deficits: Reduced availability of syntactic structures and/or of grammatical morphemes? A case study. Brain and Language.

Parisi, D. (1987). Grammatical disturbances of speech production. In M. Coltheart, G. Sartori & R. Job (Eds.), The Cognitive neuropsychology of language, London: Lawrence Erlbaum Associates.

Saffran, E. M., Schwartz, M. F. & Marin, O. S. M. (1980). The word order problem in agrammatism: II. Production. Brain and Language, 10, 263-280.

Thorndike, E. L. & Lorge, I. (1944). The teacherswork book of 30,000 words. New York, NY: Teachers College Press.

Weschler, D. (1972). The Weschler memory scale. New York, NY: The Psychological Corporation.

Yorkston, K. & Beukelman, D. (1981). The assessment of intelligibility of dysarthric speech. Tigard, OR: C.C. Publications, Inc.

APPENDIX A

Examples of M.L.'s Spontaneous Speech

Description of the "Cookie Theft" picture from the Boston Diagnostic Aphasia Examination:

"Mother washing sink...water flowing floor...running water...dishes, slopping...cookie jar...stealing cookies...toppling stool."

Description of the "Picnic picture" from the Western Aphasia Battery:

"Couple having picnic...a boy flying kite...sailboat in water...flagpole ...dog."

Telling the story of "Little Red Riding Hood":

"Grandmother...baked basket of cookies...Grandmother went...wolf dressed up...Grandmother says, 'Eat it'...Red Riding Hood caught him...caught wolf up...happily ever after."

Telling the story of "Goldilocks and the Three Bears":

"Blond...little girl blond...walking in the words...tired...goes in the house...rested...three chairs...saw some porridge...tried some...no...it was too cold...three chairs...Goldilocks tried...three chairs...up...went up the stairs...saw some...three beds...tried three beds...too soft...just right... Goldilocks fell asleep."

Re-telling the "Annie Thompson" story from the Weschler Memory Scale:

"Cleaning...Annie Thompson...Boston...got up four dollars...taken for little children...eaten...not eaten three days...touch by the story...made up purse her...for her."

Re-telling the "American Liner" story from the Weschler Memory Scale:

"A steam ship...New York...Liverpool...sixty passengers...picked up... London...got wet."

... = pause

APPENDIX B

Examples of M.L.'s Spontaneous Writing

Description of the "Cookie Theft" picture from the Boston Diagnostic Aphasia Examination:

> The drying dishes mother is
> water running
> the fall stool
> the boys falling over on to stool

Description of the "Picnic picture" from the Western Aphasia Battery:

> Couple having picnic
> Boy kite flying
> Playing in the water
> A sailboat
> flagpole, dog
> The boat is down water
> Dog watch boy.

In M.L.'s own spelling:

> Cople having pinnic
> Boy kite flying
> Plaing in th water
> A sial boat
> flagaplo, dog
> The boat is down water
> Dog watch boy.

NOTES

[1] For the moment we leave aside the issue of whether selective damage at the level of positional level processing predicts other types of errors in addition to those with the closed-class vocabulary. We take up this issue in the Discussion section.

[2] Using pauses to separate phrases may present both theoretical and methodological problems (see Parisi, 1987, for discussion). One objection raised, concerning the arbitrary selection of a pause length was not critical in our analyses, because all of M.L.'s pauses were quite long--all longer than the 2 second minimum we selected. Also, others (e.g., Goodglass,

Quadfassel, & Timberlake, 1964) have found it necessary to use additional criteria other than pauses, to account for sentences that begin without a suprathreshold pause. We did not encounter this difficulty, because M.L. never began a "sentence" (a new verb construction) without pausing. However, the validity of this measurement may be questioned, since a pause may separate words in the same sentence construction attempt. Re-analysis of the speech samples using Parisi's criterion of counting adjacent words as part of the same phrase when there are semantic or syntactic cues for doing so, yields a phrase length of 2.18 content words (considerably below the 6.50 reported for non-aphasic controls; Parisi, 1987), or 2.78 words. It would appear that by any measure of phrase length M.L.'s speech consists of very short, simple constructions.

[3] The noted limitation is not intended to specifically isolate Garrett's model for criticism. We have already pointed out that this model is among the best developed and clearly motivated models in the psycholinguistic literature. Rather, our point is simply that the computational inexplicitness of Garrett's model reflects the current level of theoretical development in cognitive psychology: The bemoaned limitation is a pervasive feature of current theorizing in cognitive psychology.

[4] We leave aside the very difficult question of whether the notion "closed-class vocabulary" can be given independent theoretical motivation. The crucial question is: Why are we grouping together articles with prepositions, auxiliary verbs with pronouns, or conjunctions with inflections? Is there some motivated reason for grouping all these items under the category label "closed-class vocabulary"? Garrett is fully aware of this problem. He cites the case of (some) prepositions which on strictly linguistic criteria pattern like major lexical items; for example, prepositions, like major lexical items, can be the head of a phrase. Garrett's attempted solution for this specific problem was to appeal to Kean's (1977; 1980) analysis of closed-class vocabulary in terms of their phonological status in sentences (i.e., they pattern together as phonological nonwords--non stress bearing elements). The reasoning (and the implied process) involved in motivating Garrett's analysis is not simple. It requires "demoting" a lexical item that has the potential status of 'phonological word' at the functional level of representation to the status of 'phonological nonword' at the positional level of representation. Aside from this difficulty, it must be pointed out that this solution will not lead to a well-defined criterion of closed-class vocabulary that will work for all cases: polysyllabic function words can be stress bearing elements. Nonetheless, for present purposes we will have to do with a category whose principal motivation is strictly empirical--the distribution of speech errors.

[5] Of course, word-order errors may dissociate from production errors of the closed-class vocabulary because of selective damage to other components of the complex process that determines positional level representations. Thus, for example, the dissociation in question may reflect differential damage to the process that Garrett has labeled "retrieval of lexical forms," either because this process distinguishes between routines for retrieving open- and closed-class words and these subroutines may be damaged selectively or because the information in a phrasal frame needed to specify a particular closed-class item is selectively damaged.

[6] Actually the situation is not nearly as simple as we have made it appear here. One could argue that in the absence of any positive evidence for a dissociation of word-order and closed-class vocabulary errors, we would be encouraged to entertain the hypothesis that a single, indifferentiable process subserves both the specification of the phrasal geometry of a sentence and the closed-class vocabulary associated with that frame.

[7] The reason for choosing to compare M.L.'s performance to that of Mr. Clermont is based strictly on the availability of relevant performances for comparison. The two patients have been tested with very similar sets of tasks making it possible to compare their performance across tasks.

[8] We recognize the danger of using notions such as "severity" in attempts to explain patterns of impaired performance--this notion is not sufficiently well defined (but not much less than the notion "damage") to do very much work for us. Nonetheless, in the present context the intended gloss for "severity" should be as either: 1) extent--understood as 'number of'--of damage to the various subprocesses that comprise the complex process assumed to generate positional level representations; or, 2) extent--understood as 'degree of'--of damage to some specific aspect or aspects of the complex process assumed to generate positional level representations. At this point of theoretical development of our field we are unable to distinguish between the two senses of severity considered here.

[9] This last point is worth stressing since it has been noted (Berndt, 1987) that previous reports of dissociation between comprehension and production impairments--clinical symptoms of so-called agrammatism with unimpaired sentence comprehension--involved patients whose production could be characterized as having atypically long MLU's for "agrammatic" patients. This atypicality does not apply to M.L. whose MLU was very reduced. It would appear, then, that comprehension performance can be spared even in the face of "severely agrammatic" patients.

CHAPTER TWELVE

VARIATION IN THE PATTERN OF OMISSIONS AND SUBSTITUTIONS OF GRAMMATICAL MORPHEMES IN THE SPONTANEOUS SPEECH OF SO-CALLED AGRAMMATIC PATIENTS

INTRODUCTION

Historically, aphasia research has attempted to answer questions of the following sort: What are the neuroanatomical structures associated with such and such a syndrome? Or, what are the cognitive/linguistic mechanisms that are damaged in such and such a syndrome? This approach to the study of aphasia, as the basis for inferring the structure of normal language processing, has recently been challenged on the grounds that it cannot lead to meaningful, theoretically interpretable results (Caramazza, 1984; 1986; Marshall, 1986). The principal objection concerns the dependence of this approach on the notion "syndrome." Research based on this approach requires that the clinically identified syndromes constitute natural-kind categories which can serve as the basis for the a priori description and selection of the exemplars of such categories. Clinical syndromes cannot play such a role, however.

It has recently been shown that valid inferences about the structure of normal cognitive processing from impaired performance crucially depend on the prior identification of the *functional lesion(s)* in a damaged cognitive system. But the identification of a functional lesion to a damaged cognitive system is only possible **a posteriori**, that is, on the basis of all the theoretically relevant evidence for each brain-damaged patient. On this account, there is no arbitrarily large subset of a patient's performance, short of all the theoretically relevant evidence, which can serve as the basis for the identification of a functional lesion to a cognitive system (Caramazza, 1986). A major implication of this analysis is that variation in performance within a clinical type cannot be assumed, **a priori**, to be theoretically unimportant. Consequently, clinical categories such as Broca's aphasia, deep dyslexia, phonological dysgraphia, and so forth, cannot serve as the basis for theoretically meaningful research.

The implications of these metatheoretical developments were extensively analyzed in Badecker and Caramazza (1985; see also Caramazza, in press) specifically for the case of agrammatism. These authors argued that the clinical category agrammatism cannot serve as the basis for theoretical statements about the nature of normal language processes nor for claims about the nature of the language mechanisms that are presumably damaged in so-called agrammatics. An important part of their argument revolved about the issue of performance variability in clinically classified agrammatic patients. Specifically, Badecker and Caramazza argued that agrammatism is an ill-defined concept which does not allow the specification of an homogeneous patient population (or the selection of an homogeneous patient group) over which we may base theoretical claims.

The conclusion reached by Badecker and Caramazza (1985) has been challenged by Caplan (1986), who maintains that the variation in performance that characterizes the (putative) category of agrammatism "... actually constitutes evidence *in favor* of a general syndrome of agrammatism, since the variation they (Badecker & Caramazza) cite can largely be explained ..." (pg. 266; his emphasis). Caplan appeals to Kean's (1977) and Lapointe's (1985) work in support of his contention that significant aspects of the clinically classified agrammatic's variation in speech performance can be explained within a general theory of "agrammatism." However, the latter two authors were only concerned with the putative existence of a hierarchy of production difficulty for different grammatical morphemes; they were not concerned with performance variability across types of grammatical morphemes in different patients of the putatively same category--i.e., these authors were not directly concerned with the issue Caplan identifies as the problem of "profiles of agrammatism." Caplan recognizes that the existence of this latter type of variability presents a major problem for the view that "agrammatism" constitutes a theoretically coherent cognitive category. Nonetheless, he goes on to appeal to the abstract notion of "adaptation/compensatory mechanisms" to explain this variability. This latter appeal remains without force, however, since it is unaccompanied by any concrete proposal concerning the nature of these compensatory mechanisms.

But, what *is* the range of performance variation that must be accounted for by any proposal that posits "agrammatism" as a coherent cognitive category? Important as this question is for any serious account of the putative category "agrammatism," there is surprisingly a dearth of adequate information (with some notable exceptions, e.g., de Villiers, 1978) on which to base informed discussion of this issue. The principal scope of this paper is to remedy this situation--that is, to consider the range of production deficits involving the omission or substitution of grammatical morphemes in patients clinically classified as agrammatic.

Since the principal issue under consideration in this paper concerns the contentious issue of performance variability across a putatively coherent patient category, it is crucial that the criteria for the selection of the patients to be analyzed be above suspicion; that is, the patients included in the analysis must be manifestly agrammatic on current criteria for identification of this disorder. Furthermore, since language differences (e.g., whether or not inflections attach to words or stems) may interact with the form taken by the agrammatic disorder, we have restricted our analysis to Italian patients. Finally, in order to obtain a fair representation of the variability of the disorder we have analyzed the performance of a large number of clinically classified agrammatic patients (N=20).

Agrammatism is defined as a disorder of sentence production characterized by the selective omission of free-standing and bound grammatical morphemes. This definition of the disorder, in particular that aspect concerning the omission of bound grammatical morphemes, while appropriate for a language like English, which attaches inflections to words, is not adequate for a language like Italian, which attaches inflections to stems. For languages of the latter type the omission of a word's inflection would result in a nonword (compare walking → walk vs. portare (to carry) → *port, where walk is a word of English but port is not a word in Italian). Indeed, there are no reports of Italian patients who systematically omit bound morphemes and produce uninflected nonwords. In light of this language-specific feature of Italian the definition of agrammatism used to select patients for the study reported here was modified as follows: Agrammatism is a disorder of sentence production characterized by the omission of free-standing grammatical morphemes *with or without* the substitution of bound grammatical morphemes.

SUBJECTS

Right-handed brain-damaged patients in stable neurological condition, without disorders of "consciousness," with a history of acute disturbance of language functions, without neuropsychological signs of diffuse mental deterioration and who had received a formal education for at least 5 years were considered for inclusion in the present study.

Of the subjects who fulfilled the general requirements detailed above, only those who conformed to a clinical (intuitive) characterization of agrammatism as presented in the literature were included. The linguistic criterion for inclusion in the present research was the production of grammatically ill-formed sentences, containing omissions of free-standing grammatical markers with or without substitutions of bound grammatical markers in spontaneous speech.

Of the 20 subjects included in the present research, one is a crossed aphasic (C.S.). Patients G.G. and T.F. have already been described in

Miceli, Mazzucchi, Menn and Goodglass (1983); patients C.D.A. and F.G. have been described in Miceli and Mazzucchi (in press), where they are referred to as Mr. Rossi and Mr. Verdi, respectively; patients F.S. is described in Miceli and Caramazza (in press).

In addition to the aphasic patients, 10 control subjects, roughly matched for age and education to the aphasic patients, were asked to collaborate in the study. The control subjects were either outpatients at the Clinica Neurologica del Sacro Cuore, Rome, or spouses of the patients who participated in this study.

The essential biographic information and lesion data for the 20 patients who participated in the present study are presented in Table 1. The subjects are indicated by their initials. They are listed in alphabetical order according to the second letter of their initials, which corresponds to their last name.

Table 1. Essential biographical information on the patients included in the study (see also Appendix).

Subject	Age at onset	Years of formal education	Etiology	Lesion site	Time Post onset
A.A.	34	7	aneurysm	-	1 yr.
F.A.	63	8	meningioma	F	5 yrs.
F.B.	24	14	trauma	F (P)	3 yrs.
C.D.	59	11	CVA	deep F	4 yrs.
F.D.	59	19	CVA	T (bilat)	1 yr.
C.D.A.	45	17	aneurysm	T-P	2 yrs.
G.D.C.	50	5	CVA	FTP	8 yrs.
E.D.U.	59	17	CVA	-	1 yr.
G.F.	58	19	CVA	TP	3 wks.
T.F.	38	5	CVA	deep P	1 day
F.G.	21	15	CVA	deep FP	2 yrs.
G.G.	58	8	CVA	F	1 yr.
M.L.	35	13	cardiac arrest	neg CT	7 yrs.
A.M.	53	8	CVA	TP	4 yrs.
M.M.	50	5	CVA	-	1 yr.
B.P.	49	8	CVA	FTP	9 yrs.
C.S.	68	13	CVA	right FP	1 yr.
F.S.	57	17	CVA	deep FT	5 yrs.
L.S.	37	5	meningioma	F	1 yr.
M.U.	47	13	CVA	-	1 yr.

MATERIALS AND METHODS

The speech corpora analyzed for this paper were collected by asking our subjects to produce the following narratives: History of illness, Activities of daily life, The Little Red Riding Hood, descriptions of the Cookie Theft picture (Goodglass and Kaplan, 1972). Patients F.B., G.D.C., C.D.A., F.G., C.D. and A.M., and 4 normal controls also provided a description of the four stories of the original Wechsler-Bellevue Test.

The examiner asked each patient (and each control subject) to produce a given narrative. Once the patient began producing a narrative, communication on the examiner's part was limited to nods. Severely impaired patients were encouraged if they appeared to be too frustrated by the task, or, if necessary, were asked open questions of the type "Could you tell me more?"

Speech samples, collected over several sessions, were tape-recorded on high-quality cassettes. The tapes were independently transcribed by two of the authors of the present study. The few disagreements between the two transcriptions were adjudicated by a third person who independently listened to the problematic taped sequence. Sequences which could not be resolved unambiguously were omitted from the final transcript.

Phonetic and phonemic distortions were ignored--the "intended" target response was transcribed. If the patient made more than one attempt at producing a word, only the last attempt was transcribed. This criterion was used both for content words and function words. Fillers ("Well," "Let's see," "Wait," etc.) and stereotyped sentences used to fill word-finding pauses ("I don't know", "What's its name," etc.) were excluded from word counts.

SCORING PROCEDURES

The quantitative measures used in the present study are reported and described below.

Agrammatic speakers frequently produce fragmented utterances, i.e., strings of words in which the intended grammatical structure cannot be reconstructed. In order to quantify this feature of our patients' speech, the *proportion of words produced in fragmented utterances* was calculated for each subject. It was decided to consider as fragmented utterances all false starts and all those sequences of words that could not unambiguously be considered as attempts to produce a sentence. An example of the latter type of Fragmented Speech produced by a patient who was trying to tell the History of illness is the following (ellipses in the transcript stand for pauses of more than 3 seconds):

"Comune...invece...aspetta, eh...carta...scritto...medico..."

"Town Hall...instead...wait, eh...paper...written...doctor..."

The quantitative incidence of fragmented speech is expressed as the ratio of the number of words produced without a recoverable grammatical structure to the total number of words in the sample (produced either correctly or incorrectly, with or without a recoverable grammatical structure). Small values of this ratio indicate a relative paucity of fragmented speech.

The mean length of utterance (MLU) was calculated on the corpus retained after elimination of Fragmented Speech, according to two distinct criteria: a Lexical and a Morphological criterion (MLU-Lexical and MLU-Morphological, respectively). MLU-Lexical corresponds to the number of major-class items produced by the patient in an uninterrupted, syntactically correct string. The end of an utterance according to this criterion was marked by the omission of a major-class lexical item, by prosodic criteria (only in patients whose prosody was not flat), or by a major pause (longer than 3 seconds). MLU-Morphological was calculated on the basis of the number of uninterrupted, syntactically *and* morphologically well-formed strings of words. The end of an utterance according to this criterion was marked by the omission of a major-class lexical item, by prosodic criteria, or by a major pause, as in the case of MLU-Lexical, but also by the omission or substitution of a free-standing grammatical marker, or by the substitution of a bound grammatical marker. Take for example a sentence like "Tre volte [a] settimana io scrive una lettera" (roughly corresponding in English to the sentence "Three times [a] week I writes a letter"). For the MLU-Lexical count, this sentence would count as one utterance of length 7. For the MLU-Morphological count, however, the sentence would count as three utterances of length 2, 3 and 2, due to the omission of a free-standing grammatical morpheme (in square parenthesis) and to the substitution of a bound grammatical morpheme ("scrive" is the Present Indicative, 3rd singular form, and was produced in a context where the 1st singular form was called for).

Filler sentences or frozen expressions, of the type "I do not know," "What's its name," and the like were not counted when calculating MLU's.

a. Single-word level analyses. Several counts were conducted to quantify the disorder of grammatical morphemes and content word production in our patient sample.

The set of content words included Nouns, Adjectives and main (lexical) verbs. Adverbs were excluded from the counts of content words, because only few of the patients retained the ability to produce them. When a verb was of the form *aux + V-ato*--the perfect tense composed of the *have* or *be* plus past participle as in "Ho parlato" (I have spoken)--aux was scored as a function word (see below), and *V + ato* as a main verb.

Several measures were considered. The first, *Content Word Omission Rate*, is an index which captures the rate of omission of major class lexical items in obligatory context. Some examples will clarify this criterion. Instances of missing arguments without indications of anomic difficulties (such as long pauses or intervening "I don't know" sentences) were counted as omissions of a major-class lexical item. Two examples of this type of speech production errors are the sentences "Il bambino dà alla bambina" (The boy gives to the girl), or "Il bambino mette" (The boy puts). By the same token, instances of non-permissible subject deletion were considered as omissions of a content word (e.g., "Il grano cresce e guarda il punto di maturazione" (The corn grows and watches the degree of maturation), where the context unequivocally establishes that "il contadino" (the farmer) is the subject of "guarda" (watches)). Instances where sequences of two or more nouns were produced without an intervening main verb, but where the nouns were obviously related to each other as indicated by context, prosodic features, or by gestures made by the patient, were counted as verb omissions. By contrast, clear cut instances of word-finding difficulty, like: "Il cane mangia la...come si dice?" (The dog eats the...what's its name?") were not counted as omissions of a noun, but were considered as interruptions of (otherwise well-formed, in this case) syntactic strings. This last type of error was infrequent in our samples.

The set of *Bound Grammatical Morphemes* included nominal, adjectival and verbal inflections. The *Bound Grammatical Morpheme Substitution Rate* was based on the occurrences of incorrect nominal, adjectival and verbal inflections.

The set of *Free-Standing Grammatical Morphemes* included prepositions, definite and indefinite articles, clitics and auxiliaries. This set of words did not include the following items:
1) subordinate conjunctions, because only some patients retained the ability to produce them, and we wanted to compare the patients on the ability to produce a subset of grammatical markers that they were all able to use;
2) indefinite pronouns, possessive pronouns and quantifiers, partly for the same reasons as 1), partly because in Italian it is very hard to establish the occurrence of an obligatory context for these items;
3) strong pronouns, because of the disagreement regarding their placement in the category of grammatical morphemes; and
4) main Have/Be verbs.

For Free-standing Grammatical Morphemes, the following measures were obtained: *Free-standing Grammatical Morpheme Omission Rate*: omissions of free-standing grammatical morphemes in obligatory context;

Free-standing Grammatical Morpheme Substitution Rate: substitutions of free-standing grammatical morphemes in obligatory context.

b. Analyses of agreement relations. Given the complexity of its morphological system, Italian offers an excellent opportunity to evaluate the incidence and the qualitative aspects of disorders of grammatical agreement in patients with disorders of speech production. We assessed the following agreement violations:

i. Violations of determiner-noun agreement: Only mismatches between determiner and Noun were counted, i.e., instances where det and Noun did not agree for gender and/or number (e.g., il bambina--the (m.sg.) girl (f.sg.); il bambini--the (m.sg.) boys; il bambine--the (m.sg.) girls (f.pl.). The few instances in which the lexical gender and/or number of the noun was incorrect, but the determiner agreed with the incorrect gender and/or number, were counted as instances of correct agreement (e.g., la studia*-- the (f.sg.) office (f.sg.*), where the correct form would have been lo studio --the (m.sg.) office (m.sg.); i bambini--the (m.pl.) boys (m.pl.), in a context where "il bambino"--the (m.sg.) boy (m.sg.)--should have been produced). Substitutions of the incorrect for the correct allomorph of the definite article were counted separately, and were not considered as agreement violations (e.g., "lo rubinetto" for "il rubinetto" (the faucet), where both "il" and "lo" are m.sg. definite articles but are used in different phonological contexts--"lo" is used with nouns and adjectives that begin with a vowel sound or certain consonant clusters).

ii. Violations of noun-adjective agreement: The same general principles as in i. were applied, i.e., only mismatches between nominal and adjectival inflection were considered to be instances of agreement violation. Again, for the few cases where lexical gender and/or number of the noun was incorrect, but the adjective carried the inflection appropriate for the incorrect noun suffix, these were not considered as errors of agreement. Thus, for example, "il bambino bionda" (the boy-m.sg. blonde-f.sg.) and 'il bambino biondi" (the boy-m.sg. blonde-m.pl.) were instances of agreement violation, whereas "la mia studia*" (the my-f.sg. office-incorrect f.sg., should be "studio," m.sg.) and "i miei studi" (the my-m.pl. offices-m.pl., in a context where the m.sg. would be required) were not scored as agreement errors. Furthermore, NP's containing cardinal numeral adjectives were excluded when scoring agreement violations. This step was taken because only some patients (but not others) made extensive use of these adjectives.

iii. Subject-verb agreement: Verb inflections inappropriately marked for person and/or number were scored as agreement errors. However, analogously to i. and ii., if the subject was produced in the incorrect number and the verb agreed in person with the subject, this was not considered as an agreement error. Thus, utterances like "Il bambino corrono" (The boy run-3 pl., number error) and "Il bambino corri" (The boy run-2 sg., person error) were considered as agreement errors, whereas "Cappuccetti Rossi corrono" (The Little Red Riding Hoods run-3 pl.) was not. Errors in the production of verb aspect and/or tense were considered separately from agreement errors. Aspect and tense errors were grouped under the category "verb morphology errors." We recognize the arbitrary nature of the distinction drawn here--although tense and aspect errors cannot be agreement errors, the errors we have labeled agreement errors need not result from an inability to appreciate agreement relations but may only reflect difficulties in selecting the proper inflectional form (just like the other "verb morphology" errors).

ANALYSIS OF RESULTS

The size of the speech sample collected from each subject, speech rate (measured as the number of words per minute produced by the patient), and the presence or absence of dysarthria (assessed solely on clinical criteria) are reported in Table 2. Table 2 also reports information on sample size and speech rate for normal controls. For normal controls only, average values and ranges are reported.

Estimates of patients' speech rates were obtained by averaging over several one-minute samples selected through quasi-random sampling of each patient's speech corpus. Two constraints were respected in the sampling procedure: 1) the chosen sample was free of interruptions by the examiner (with questions or comments) and, 2) the sample was free of clear anomic pauses. All the words produced by the patient in each section were counted, including frozen expressions and words produced out of grammatical context (see Incidence of fragmented speech below).

The results reported in Table 2 are relevant to the classical concern with the relationship that may obtain among agrammatism, dysarthria and reduced speech rate. It has traditionally been held that the three disorders co-occur. The putative co-occurrence of these deficits provided the empirical basis for the "economy of effort" hypotheses of "agrammatism," from Isserlin (1922) to Lenneberg (1967)--speech articulation is so laborious in these patients that they reduce their output to just the most essential, communicative elements, thus avoiding "unnecessary" words, i.e., free-standing grammatical markers. The results in Table 2 demonstrate that, although the co-occurrence of agrammatism (defined as the omission of free-standing grammatical morphemes), reduced speech rate (measured by the number of words produced per minute) and dysarthria (clinically defined as the simplification of consonant clusters in words) reflect a statistical effect, the putative co-occurrence is **not** functionally necessary. Although in a number of our patients (A.A., F.A., C.D., C.D.A., G.D.C., F.G., G.G., B.P., C.S., F.S.) agrammatism, reduced speech rate and dysarthria are associated, other patients in our series display a behavioral pattern that is at variance with the classical description. Patient A.M., for example, displays a severely reduced speech rate (20 words per minute) and a fairly high rate of omission of free-standing grammatical markers, but no dysarthria at all--in fact, he speaks with an impeccable, standard Italian pronunciation; patient F.B. presents with a similar pattern of performance, although her speech rate (55 words per minute) is less reduced than A.M.'s. Patients T.F. and G.F. show the most interesting dissociation: a very high rate of omission of free-standing grammatical morphemes with a total absence of dysarthria and a speech rate (96 and 81 words per minute, respectively) that is not far from the normal range. Indeed, when we consider that the word count for these patients consisted primarily of content words, which on the average are longer than function

Table 2. Size of the speech corpus collected from each patient; presence of dysarthria; speech rate.

Subject	Sample size	Dysarthria	Speech rate
A.A.	118	+	49
F.A.	313	+	66
F.B.	394		55
C.D.	1214	+	52
F.D.	1123		73
C.D.A.	708		23
G.D.C.	197	+	34
E.D.U.	780		84
G.F.	362		81
T.F.	460		96
F.G.	488	+	29
G.G.	328	+	23
M.L.	390	+	81
A.M.	481		20
M.M.	433		38
B.P.	227	+	32
C.S.	199	+	54
F.S.	749	+	67
L.S.	270		44
M.U.	328	+	61
Norm (range)	526-936		108-122
Norm (avrg)	697		117

words, the discrepancy in speech rate between these two patients and the normal controls is further reduced.

One pattern of performance--the co-occurrence of dysarthria and reduced speech rate without omission of free-standing grammatical morphemes--could not be found in our patient series because we only considered patients who omitted function words in spontaneous speech. However, the dissociation has been reported in the literature (see Schiff, Alexander, Naeser and Galaburda, 1983, for a review). The dissociations we have reported together with those already described in the literature conclusively demonstrate, if there still was any need, that the co-occurrence of agrammatism, reduced fluency and dysarthria, although not infrequent, is by no means functionally necessary.

1. Incidence of Fragmented speech in our Agrammatic Speakers

A common feature of so-called agrammatic speech is the presence of "fragmented speech"--operationally defined here as those utterances for which it is not possible to recover the intended grammatical structure. The presence of fragmented utterances in these patients' speech considerably complicates the analysis of the grammatical structure of their speech, and for this reason speech samples were pruned of fragments prior to further analysis. The incidence of fragmented speech in each patient is shown in Table 3.

The proportion of fragmented utterances in the speech of our patients varied considerably. To mention only extreme examples, the proportion of fragmented utterances in the speech of patients F.D., T.F. and F.G. fell within the range observed in normal controls (and the value for patient G.G. was only marginally higher). By contrast, in the case of patients A.S. (.40), B.P. (.39), G.D.C. (.33) and M.U. (.32), the proportion of fragmented utterances was very high. It is unclear to us what weight to assign to the extreme differences in the production of fragmented utterances in the speech of our "agrammatic" sample. We have chosen to downplay the importance of these differences and all further analyses, unless otherwise indicated, are based on the speech samples from which fragmented utterances have been removed.

2. The MLU Produced by Our Agrammatic Speakers

Mean Length of Utterance (MLU) may be taken as a gross index of a patient's sentence production. However, as we have argued elsewhere (Badecker & Caramazza, 1986; Miceli & Mazzucchi, in press) this measure is of suspect theoretical import, as its value can be determined by a number of totally independent impairments of the speech production system (phonological, lexical, syntactic, morphological). Nonetheless, we have chosen to report MLU information as a descriptive means to capture some of the gross differences in our patients' speech.

Table 3. Incidence of fragmented speech observed in each patient (expressed as number of words produced without a recoverable grammatical structure/total number of words in the speech sample).

Subject	F.S.R.
A.A.	.40
F.A.	.08
F.B.	.18
C.D.	.04
F.D.	.01
C.D.A.	.09
G.D.C.	.33
E.D.U.	.06
G.F.	.10
T.F.	.01
F.G.	.01
G.G.	.02
M.L.	.06
A.M.	.06
M.M.	.20
B.P.	.39
C.S.	.18
F.S.	.04
L.S.	.21
M.U.	.32
Normals (range)	.00-.01
Normals (avg.)	.003

As stated in the Materials and Methods Section, two different MLU's were calculated for each patient (MLU-Lexical and MLU-Morphological). MLU-Lexical is an index of the mean number of "syntactically-appropriate," consecutively produced words, ignoring errors of morphology (e.g., agreement errors); MLU-Morphological refers to the mean length of word strings which are both syntactically *and* morphologically correct.

The MLU's reported here were obtained from the analysis of the syntactically structured speech produced by each patient--that is, excluding fragmented utterances. The values of MLU-Lexical and of MLU-Morphological obtained for each patient are shown in Table 4.

Table 4. Mean length (lexical and morphological) of the utterances produced by the patients included in the study, and ratio of the mean length of lexically vs. morphologically intact strings.

Subject	M.L.U.- Lexical	M.L.U.- Morphological	Ratio
A.A.	3.10	2.40	0.78
F.A.	6.06	3.69	0.61
F.B.	4.15	3.74	0.90
C.D.	7.32	4.72	0.64
F.D.	6.55	4.07	0.62
C.D.A.	3.25	2.33	0.72
G.D.C.	3.14	2.13	0.68
E.D.U.	6.65	4.21	0.63
G.F.	4.55	2.46	0.54
T.F.	10.50	3.60	0.34
F.G.	4.69	3.69	0.79
G.G.	4.40	2.90	0.66
M.L.	7.44	6.06	0.81
A.M.	3.37	2.67	0.79
M.M.	4.68	3.45	0.74
B.P.	3.95	2.18	0.55
C.S.	4.26	3.38	0.79
F.S.	6.11	3.16	0.52
L.S.	4.00	2.71	0.68
M.U.	4.70	3.50	0.74
Normals (range)	6.70-13.01	6.65-13.01	0.96-1
Normals (avg.)	8.39	8.35	0.99

Patients' speech production performance as indexed by MLU-Lexical and MLU-Morphological is extremely variable. Thus, when considering MLU-Lexical, three of our 20 subjects (C.D., T.F., and M.L.) fall within the normal range, with T.F. scoring in the upper normal range, whereas the four most impaired subjects (A.A., G.D.C., C.D.A. and A.M.) obtained MLU-Lexical values in the range 3.10 to 3.37 words, considerably below the normal range. As expected, none of our agrammatic speakers are within the normal range for MLU-Morphological. M.L. is the only patient whose MLU-Morphological value is reasonably close to the values obtained by normal subjects--6.06 vs. 6.65; furthermore, 8 of our subjects display a MLU-Morphological of less than 3.0 words.

Our selection criteria for inclusion of patients in this study necessarily requires that patients' MLU-Morphological be shorter than their MLU-Lexical--after all, patients were included in the study *only* if they omitted free-standing grammatical morphemes. Thus, the mere discrepancy between MLU-Morphological and MLU-Lexical scores is not informative.

The *relative* difference between these scores is not unimportant, however--it represents a gross index of sentence processing difficulty. That is, we may take a large discrepancy between MLU-Lexical and MLU-Morphological as an index of the degree of difficulty a patient presents with in the production of context-appropriate morphology. Inspection of the ratio of MLU-Morphological to MLU-Lexical values reveals major differences. Some patients (F.B., M.L., A.M., C.S., A.A.) obtained ratios ranging from 0.78 to 0.90, reflecting minimal morphological processing difficulties. By contrast, patient T.F., and to a lesser extent patients F.S., G.F., and B.P., present with severe difficulties in morphological processing (ratios of 0.34, 0.52, 0.54 and 0.55, respectively). This observation clearly indicates that our patients differ in the extent to which their ability to use free-standing and bound grammatical morphemes in spontaneous speech is impaired. The remainder of this paper will focus on the quantitative and qualitative analysis of these individual differences in grammatical morpheme production.

3. Patterns of Errors on Freestanding Grammatical Morphemes

The crucial, distinguishing feature of agrammatism is the relative omission of free-standing grammatical morphemes. The patients included in our study all presented with this latter feature in their spontaneous production. The issues considered in this section concern, first, the relationship between omissions and substitutions of function words and, second, the extent and type of variation in the omission and substitution of function words in our sample of agrammatic speakers. The objective is to explore the patterns and range of variation in the omission and substitution of free-standing grammatical morphemes when we ignore various other aspects of patients' performance such as substitutions of bound grammatical morphemes and omissions of major lexical items. This analysis shows that the observed variation is such that it cannot easily be accounted for by extant models of the putative category of "agrammatism."

The analysis considers the incidence and distribution of omission and substitution errors on free-standing grammatical morphemes as a whole and the patterns of omission and substitution errors observed in each patient for each of five subsets of morphemes--definite and indefinite articles, prepositions, clitic particles and auxiliary verbs. The results of these analyses are shown in Tables 5-8.

Table 5. Incidence and distribution of omission and substitution errors on free-standing grammatical morphemes considered as a whole and cumulative error rate on the same items.

Subject	% Omission Errors	% Substitution Errors	% Overall Errors
A.A.	25.0	7.7	32.7
F.A.	19.2	1.7	20.9
F.B.	9.7	2.8	12.5
C.D.	7.2	5.2	12.4
F.D.	21.4	7.5	28.9
C.D.A.	24.3	7.4	31.7
G.D.C.	40.4	7.4	47.8
E.D.U.	7.4	8.4	15.8
G.F.	49.6	2.4	52.0
T.F.	50.0	0.6	50.6
F.G.	9.9	4.3	14.2
G.G.	24.6	0.8	25.4
M.L.	5.3	3.8	9.1
A.M.	32.7	4.7	37.4
M.M.	19.8	4.3	24.1
B.P.	28.6	10.5	39.1
D.S.	12.7	3.2	15.9
F.S.	22.3	19.8	42.1
L.S.	19.3	14.8	34.1
M.U.	20.0	9.5	29.5
Norm (range)	0-1.6%	0-1.3%	0-2.9%
Norm (avrg)	0.27%	0.26%	0.5%

Table 5 presents the percentage omission and substitution rates of free-standing grammatical morphemes for each patient and a normal control group. It is clear from these data that patients vary considerably in the extent to which they omit function words in sentence production. Some patients only omitted about 10% while others omitted up to 50% of function words in obligatory contexts. However, these numbers are quite uninformative on their own as they may reflect no more than the severity of deficit in patients with the same underlying disorder. A more informative analysis for our purposes concerns the comparison of omission and substitution rates. As is the case with omissions, substitution errors on free-standing grammatical morphemes show a wide range of variation (compare T.F. (0.6%) and G.G. (0.8%) with F.S. (19.8%) and L.S. (14.8%)). However, there appears to be little relationship between the incidence of omissions and substitutions of function words in the same patient. Patients T.F., G.F., G.G. and F.A. demonstrate a very high omission rate and a very low substitution rate (T.F.: 50% vs. 0.6%; G.F.: 49.6% vs. 2.4%; G.G.:

24.6% vs. 0.8%; F.A.: 19.2% vs. 1.7%), whereas subjects F.S., E.D.U., L.S. and C.D. show a comparable percent incidence of omissions and substitutions (F.S.: 22.3% vs. 19.8%; E.D.U.: 7.4% vs. 8.4%; L.S.: 19.3% vs. 14.8%; C.D.: 7.2% vs. 5.2%). Furthermore, no relationship exists between absolute levels of omission and substitution rates across patients; thus, for example, patients F.S. and G.G. make approximately the same percentage of omission errors (22.3% and 24.6%), yet F.S. makes a very high proportion of substitution errors (19.8% of the free-standing grammatical morphemes are substituted), whereas G.G. makes essentially no errors of this type (0.8%). The clearest dissociation of the two types of errors is observed in patients T.F. and G.F., who display the highest omission rates in our sample (50% and 49.6%, respectively), but make virtually no substitution errors (0.6% and 2.4%, respectively).

The significance of these results is not immediately apparent. Traditionally, substitution errors of function words have been considered to reflect a different underlying deficit from that which results in the omission of these words. While this intuitive distinction may prove to be correct, it does not help us in deciding whether or not patients who in addition to omission errors also produce substitution errors should be considered as being agrammatic. We will take up this issue in the discussion section.

Distribution of errors across different function words: Table 6 shows the incidence of errors (combined omissions and substitutions) in the production of the five types of function words included in our analysis-- prepositions, definite and indefinite articles, clitics, auxiliary verbs. Once again we note striking variations in error patterns: No consistent rank of difficulty can be observed, and different subjects show different error patterns. The clearest instances of such lack of consistent patterns are patients C.D.A.: errors on 61.5% of the clitic particles, but on only 6.2% of the auxiliary verbs; E.D.U.: errors on 52.6% of the auxiliary verbs but on only 5.3% of the indefinite articles; T.F.: errors on 100% of the clitic particles but on 20.3% of the prepositions; F.G.: errors on 50% of the auxiliary verbs but on only 7.9% of the definite and 7.1% of the indefinite articles; G.G.: errors on 34.6% of the definite and 37.5% of the indefinite articles, but no errors on auxiliaries; M.M.: errors on 80% of the clitic particles, but on only 11% of the definite articles, and error-free performance on indefinite articles; M.U.: 44.4% errors on clitics and no errors on auxiliaries and indefinite articles. From these data it is clear that no consistent pattern of impairment in the production of free-standing grammatical morphemes is found in our patient series. It may turn out that there is a principled account that could explain the observed variation. However, if nothing else, it should be abundantly clear that the observed variation is not "largely explainable" by current accounts of "agrammatism" --Principles such as the sonorance hierarchy, morphological paradigms, or "processing" considerations cannot account for the varied forms of relative error patterns of function word errors (omissions and substitutions).

Table 6. Cumulative error rate in each of the five categories of free-standing grammatical markers (N = number of obligatory contexts).

Subject	Prepositions N	%Errors	Definite Articles N	%Errors	Indefinite Articles N	%Errors	Clitics N	%Errors	Auxiliaries N	%Errors
A.A.	9	66.7	28	25.0	6	--	5	--	4	100.0
F.A.	32	34.3	48	8.3	6	--	15	46.7	9	33.3
F.B.	65	15.3	57	3.5	2	--	11	18.2	13	30.8
C.D.	149	10.8	136	7.5	24	25.0	114	16.7	23	17.4
F.D.	148	33.1	92	26.1	21	42.8	62	24.2	44	29.6
C.D.A.	85	40.0	121	29.8	4	25.0	13	61.5	32	6.2
G.D.C.	18	83.3	56	33.9	9	55.6	9	44.4	2	100.0
E.D.U.	110	10.9	109	12.8	19	5.3	40	25.0	19	52.6
G.F.	52	44.3	41	58.5	3	33.3	11	36.4	18	72.2
T.F.	59	20.3	50	64.0	9	33.3	15	100.0	30	73.3
F.G.	60	16.6	51	7.9	14	7.1	28	14.3	8	50.0
G.G.	41	18.5	52	34.6	8	37.5	13	15.4	8	--
M.L.	37	5.4	33	18.2	11	--	32	9.4	20	5.0
A.M.	36	38.9	44	56.8	6	33.3	36	16.6	28	32.2
M.M.	58	29.3	100	11.0	5	--	15	80.0	9	55.5
B.P.	30	53.3	58	27.5	2	--	7	57.2	8	62.5
C.S.	6	--	33	15.4	2	--	16	25.0	6	16.7
F.S.	75	54.7	98	35.7	40	25.0	24	50.0	5	80.0
L.S.	28	21.4	31	38.7	6	50.0	15	33.3	8	50.0
M.U.	30	40.0	49	16.3	6	--	18	44.4	2	--

It might be objected that the observed variations in error patterns only result because of our conflation of omissions and substitutions of function words. But, this is not the case. Equally diverse patterns of function word errors emerge when we consider separately omissions and substitutions of function words. Table 7 presents separately the relative omission and substitution rates of the various free-standing grammatical morphemes observed in our patient sample. For example, A.A. makes substitution and omission errors with definite articles (10.7% and 14.3%, respectively), otherwise she makes only omission errors with prepositions (66.7%) and no errors at all with indefinite articles and clitics (the number of obligatory contexts for auxiliary verbs is too small to draw any conclusions on A.A.'s behavior on these items). Patient G.D.C. makes substitution errors only with articles--with other function words his errors consist only of omissions. Patient F.S. produces a high number of omission and substitution errors on prepositions and articles (17.8% and 22.5%, respectively), but all his errors on clitic particles and auxiliary verbs take the form of omissions (55.2%).

Table 7. Incidence and distribution of omission and substitution errors in each category of free-standing grammatical markers.

Subject	Prepositions %Om.	Prepositions %Sub.	Definite Articles %Om.	Definite Articles %Sub.	Indefinite Articles %Om.	Indefinite Articles %Sub.	Clitics %Om.	Clitics %Sub.	Auxiliaries %Om.	Auxiliaries %Sub.
A.A.	66.7	--	14.3	10.7	--	--	--	--	75.0	25.0
F.A.	28.1	6.2	8.3	--	--	--	46.7	--	33.3	--
F.B.	13.8	1.5	3.5	--	--	--	--	18.2	23.1	7.7
C.D.	7.4	3.4	6.0	1.5	12.5	12.5	7.0	9.7	8.7	8.7
F.D.	22.3	10.8	20.7	5.4	33.3	9.5	16.1	8.1	27.3	2.3
C.D.A.	27.1	12.9	24.8	5.0	25.0	--	53.8	7.7	3.1	3.1
G.D.C.	83.3	--	25.0	8.9	33.3	22.2	44.4	--	100.0	--
E.D.U.	7.3	3.6	5.5	7.3	--	5.3	10.0	15.0	21.0	31.6
G.F.	38.5	5.8	58.5	--	33.3	--	36.4	--	72.2	--
T.F.	18.6	1.7	64.0	--	33.3	--	100.0	--	63.3	10.0
F.G.	8.3	8.3	5.9	2.0	--	7.1	14.3	--	--	50.0
G.G.	18.5	--	32.7	1.9	37.5	--	15.4	--	--	--
M.L.	2.7	2.7	15.2	3.0	--	--	--	9.4	5.0	--
A.M.	38.9	--	50.0	6.8	33.3	--	8.3	8.3	28.6	3.6
M.M.	27.6	1.7	6.0	5.0	--	--	80.0	--	33.3	22.2
B.P.	43.3	10.0	24.1	3.4	--	--	14.3	42.9	25.0	37.5
C.S.	--	--	12.1	3.3	--	--	18.7	6.2	16.7	--
F.S.	30.7	24.0	11.2	24.5	10.0	15.0	50.0	--	80.0	--
L.S.	14.3	7.1	22.6	16.1	--	50.0	20.0	13.3	37.5	12.5
M.U.	20.0	20.0	14.3	2.0	--	--	33.3	11.1	--	--

To sum up this section, our analyses demonstrate that there is extreme variation in the rate of omission of free-standing grammatical markers and that omissions are not distributed homogeneously across subsets of grammatical morphemes. A surprisingly high incidence of substitution errors was found in most (but by no means in all) patients in our sample; once again, however, no consistent relationship existed between omission and substitution rates, and substitution rates differed across subsets of free-standing grammatical morphemes. These results cannot be accommodated within extant characterizations of the mechanisms underlying the processing of free-standing grammatical morphemes. Indeed, it is not even clear what data patterns should be taken as the basis for an explanatory effort--it does not appear possible to specify a level of abstraction from these data (short of a useless definitional approach--see

Badecker & Caramazza, 1985) which would serve as the basis for making claims about the nature of the underlying disorder in these patients we have classified as agrammatic.

4. Errors on Bound Grammatical Markers and Their Relationships to Errors on Freestanding Grammatical Markers

In the introduction we defined agrammatism as a disorder of sentence production characterized by the *omission* of free-standing grammatical morphemes and the *omission or substitution* of bound grammatical morphemes. The need for including substitution of bound grammatical morphemes in our definition is dictated by specific properties of Italian, which unlike English does not permit the mere omission of an inflection without resulting in a nonword. It is important, therefore, to consider the pattern of substitutions of inflections in our patients.

The relative incidence of errors in the production of bound grammatical morphemes for our patients is reported in Table 8. Before considering these results further it is worth stressing right at the outset that not one of our patients made errors which could be interpreted as omissions of a bound grammatical morpheme. All the errors in the production of these items observed in our corpora (n=434) can be unambiguously interpreted as substitution errors.

The comparison between the errors made by our subjects in the production of free-standing vs. bound grammatical morphemes can be made by considering different indices of impairment.

A first comparison was made by contrasting the combined incidence of substitution and omission errors on free-standing grammatical morphemes with the incidence of bound grammatical morpheme substitutions. Although there appears to be a correlation between error rates on the two types of morphemes (r=.84, p<.01) there are also some interesting deviations from this pattern. Thus, for example, patients C.D. and A.M. display roughly the same incidence of substitutions of bound grammatical morphemes (5.8% and 6.5%, respectively); however, C.D. makes errors on only 12.4% of the free-standing grammatical morphemes, whereas A.M. produces incorrectly 37.4% of these items. Conversely, patients F.G. and E.D.U. make approximately the same percentage of errors on free-standing grammatical morphemes (14.2% and 15.8%, respectively), yet F.G. substitutes only 0.8% of the bound grammatical morphemes while E.D.U. displays a much higher rate of substitution of these items (8.6%).

Essentially the same results are obtained if the rate of omission of free-standing grammatical morphemes is compared to the rate of substitution of bound grammatical morphemes: A general correlation exists (r=.77, p<.01) but clear exceptions are also present. The same contrast as in the previous paragraph is observed if patients C.D. and A.M. are considered again: C.D. omits only 7.2% to A.M.'s 32.7% of the free-standing grammatical morphemes. The opposite contrast is demonstrated by patients C.D.A. and G.G., as opposed to patient F.S. These three patients omit approximately the same percentage of free-standing grammatical morphemes (24.3%, 24.6% and 22.3%, respectively), but C.D.A. and G.G. demonstrate a rather low substitution rate on bound grammatical morphemes (5.7% and 4.7%, respectively) compared to F.S.'s 20.4% incorrect production.

Table 8. Incidence and distribution of omission and substitution error on free-standing grammatical morphemes considered as a whole and cumulative error rate on the same items (as in Table 5); incidence and distribution of substitution errors on bound grammatical markers.

Subject	Free-Standing Grammatical Morphemes			Bound Grammatical Morphemes
	Overall Errors	Omission Errors	Substitution Errors	Substitution Errors
A.A.	32.7%	25.0%	7.7%	9.6%
F.A.	20.9%	19.2%	1.7%	9.9%
F.B.	12.5%	9.7%	2.8%	1.7%
C.D.	12.4%	7.2%	5.2%	5.8%
F.D.	28.9%	21.4%	7.5%	5.7%
C.D.A.	31.7%	24.3%	7.4%	5.7%
G.D.C.	47.8%	40.4%	7.4%	15.3%
E.D.U.	15.8%	7.4%	8.4%	8.6%
G.F.	52.0%	49.6%	2.4%	24.2%
T.F.	50.6%	50.0%	0.6%	21.1%
F.G.	14.2%	9.9%	4.3%	0.8%
G.G.	25.4%	24.6%	0.8%	4.7%
M.L.	9.1%	5.3%	1.8%	3.7%
A.M.	37.4%	32.7%	4.7%	6.5%
M.M.	24.1%	19.8%	4.3%	4.1%
B.P.	39.1%	28.6%	10.5%	17.8%
C.S.	15.9%	12.7%	3.2%	3.4%
F.S.	42.1%	22.3%	19.8%	20.4%
L.S.	34.1%	19.3%	14.8%	7.3%
M.U.	29.5%	20.0%	9.5%	8.4%
Norm (range)	0-2.9%	0-1.6%	0-1.3%	0-2.2%
Norm (avrg)	0.5%	0.27%	0.26%	0.22%

We also compared the rate of substitution of bound grammatical morphemes with the rate of substitution of free-standing grammatical morphemes. In this case too, obvious differences in performance are observed across patients (r=.25, n.s.). Cases G.G. and T.F. show the same, negligible incidence of free-standing grammatical morpheme substitution (0.8% and 0.6%, respectively), and yet G.G. substitutes 4.7% bound grammatical morphemes to T.F.'s 21.1%. Similarly, F.B. and G.F. produce a comparable number of substitutions of free-standing grammatical morphemes (2.8% and 2.4%, respectively), and a very different number of substitutions of bound grammatical morphemes (1.7% and 24.2%, respectively). Conversely, T.F. and F.S. substitute bound grammatical morphemes at approximately the same rate (21.1% vs. 20.4%, respectively), yet T.F. almost never substitutes free-standing grammatical morphemes, whereas F.S. makes very frequent substitution errors (0.6% vs. 19.8%). In our sample there are no instances of patients who make substitution errors on free-standing, but not on bound grammatical morphemes.

The results of our analyses of the relationship between errors on free-standing and on bound grammatical morphemes can now be briefly summarized. In all the comparisons we noted a relationship between errors on free-standing and bound grammatical morphemes, however, clear-cut deviations from the general pattern were observed. In each comparison we carried out we found patients who show comparable impairment on one set of items, but very different impairment in the production of items from the other set. Only when the comparison was restricted to substitution errors did we find that in our sample there are no patients who display a high incidence of substitutions of free-standing grammatical morphemes and a low (or very low) incidence of bound grammatical morpheme substitutions. One conclusion that is possible from these results is that the difficulties in the production of free-standing and of bound grammatical morphemes in our patient sample are largely independent--damage to separate mechanisms is responsible for the two types of grammatical morphemes.

5. Analysis of the violations of agreement relations

Thus far, we have considered grammatical morphemes in isolation. However, both free-standing and bound grammatical morphemes enter into agreement relations. Thus, for example, articles are involved in nominal agreement, auxiliary verbs are part of complex verbal relations, and inflections, be they nominal, adjectival or verbal, all enter into agreement relations. For this reason, the scope of our analysis was further broadened. The performance obtained by our group of agrammatic speakers on all grammatical morphemes was evaluated by considering the following agreement relations: det-Noun, Noun-Adjective, and Subject-Verb.

Before we present our data, some clarifications concerning the scoring procedure should be made. In the evaluation of det-Noun agreement, instances where the article was omitted were not counted. The incidence of det-Noun agreement violations was evaluated on the basis of those instances where an article was produced (correctly or incorrectly). Some NP's containing a det-Noun combination, which had been excluded from previous analysis because they had been produced in the absence of a recoverable grammatical structure, where included in this count.

The incidence of Noun-Adjective agreement violations was evaluated using as a data base all sequences that included inflected Adjectives. The incidence of Subject-Verb agreement violations was calculated on the basis of all the instances where the subject of the sentence, whether present or (as it is very often the case in Italian) absent from the surface structure, could be unambiguously identified. Agreement errors were scored both if they appeared in the production of lexical verbs and if they occurred in the production of the auxiliary verb (which, in Italian, is inflected just like any other verb).

The results of this analysis are shown in Table 9. Inspection of Table 9 reveals the existence of two distinct patterns of impairment, as well as intermediate patterns between the two extremes. The first pattern is observed most clearly in patients F.S. and L.S., but is also present in patients F.A., G.D.C., B.P. and M.U. In these patients, all types of agreement are impaired. Not surprisingly, Subject-Verb agreement is usually the most impaired, probably due to the fact that in Italian the inflectional paradigm of verbs is much more complex than that of nouns and adjectives (approximately 40 inflections for verbs, as opposed to 2, or exceptionally 4, for nouns and 4, or less frequently 2, for adjectives). The other relevant pattern is observed in patient T.F., and consists of the complete sparing of nominal and adjectival agreement, in the presence of a very severe deficit of verbal agreement--in fact, T.F. is the patient in our sample who shows the most severe impairment of verb agreement. The same pattern of impairment, although in a slightly less pure form, is observed in patients G.F. and G.G. Patient G.F. makes only 1 error in 18 instances of det-Noun agreement (5.6%), no errors of Noun-Adjective agreement, and 55 violations of Subject-Verb agreement out of 100 instances (55%). Patient G.G. makes no errors of det-Noun agreement, only 1 error in 26 instances of Noun-Adjective agreement (3.8%), and 10 violations out of 54 instances of Subject-Verb agreement (18.5%).

Table 9. Incidence and distribution of violations of det-Noun, Noun-Adjective and Subject-Verb agreement.

Subject	Determiner-Noun		Noun-Adjective		Subject-Verb	
	N	%Violation	N	%Violation	N	%Violation
A.A.	25	8.0	8	--	23	43.5
F.A.	71	5.6	45	11.1	81	29.6
F.B.	63	--	9	11.1	86	3.5
C.D.	127	0.8	57	7.0	194	6.7
F.D.	67	1.5	78	14.1	193	11.9
C.D.A.	95	4.2	38	--	100	16.0
G.D.C.	70	5.7	9	22.2	46	43.5
E.D.U.	99	2.0	32	6.2	152	18.4
G.F.	18	5.6	28	--	100	55.0
T.F.	18	--	56	--	101	64.4
F.G.	73	1.4	32	3.1	114	4.4
G.G.	65	--	26	3.8	54	18.5
M.L.	34	2.9	25	4.0	52	3.9
A.M.	18	11.1	20	--	85	15.3
M.M.	110	4.5	26	--	61	14.7
B.P.	43	9.3	26	3.8	46	52.2
C.S.	20	--	10	--	33	9.1
F.S.	138	14.5	50	20.0	88	47.7
L.S.	32	12.5	7	28.6	51	19.6
M.U.	61	3.3	12	8.3	63	12.7

A more detailed analysis of error patterns in agreement relations was undertaken for verbal agreements. Verb agreement errors were divided in two broad categories: those which resulted in the production of the citation form of the verb, and those which resulted in the production of other incorrect verb forms. For this analysis we considered both the infinitive and the past participle as citation forms. Table 10 reports the results of this analysis. The results unequivocally show that three patients (T.F., G.F. and G.G.) can be confidently set apart from the other subjects in our sample. If we consider only those patients who produced at least 10 instances of verb agreement errors, we find that the citation form of the verb constitutes the overwhelming majority of the errors only in the case of patients T.F. (95.4%), G.F. (96.4%) and G.G. (100%). In the other patients of our group, the percentage incidence of this error type is much lower. By striking contrast to G.G., G.F. and T.F., other subjects in our sample display a very high incidence of incorrectly inflected verb forms which are not citation forms. The highest number of these errors was produced by patients C.D.A. (87.5%), C.D. (83.3%) and E.D.U. (82.1%).

Table 10. Subject-Verb agreement errors: distribution of distribution of errors consisting of the production of citation forms vs. other incorrectly inflected forms.

Subject	Number of violations	Citation form		Other incorrect verb forms	
		N	%	N	%
A.A.	10	6	(60.0)	4	(40.0)
F.A.	24	7	(29.2)	17	(70.8)
F.B.	3	2	(66.7)	1	(33.3)
C.D.	12	2	(16.7)	10	(83.3)
F.D.	23	15	(65.2)	8	(34.8)
C.D.A.	16	2	(12.5)	14	(87.5)
G.D.C.	20	6	(30.0)	14	(70.0)
E.D.U.	28	5	(17.9)	23	(82.1)
G.F.	55	53	(96.4)	2	(3.6)
T.F.	65	62	(95.4)	3	(4.6)
F.G.	5	3	(60.0)	2	(40.0)
G.G.	10	10	(100.0)	0	
M.L.	2	1	(50.0)	1	(50.0)
A.M.	13	7	(53.8)	6	(46.2)
M.M.	9	2	(22.2)	7	(77.8)
B.P.	24	11	(45.8)	13	(54.2)
C.S.	3	2	(66.7)	1	(33.3)
F.S.	42	23	(54.8)	19	(45.2)
L.S.	10	3	(30.0)	7	(70.0)
M.U.	8	6	(75.0)	2	(25.0)

DISCUSSION

A crucial issue in neuropsychology concerns the role of clinically defined aphasic patient categories as a basis for making claims about normal language processing. In previous publications we have argued that it is impossible to draw theoretically meaningful conclusions about language processing from research based on clinically defined patient categories, and that it is impossible to make theoretically meaningful claims about the nature of the language disorder in such patient categories (Badecker & Caramazza, 1985; Caramazza, 1984; 1986; Caramazza & McCloskey, in press; McCloskey & Caramazza, in press). Much of the discussion on this issue has focused on the putative category "agrammatism," although our claim extends to all *a priori* patient categories (e.g., deep dyslexia, phonological agraphia, transcortical aphasia, and so forth). Despite the many discussions of this issue, it is far from being resolved. A particularly contentious issue concerns the empirical facts that should be considered in any attempted resolution of the problem. Contrasting claims have been made about the empirical facts concerning the clinical category agrammatism. Consequently, the principal objective of this research was to explore the range of variation in the production of grammatical morphemes in clinically classified agrammatic patients. The detailed and extensive data base obtained could then serve as the basis for an **informed** discussion of whether or not the clinical disorder identified as agrammatism constitutes a cognitively homogeneous category. We consider the results we have reported in this paper as *prima facie* evidence against extant claims of homogeneity for the category of "agrammatism." The rest of this discussion is devoted to a defence of this conclusion.

Before undertaking a discussion of the reported results we should consider, even if only briefly, the general problem of determining the boundaries of the agrammatic deficit; that is, we should attempt to answer the question: Which features of agrammatic patients' performance should figure in the present analysis? We have chosen to adopt a narrow definition of the disorder. We have considered only that form of agrammatism which is defined as a disorder of sentence production characterized by the omission of free-standing grammatical morphemes and the omission or substitution of bound grammatical morphemes. We have ignored other putative features of this disorder such as "asyntactic" comprehension and word order processing difficulties. The inclusion of the latter performance features would only have complicated our discussion and, in any case, it is well established that these symptoms dissociate from difficulties in the production of grammatical morphemes (Caramazza & Hillis, 1987; Kolk, van Grunsven & Kuper, 1985; Miceli, Mazzucchi, Menn & Goodglass, 1983; Nespoulous, Dordain, Perron, Ska, Bub, Caplan, Mehler & Lecours, in press; see also Caramazza & Berndt, 1985, for review). The advantage of restricting the focus of our investigation to difficulties in the production of grammatical morphemes is that this symptom (or symptom complex) is unarguably the central feature, if not the only relevant one on all accounts, of agrammatism.

Even with this restriction in the focus of our investigation, there remain non-negligible problems in determining which aspects of the performance of clinically agrammatic patients should be considered in our analysis. Thus, for example, what status should function word substitution errors be accorded in the analysis of agrammatic production? Are these errors a reflection of the "agrammatic" disorder? Should substitution errors of inflections be considered on a par with omissions of function words in the analysis of agrammatic patients? Obviously, if we cannot answer questions of this type it will be futile to pretend that the issue under consideration is an empirical one; not only will we not know who is to be considered as an agrammatic patient but we also will not know what aspects of a patient's performance are theoretically relevant for the analysis of agrammatism. Indeed, a major criticism we have leveled against the use of patient categories in neuropsychological research is that the boundaries of patient categories such as agrammatism are not sufficiently well-specified to permit meaningful investigation of the putative categories of deficit (Badecker & Caramazza, 1985; Caramazza, in press). This latter problem aside, we can take a boot-strap approach to an evaluation of the variation in agrammatic performance by considering, in turn, various definitions of the disorder. Even on such a weak definition of agrammatism (ultimately too weak to be of much theoretical interest), the observed variability in patients' performance undermines any pretension of an empirically based coherence for the category of "agrammatism."

Variation in the Omission (and Substitution) of Function Words

The central, defining feature of agrammatism is the omission of free-standing grammatical morphemes in spontaneous speech (Caplan, 1986; Goodglass, 1976; Kean, 1977). The analysis of this performance variable in our set of agrammatic patients brings to the fore a series of interesting problems. Let us consider first the pattern of variation among function word omissions. Our analysis of the pattern of omissions of these words failed to reveal a consistent hierarchy of omission rates for five types of function words. Obviously, in such a case it is difficult to maintain the position that there is a principled (unitary) linguistic account which could explain the observed variation (Caplan, 1986). Indeed, the patterns of variation are so large that it is difficult to imagine what could be gained by considering the patients included in the sample as all having a common functional lesion at some level of language processing. Thus, consider the following contrasts (see Table 7). Patients F.A. and A.M. show contrasting patterns of omissions of definite articles and clitics (8% vs. 47% and 50% vs. 8%, respectively); patients C.D.A. and F.B. show contrasting patterns of omissions for clitics and auxiliaries (54% vs. 3% and 0% vs. 23%, respectively); and, patients G.D.C. and T.F. show contrasting patterns of omissions for prepositions and definite articles (83% vs. 25% and 19% vs. 64%, respectively). Of course, one could always appeal to some unspecified, non-linguistic, "processing" principle which may be assumed to account for the observed variability. However, such a move remains vacuous unless one could articulate the putative "processing" principles that are assumed to be responsible for the variation in question. To our knowledge no interesting proposal has been offered in this regard. And, in any case, this move is a dangerous one, as we will see below.

The picture is further muddied when we consider the relationship between the omission and substitution of free-standing grammatical morphemes. Our results show that there is no consistent relationship between the overall rates of omission and substitution errors for function words. More interestingly, we found contrasting patterns of omission versus substitution error rates for different types of function words. Thus, for example, patient F.S.'s errors for prepositions and articles consist of substitutions and omissions but only of omissions for clitics and auxiliaries; analogously, patient G.D.C.'s errors for prepositions, clitics, and auxiliaries consist entirely of omissions while his errors for articles (definite and indefinite) include nonnegligeable proportions of substitutions. Once again we find that the patterns of errors for free-standing grammatical morphemes do vary along apparently inexplicable dimensions at least with respect to linguistic considerations.

Our decision to inject consideration of function-word substitution errors in a discussion of "agrammatism" may be challenged on the grounds that this latter type of error does not form part of the symptom complex of agrammatism. On this account, function-word substitution errors are considered symptomatic of "paragrammatism" and not "agrammatism" and, therefore, should be excluded from analysis of the latter disorder. There are two reasons for considering this counterargument as inadequate for the present discussion. One reason involves the problem of distinguishing between "agrammatism" and "paragrammatism" as distinct, cognitively coherent disorders; the other reason involves the failure to provide a linguistically motivated distinction between omission and substitution of function words.

Suppose that we were to agree that the omission and the substitution of function words could be taken as symptomatic of distinct disorders-- "agrammatism" and "paragrammatism," respectively. We would then be confronted with the problem of having to decide which of our patients are agrammatic and which are paragrammatic, or, alternatively, we would have to decide the extent to which each of our patients presents with a mix of agrammatism and paragrammatism. Thus, which of our patients are "true" agrammatics given that they all substitute function words to some extent or other? And, if we take the presence of function-word substitution as symptomatic of "paragrammatism," should we conclude that each of our agrammatic patients also presents with a paragrammatic disorder? Clearly, the empirical facts are such that it does not appear that we can distinguish between the putative categories of "agrammatism" and "paragrammatism," even when we restrict the analysis of speech production impairment to errors with free-standing grammatical morphemes.

There is a more fundamental reason for considering "agrammatism" as a theoretically vacuous category. The most important (defining) feature of agrammatism is taken to be the omission of function words in spontaneous speech. But, is there a principled basis for distinguishing between the **omission** and the **substitution** of function words? The principal argument given for considering "agrammatism" as a theoretically coherent category, as opposed to merely an empirical category without theoretical motivation, is that this category is defined by appeal to a linguistically motivated distinction--function words can be given an independent linguistic characterization (Caplan, 1986; Kean, 1977). However, even if one were to accept this argument as sufficient motivation for distinguishing patients with a deficit to this class of words from patients with deficits to other linguistic units, the argument would not be sufficient for distinguishing between patients who **omit** and patients who **substitute** these words. Thus, the distinction between omission and substitution of function words does not receive its motivation from linguistic theory and, therefore, we do not have a linguistically motivated basis for the putative distinction. If we wish to consider the omission and the substitution of function words as symptomatic of different deficits to the language system we must appeal not to linguistic theory but to processing principles.

Suppose, then, that we were to assume that the distinction between omission and substitution of free-standing grammatical morphemes reflects different forms of processing deficit to this class of items. This assumption is not implausible, but it is equally unmotivated. Note that the distinction is not made on considerations based on one or another processing theory but on strictly intuitive grounds--it feels like omissions and substitutions should result from different kinds of processing deficits. This intuition may ultimately prove to be correct. However, until a motivated processing account is given for the omission/substitution distinction we must recognize its **arbitrary** nature and give up any pretense of having a theoretically motivated basis for the category of "agrammatism."

A final comment on the arbitrary nature of the classificatory criteria used for defining agrammatism is in order, especially in light of the analyses reported in this paper. Recall that at an earlier point we noted that the patients in this study differed considerably in terms of their patterns of omissions of five types of function words. The patterns of variation were such that they could not be accounted for on the basis of linguistic principles. In order to maintain that the patients tested should nonetheless all be considered to be agrammatics, one has to assume that the observed differences can be explained by some as yet unspecified processing differences among our patients. In this case a linguistic criterion--errors in the production of function words--independently of differences in processing deficits, is sufficient to specify category membership. By contrast, the same linguistic criterion is not sufficient for determining category membership when the processing difference involves the contrast between omission and substitution of words (i.e., the difference between "agrammatic" and "paragrammatic" function-word errors). Clearly, the decision of when a linguistic or processing criterion is sufficient for determining the patient category of agrammatism is totally arbitrary.

Variation in the Substitution of Bound Grammatical Morphemes and Violations of Agreement Relations

Patients' performance in the production of bound grammatical morphemes varied extensively, and independently of their performance with free-standing grammatical morphemes. Although we did find a quantitative relationship between omission rate of function words and substitution rate for bound grammatical morphemes, the relationship was not a necessary one as there were a number of clear "dissociations" between error rates for the two classes of grammatical morphemes. That is, we found that some patients presented with striking discrepancies between their rate of substitution errors for bound grammatical morphemes and the rate of function word omissions or substitutions. Furthermore, when we considered the types of substitution errors made by the patients we found as much variability among error types as we had found for omissions of different types of function words. Thus, for example, we found that some patients almost always produced the citation form when they made a verb inflection error, whereas other patients almost always produced the non-citation form when they made a verb error. Equally extreme variations in performance were obtained in the patterns of agreement errors where some patients produced many errors of subject/verb agreement but almost never made errors for within noun phrase agreements--both det/noun and adjective/noun agreements; other patients, by contrast, were as likely to make within noun phrase errors as they were to make subject/verb agreement errors.

Once again we find that the "empirical facts" belie all claims of an obvious performance homogeneity among patients who would be clinically classified as agrammatic. The extensive performance variability we found among our agrammatic patients presumably reflects major differences in the deficits to language-specific processes (or related cognitive processes) which underlie each patient's performance. In light of the results and arguments presented here we find no grounds on which to support the claim that "agrammatism" constitutes a "natural kind" category representing those patients with deficit to a single, well-defined component of the language processing system (or even common and equivalent deficits to multiple components). Instead we are led once again to conclude that the variability among the putative cases of agrammatism we tested appears to be no less important in determining the precise nature of the functional lesion in thus-classified patients, than the variability that distinguishes among any **randomly** selected aphasic patients.

In concluding it is important to stress one final point. The results we have reported belie the claim of significant homogeneity among so-called agrammatic patients **even when** the analysis is restricted to just those features of patients performance--errors in the production of grammatical morphemes--which are considered to be defining of the patient category. The situation is equally bad when we consider variation among other dimensions of language processing; that is, when we consider such features as major-class lexical omissions and phrase length in sentence production, comprehension performance, and grammaticality judgments. For here we find that each of these indices of language processing dissociate from one another and from difficulties in the production of grammatical morphemes (see Caramazza & Berndt, 1985, for review). Thus, in our sample of agrammatic patients we found that some of them have major problems in producing main verbs (rate of omission of the main (lexical) verb in obligatory context: A.A.: 36.7%; C.S.: 26.2%; C.D.A.: 24.8%; B.P.: 21.7%) while others present with little or no difficulty in this area (G.F.: 0%; T.F.: 1.2%; M.L.: 1.9%; E.D.U.: 2%); we found that some patients are able to produce very long sentence constructions (MLU-Lexical: T.F.: 10.5; M.L.: 7.44; C.D.: 7.32; E.D.U.: 6.65) while others have their output reduced to three-word sentences (MLU-Lexical: A.A.: 3.1; G.D.C.: 3.14; C.D.A.: 3.25; A.M.: 3.37); and, as is now well established, sentence comprehension difficulties dissociate from sentence production difficulties (Caramazza & Hillis, 1987; Kolk et al., 1985; Miceli et al., 1983; Nespoulous et al., in press) and the ability to judge the grammaticality of sentences (Linebarger, Schwartz & Saffran, 1983). These empirical facts can no longer be ignored just for the obstinate protection of a fictional category of dubious theoretical value. There are not only metatheoretical and methodological reasons for doing away with patient categories such as agrammatism, but also empirical demonstrations of the futility of holding on to such categories. Here we have provided one such demonstration.

ACKNOWLEDGEMENTS

The research reported here was supported in part by a grant from the Consiglio Nazionale delle Ricerche, Italy, and NIH Grant NS23836 to The Johns Hopkins University. We would like to thank Chris Barry for helpful comments on an earlier version of this paper and Kathy Yantis for her help in the preparation of the manuscript.

REFERENCES

Badecker, W. & Caramazza, A. (1985). On considerations of method and theory governing the use of clinical categories in neurolinguistics and cognitive neuropsychology: The case against agrammatism. Cognition, 20, 97-125.

Badecker, W. & Caramazza, A. (1986). A final brief in the case against agrammatism: The role of theory in the selection of data. Cognition, 24, 277-282.

Caplan, D. (1986). In defense of agrammatism. Cognition, 24, 263-276.

Caramazza, A. (1984). The logic of neuropsychological research and the problem of patient classification in aphasia. Brain and Language, 21,-9 20.

Caramazza, A. (1986). On drawing inferences about the structure of normal cognitive systems from the analysis of patterns of impaired performance: The case for single-patient studies. Brain and Cognition, 5, 41-66.

Caramazza, A. (in press). When is enough, enough? A comment on Grodzinsky and Marek's "Algorithmic and heuristic processes revisited." Brain and Language.

Caramazza, A. & Berndt, R. S. (1985). A multicomponent deficit view of agrammatic Broca's aphasia. In M.-L. Kean (Ed.), Agrammatism, 21-63. Orlando, FL: Academic Press.

Caramazza, A. & Hillis, A. (1987). The disruption of sentence production: A case of selective deficit to positional level processing. Reports of The Cognitive Neuropsychology Laboratory, The Johns Hopkins University.

Caramazza, A. & McCloskey, M. (in press). The case for single-patient studies. Cognitive Neuropsychology.

De Villiers, J. G. (1978). Fourteen grammatical morphemes in acquisition and aphasia. In A. Caramazza & E. B. Zurif (Eds.), Language acquisition and language breakdown: Parallels and divergences, pp 121-144. Baltimore, MD: The Johns Hopkins University Press.

Goodglass, H. (1976). Agrammatism. In H. Whitaker & H.A. Whitaker (Eds.), Studies in neurolinguistics, Vol. 1. New York, NY: Academic Press.

Goodglass, H. & Kaplan, E. (1972). The Assessment of aphasia and related disorders. Philadelphia, PA: Lea and Febiger.

Isserlin, M. (1922). Uber Agrammatismus. Zeitschria fur die Gesamte Neurologie and Psychiatrie, 75, 332-416.

Kean, M.-L. (1977). The linguistic interpretation of aphasia syndromes: Agrammatism in Broca's aphasia, an example. Cognition, 5, 9-46.

Kolk, H. H. J., Van Grunsven, M. J. F. & Kuper, A. (1985). On parallelism between production and comprehension in agrammatism. In M.-L. Kean (Ed.) Agrammatism, 165-206. Orlando, FL: Academic Press.

Lapointe, S. (1985). A theory of verb from use in the speech of agrammatic aphasics. Brain and Language, 24, 100-155.

Lenneberg, E. H. (1967). Biological foundations of language. New York, NY: John Wiley & Sons.

Linebarger, M., Schwartz, M. & Saffran, E. (1983). Sensitivity to grammatical structure in so-called agrammatic aphasics. Cognition, 13, 361-392.

Marshall, J. C. (1986). The description and interpretation of aphasic language disorder. Neuropsychologia, 24, 5-24.

McCloskey, M. & Caramazza, A. (in press). Theory and methodology in cognitive neuropsychology. Cognitive Neuropsychology.

Miceli, G. & Caramazza, A. (in press). Dissociation of inflectional and derivational morphology. Brain and Language.

Miceli, G. & Mazzucchi, A. (in press). The speech production deficit of so-called agrammatic aphasics: Evidence from two Italian patients. In L. Menn, L. K. Obler, & H. Goodglass (Eds.), Agrammatic aphasia: Cross-language narrative source book. Baltimore, MD: John Benjamins.

Miceli, G., Mazzucchi, A., Menn, L. & Goodglass, H. (1983). Contrasting cases of Italian agrammatic aphasia without comprehension disorder. Brain and Language, 18, 65-97.

Nespoulous, J.-L., Dordain, M., Perron, C., Ska, B., Bub, D., Caplan, D., Mehler, J. & Lecours, A. R. (in press). Agrammatism in sentence production without comprehension deficits: Reduced availability of syntactic structures and/or of grammatical morphemes? A case study. Brain and Language.

Schiff, H. B., Alexander, M. P., Naeser, M. N. & Galaburda, A. M. (1983). Aphemia. Clinical-Anatomic Correlations. Archives of Neurology, 40, 720-727.

Foreword to Appendices

Since in order to make the case that agrammatism is not a cognitively homogeneous category we must test patients who satisfy accepted criteria for classification as agrammatics, we provide in Appendix 1 patient histories (when available) and in Appendix 2 samples of their spontaneous production.

KEY TO APPENDIX 1

Some of the patients have been described in detail elsewhere (patients G.G. and T.F. in Miceli, Mazzucchi, Menn & Goodglass (1983), patients C.D.A. and F.G. in Miceli & Mazzucchi (in press), where they are referred to as Mr. Rossi and Mr. Verdi, respectively, and patient F.S. in Miceli & Caramazza (in press). For patient F.A., who was tested thanks to the courtesy of Dr. Sergio Carlomagno, only partial information is available. For patients G.D.C., M.M., L.S. and M.U., whose spontaneous speech was made available to us by Prof. Anna Mazzucchi, only the details provided in Table 1 are known.

The patients were all submitted to an extensive screening battery for aphasia. The results of only some tasks are described here. The "production" tasks considered concern transcoding (word, nonword and sentence reading, repetition and writing to dictation) and naming tasks (of objects and actions, oral and writen) are reported. The following "reception" tasks are reported:

1) Phoneme discrimination and auditory-visual phoneme matching, explored by means of minimal pairs of phonemes (stop consonants) embedded in natural CV syllables;

2) Single-word comprehension tests. The patient is asked to match a stimulus (presented auditorily or visually by the examiner) to one of two pictures (the correct response and a foil which is related to the stimulus either semantically or phonemically (auditory presentation)/ (visual presentation)). Examples: gamba--braccio (leg--arm); martello--mantello (hammer--cape);

3) Auditorily and visually presented grammaticality judgement tasks;

4) Reversible sentence comprehension test. The patient is asked to match a stimulus sentence (presented auditorily or visually by the examiner) to one of two pictures (the correct response and a foil). Three types of foils are used, depicting the reversal of thematic roles, a morphologically-related alternative or a semantically-related alternative (in the last case the semantically-related item portrays either a related action or a related object). Half of the sentences are presented in the

active, half in the passive voice. Examples: Il ragazzo insegue la ragazza--La ragazza insegue il ragazzo (The boy is chasing the girl--The girl is chasing the boy); Il ragazzo insegue la ragazza--Il ragazzo insegue le ragazze (The boy is chasing the girl--The boy is chasing the girls); Il ragazzo insegue la ragazza--Il ragazzo insegue la donna (The boy is chasing the girl--The boy is chasing the woman).

KEY TO APPENDIX 2

Line 2 of the transcript is a verbatim transcription of the patient's speech. Words with incorrect inflectional endings are underlined, words omitted are in square parentheses.

Line 1 reports the correct target for the words produced incorrectly by the patient.

Line 3 is a verbatim English translation of the patient's output. Omitted words are in square parentheses. Words produced incorrectly in Italian are followed by indications on the correct number (sg., pl.), gender (m., f.) and person (1st, 2nd, 3rd).

Line 4 is an attempt at giving a sense of what the patient's speech would sound like in English.

(In each sample, the narrative from which the sequence was taken is indicated to the right of the patient's name. The following abbreviations are used: A.D.L. = Activities of daily life; H.O.I. = History of illness; C.T. = Cookie Theft.)

APPENDIX 1

Patient A.A.

The patient is a right-handed housewife. She has a 5th grade education, but additionally attended a technical school for 2 years. Prior to her illness, she held a secretarial job. She suffered a ruptured aneurysm in the left middle cerebral artery territory in 1983, at age 33. CT-scan is not available. The patient was seen approximately 1 year post-onset. The neurological exam shows a very mild right hemiparesis, with occasional extinction phenomena on the right side of the body. The neuropsychological exam reveals a massive deficit of verbal and visual memory, a severely reduced digit span (span forward: 3) and a mild-to-moderate buccofacial apraxia. Language exam shows a severely non-fluent aphasia, with a mild dysarthria. Transcoding tasks are severely impaired with all materials (nonwords, words and sentences). Phoneme discrimination is severely impaired. Lexical decisions and single-word comprehension tasks are moderately impaired, more in the visual than in the auditory modality. Naming is poor. Auditory sentence comprehension performance is severely impaired (the majority of the errors are reversals or of the morphological type). Reading comprehension could not be examined, due to the severity of the reading deficit.

Patient F.A.

The patient is a right-handed man, with an 8th grade education. Prior to his illness, the patient worked as an employee for the national lotteries. A large frontal meningioma was surgically excised in 1975, when F.A. was 58. He was seen 5 years after the onset of symptoms. The neurological exam only showed a mild right-sided hemiparesis. The neuropsychological exam demonstrated a very mild difficulty in learning lists of words, but was otherwise normal. As regards language, the information is scanty. Spontaneous speech was mildly dysarthric and non-fluent. Occasional phonemic paraphasias were produced, both in spontaneous speech and in naming. Single-word comprehension was in the normal range. Sentence comprehension was mildly impaired.

Patient F.B.

This patient is a right-handed woman, a 3rd-year Ph.D. student in Architecture. She suffered from a severe, open head injury in 1982, when she was 21. She was first seen in our Service three years later. The neurological exam was negative. CT-scan showed a large hypodense area involving the superficial and deep structures of the left frontal lobe and the cortical areas of the parietal lobe. The left ventricle was enlarged. The neuropsychological exam showed only a mild deficit in a task requiring the ability to learn a list of 15 words. The language exam disclosed a severe aphasic disorder. Spontaneous speech was non-fluent, in the complete absence of dysarthria. Reading and writing to dictation were virtually abolished (for nonwords, words and sentences); repetition of words and nonwords was relatively less impaired, sentence repetition demonstrated 'agrammatic' features. Naming was moderately impaired, and action naming was remarkably more impaired than object naming. Phoneme discrimination and auditory-visual matching of phonemes were impaired. Single-word comprehension tasks were moderately impaired (semantic and phonemic errors with auditory presentation; semantic errors with visual presentation). Grammaticality judgement tasks were impaired. Sentence comprehension tasks were severely impaired (more in the visual than in the auditory modality); most of the errors were either reversals or morphologically related responses.

Patient C.D.

The patient is a right-handed man, with a 12th grade education. He had left school for financial reasons, and held an administrative job with the national railway system. At 55, after open heart surgery, he suffered from a cerebrovascular accident (in 1979). He was tested 7 years later. The neurological exam shows a severe right hemiparesis. The CT-scan shows a small lesion, involving the subcortical structures of the left frontal lobe. The neuropsychological exam demonstrates only a moderate reduction of verbal memory, with a normal digit span (span forward: 7). The language exam shows that C.D.'s speech is mildly non-fluent, dysarthric and dysprosodic, but conveys an essentially normal amount of information. Transcoding tasks are essentially normal. Naming tasks demonstrate occasional anomias and semantic or phonemic paraphasias. Phoneme discrimination, auditory-visual phoneme matching, and single-word comprehension tasks are within normal limits. C.D. demonstrates only minimal difficulties in sentence comprehension (the results are within the lower normal range).

Patient F.D.

This patient is a right-handed M.D. with a history of transient ischemic attacks, who had a right-hemisphere stroke in 1978 (at age 57) and a left-hemisphere stroke in 1979. The speech sample reported here was obtained approximately 1 year later, in 1980. At that time, the neurological exam was negative. A CT-scan showed lesions in the right and in the left temporal lobe, and in the left cingulate gyrus. The neuropsychological exam yielded abnormal results only in phonological memory tasks, and in the tasks where comprehension of an auditory input was required. The language exam showed a fluent aphasia, without articulatory or prosodic deficits. The patient showed features of the 'word deafness' syndrome. Naming was characterised by the production of infrequent phonemic paraphasias and of occasional semantic errors. Reading was normal; repetition and writing to dictation were severely impaired. Phoneme discrimination was within normal limits. Single-word and sentence comprehension were normal with visual presentation; auditory comprehension of single words was moderately impaired, and auditory sentence comprehension was severely disturbed.

Patient C.D.A.

The patient is a right-handed newspaper writer, with a Ph.D. in Education. In 1981, at age 43, he suffered from a ruptured aneurysm in the left middle cerebral artery territory. The speech sample reported here was obtained 2 years after surgery. The neurological exam demonstrates a mild right facial weakness, but is otherwise normal. The CT-scan shows a large lesion, involving the post-Rolandic (parietal and temporal) structures of the left hemisphere, both superficial and deep. The neuropsychological exam is normal, except for a reduced digit span (span forward: 3). The language exam demonstrates a severe, non-fluent aphasia, with a mild prosodic disturbance, but free from dysarthria. Naming tasks reveal anomic difficulties with occasional phonemic errors. Transcoding tasks with items presented in isolation are mildly-to-moderately impaired, word transcoding being less impaired than nonword transcoding. Most errors result in phonemic/graphemic distortions of the stimulus item. Sentence transcoding tasks demonstrate agrammatic features. Phoneme discrimination is mildly impaired. Single-word comprehension is normal. Sentence comprehension is severely impaired.

Patient E.D.U.

This patient is a right-handed woman with a Ph.D. in Humanities, who had a left hemisphere stroke at age 58. She was seen in our Service 1 year post onset. The neurological exam was normal. CT-scan was not available. Since the patient refused to undergo a full neuropsychological and language testing, the available data on higher cortical functions are largely defective. The language exam demonstrated the presence of anomic gaps and of phonemic and (very infrequently) semantic errors. Single-word comprehension was within normal limits, as well as phoneme discrimination. Sentence comprehension was impaired.

Patient G.F.

The patient is a right-handed M.D., the chief of an Orthopedic Ward in a county hospital. He suffered from a left hemisphere stroke at age 58, and was seen in the acute stage (approximately 3 weeks post onset). The neurological exam demonstrated a very mild right hemiparesis, with clear tactile extinction phenomena on the right and even more systematic visual extinction phenomena in the right visual field. The CT-scan showed a large hypodense area in the left temporal and parietal lobes. The neuropsychological exam demonstrated a severe memory disorder for auditorily-presented stimuli. The language exam showed a fluent aphasia with severely paraphasic speech, and without articulatory or prosodic disorders. Naming was impaired, with frequent phonemic substitutions, anomias and very few semantic errors. Transcoding tasks were severely impaired (more with nonwords than with words). Phoneme discrimination was moderately impaired. Single-word comprehension was mildly impaired. Sentence comprehension was severely disrupted, errors resulting mostly in reversals of thematic roles or in the choice of morphologically-related foils.

Patient T.F.

The patient is a right-handed male with a 5th grade education. When he was 38, during cardiac catheterization, he had a right-sided seizure, followed by a transient right hemiparesis. He was seen on the first day post onset. The neurological and neuropsychological evaluations were normal. The language exam showed a fluent aphasia without clinically apparent articulatory and prosodic deficits. Naming and transcoding tasks were normal. Single-word and sentence comprehension were normal. The patient's condition improved rapidly, and one month post-onset no language deficits were detectable. A CT-scan, performed two years later, showed a very small lesion involving the parietal white matter in the left hemisphere.

Patient F.G.

The patient is a right-handed male, a Ph.D. student in Biology at the time of his illness. At age 19, he suffered from an intracerebral hematoma, after a very minor closed head injury. The speech sample analysed for the present study was obtained 2 years post onset. At that time, the neurological exam showed a dense right hemiplegia, without sensory or visual defects. CT-scan demonstrated a hypodense area located in the white matter of the frontal, parietal and (to a lesser extent) temporal lobes and an enlarged left lateral ventricle. The neuropsychological exam showed only a reduced digit span (span forward: 4). The language exam revealed a non-fluent, hypophonic speech, with articulatory disorders and a flat prosody. Transcoding tasks were mildly impaired with words, moderately impaired with nonwords. Most errors resulted in phonemic/orthographic distortions of the stimulus item. Sentence transcoding tasks showed agrammatic features. Naming tasks demonstrated anomias and occasional phonemic paraphasias. Action naming was more impaired than object naming. Phoneme discrimination and single-word comprehension were within normal limits. Reversible sentence comprehension was mildly impaired, all errors consisting either of reversal of thematic roles, or of the incorrect choice of a morphologically-related picture.

Patient G.G.

The patient was a right-handed glazier, with an 8th grade education. He had a stroke at age 58, and was tested 3 months and 14 months post onset. The second speech sample was used for the present study. The neurological exam showed a very mild, right hemiparesis. A CT-scan demonstrated a lesion involving the superficial and deep structures of the left frontal lobe. The neuropsychological exam was normal. The language exam demonstrated a non-fluent speech with moderate articulatory deficits. Naming and transcoding tasks were normal, except for the presence of articulatory disorders and of phonemic distortions. Phonemic discrimination, single word comprehension and reversible sentence comprehension were flawless.

Patient M.L.

The patient is a right-handed male with a high-school education, who held an administrative position at an Italian Embassy in Africa. At age 31, he had a cardiac arrest during minor surgery and fell in a coma. A week later the patient came out of the coma, and an aphasia was discovered. M.L. was seen in our Service 4 years later. The neurological exam was negative, and serial CT-scans failed to reveal any structural abnormality. The neuropsychological evaluation revealed only a mild difficulty in a task tapping the ability to learn a list of 15 words. The language exam revealed an aphasia with articulatory deficits and a flattened prosody. Naming and transcoding tasks were normal. Phoneme discrimination, single word comprehension and reversible sentence comprehension were well within normal limits.

Patient A.M.

The patient is a right-handed male with an 8th grade education. He worked as a clerk in the largest Italian travel agency. At age 49, he had a left hemispheric stroke. He was tested for the first time 4 years post onset. The neurological exam showed a very mild right hemiparesis and moderate-to-severe right-sided extinction phenomena in the tactile and in the visual modality. A CT-scan demonstrated a large hypodense area, involving the left temporal and the parietal lobes, both superficially and deeply. The left lateral ventricle was enlarged. The neuropsychological exam showed a mild buccofacial apraxia, a difficulty in learning lists of words and a reduced digit span (span forward: 4). The language exam demonstrated a severely non-fluent aphasia, free from any articulatory and prosodic deficits. Naming was severely impaired, more so for actions than for objects. Writing to dictation was severely impaired, whereas reading aloud and repetition were only mildly disturbed. Phoneme discrimination and single word comprehension were only marginally impaired in comparison to a group of normal controls. Reversible sentence comprehension was impaired, almost all errors being thematic role reversals.

Patient B.P.

The patient was a right-handed woman with an 8th grade education who, prior to her illness, worked as a laboratory technician. She had a left hemisphere stroke at age 40. She was tested approximately 9 years post onset. The neurological exam showed a dense right hemiplegia, and mild extinction phenomena on the right side in both the tactile and the visual modality. A CT-scan revealed a massive lesion in the left hemisphere, involving the entire territory of the middle cerebral artery, and only sparing the mesial frontal and occipital areas. The neuropsychological exam showed buccofacial and limb apraxia and a severe verbal memory disorder. The language exam demonstrated a severely non-fluent aphasia with only mild articulatory disorders. Language tasks were severely impaired. B.P. was completely unable to transcode nonwords. In word reading, the patient displayed all the clinical signs of the deep dyslexia syndrome. Writing was substantially abolished, except for few, short, high-frequency words. Repetition was impaired. Naming was severely defective for objects and (even more) for actions. Phoneme discrimination, single-word and reversible sentence comprehension were severely impaired.

Patient C.S.

The patient is a right-handed female, without family history of left-handedness or of mixed hand preference. A retired high-school teacher with a Ph.D. in Education, she became aphasic at age 67, secondary to a right hemisphere stroke. She was tested approximately 1 year after the onset of her symptoms. The neurological exam showed a mild left hemiparesis and extinction phenomena on the left side of the body. The

CT-scan showed a large hypodense area, involving the superficial and deep structures of the right frontal lobe, also extending deeply into the parietal lobe. The neuropsychological exam demonstrated buccofacial apraxia, severely reduced digit span (span forward: 2), inability to learn and retain lists of words, slightly reduced visual memory, and mild signs of left-sided neglect. The language exam showed a non-fluent aphasia with hypophonic speech, a mild dysarthria and a flattened prosody. Nonword transcoding tasks were extremely impaired, whereas word transcoding tasks were relatively less defective; for both words and nonwords, repetition was less disturbed than reading and writing. In naming tasks, the patient produced some phonemic and semantic substitutions, and showed anomic behavior. Action naming and action comprehension were very severely impaired, whereas object naming and object comprehension were only mildly damaged. Phoneme discrimination was poor. Reversible sentence comprehension was markedly impaired upon auditory presentation. Visual sentence comprehension could not be tested, owing to the severe reading problem.

Patient F.S.

The patient is a right-handed male, who worked as a lawyer prior to his illness. He had a stroke in 1978, at age 52. He was seen for the first time 2 years post onset. The speech sample used for the present study was obtained 5 years post onset. The neurological exam showed a dense right hemiplegia, with tactile, visual and auditory extinction phenomena on the right. A CT-scan showed hypodensity of the superficial and deep structures of the left temporal lobe, as well as the deep structures of the parietal and of the frontal lobe. The neuropsychological exam showed a mild buccofacial apraxia and reduced verbal memory functions (span forward: 3). The language exam revealed a non-fluent aphasia with a 'foreign accent' syndrome. Reading was very mildly impaired, whereas writing to dictation and repetition showed a severe impairment with nonwords, and a moderate impairment with words. In word repetition, a substantial number of inflectional errors was produced. Naming was mildly impaired for objects, moderately for actions. Phoneme discrimination was poor. Single word comprehension was within normal limits. In reversible sentence comprehension tasks the patient produced a large number of reversal errors and of morphologically-based errors.

APPENDIX 2

Patient A.A. (A.D.L.)

                                                    lavatevi
[Chiamo] Luigi, Carla...[dico] "Su, via... lavare [vi],
[I call] Louis, Carla...[I say] "Up, away... wash [yourself]
    Louis, Carla...   "Hurry up... wash

preparate   cucino
preparare [vi], cosi'".   [Poi] cucinare. La sera   una volta una volta
prepare [yourself], so". [Then] to cook. The evening   one time one time
get ready, so."   Cook. In the evening one time one time

e mezza (*), [faccio] la terapia   e   basta.   E poi   Luigi e   Carla
and half,   [I have] the therapy and enough. And then Luigi and Carla
and a half,   therapy and that's it.   And then Luigi and Carla

[sono] sempre qua, cosi' insomma,   tutti i giorni. Cucino la sfoglia,
[are]   always here, like this in sum, all the days. I cook the pastry,
        always here, this way,   everyday.   I cook the pastry,

                                    pulisco
faccio... [tolgo]   [la] polvere, pulisci,...   insomma, tutti i
I make...[I take off] [the] dust,   clean (2nd sg),... in sum, all the
I make...   the dust,   clean (2nd sg),... in sum, all the

                                                            stiro.
giorni sono uguali... [faccio] [il] pranzo, batto i panni,   stirare.
days   are   equal... [I make] [the] lunch, I beat the clothes, to iron
days   are   the same...   lunch, I clean the clothes, to iron.

(*) Meaning: an hour, an hour and a half

Patient F.A. (H.O.I.)

Otto giorni [prima] di sposare   [mi]   [sono] sceso
Eight days [before] of to marry [myself] [I have] gone down
Eight days [before] getting married   [I had] gone out

dalla casa mia con un motorino.　　[All'] incrocio del ponte della S.
from the house my with a motorbike. [At the] corner of the bridge of
　the S.
of my house on a motorbike.　　　[At the] corner of the S. bridge

ci sta una clinica. Una signora che era la figlia di un comandante
there is a hospital. A lady who was the daughter of a commander
there is a hospital. A lady who was the daughter of a commander

usci'　　e　mi prese a destra della motorino.
came out and me took at right of the (f.sg.) motorbike (m.sg.).
came out and hit me on the right side of the motorbike.

　sono andato　　　　　　　　　　　　　　　　　sposare
Io andavo　[contro il] muro di fronte, otto giorni prima di sposato.
I was going　[against the] wall of front, eight days before of married.
I was going　　　　　　　wall in front, eight days before married.

[Mi]　　sono sposato [il]　29 settembre '62.
[Myself] am married [the] 29 september '62.
I got married　　　　　29 september '62.

　　　　　risultava　　　avevo
[A] Roma risultavo　che aveva un ematoma.
[At] Rome I resulted that he had a hematoma.
　　Rome I came out that he had a hematoma.

Patient F.B. (H.O.I.)

　　　　　eravamo andate
[Il] 20 luglio io [e] Laura andiamo a X. a mangiare.
[The] 20 July I [and] Laura go　to X to eat.
　　July 20 Laura I go　　　to X. to have dinner.

Poi di ritorno [a] Y.... Guarda, niente, neanche il papa', la mamma,
Then of return [to] Y... Look, nothing, not even the father, the mother,
Then on the way back Y..Look,nothing, not even my father,my mother,

basta, niente.   Poi [a]l'ospedale   di X. [sono stata] operata.
enough, nothing. Then [at] the hospital of X. [I am been] operated.
enough, nothing. Then X. hospital   operated.

       siamo andati
Poi andiamo a Z. [a] novembre. Dopo e' proprio carrozzina.
Then we go to Z. [at] november. Later is really wheelchair.
Then we go to Z.   november. Later it's only wheelchair.

[Ero] magra magra. E poi io la mamma e papa' a Z.[stavamo] a piangere.
[I was] thin thin. And then I the mother and dad at Z. [were] to cry.
       Very thin. And then my mother dad and I at Z.   cry.

E poi adesso [sto] bene, e poi   andiamo a Z., sempre a parlare.
And then now [I am] well, and then we go to Z,   always to talk.
And then now   well, and then we go to Z., always to talk.

Patient C.D. (H.O.I.)

 dell'
Il 17 luglio 1979 sono [stato] chiamato dai proprietari da[l] ospedale (*)
The 17 July 1979 I am   called   by the owners from [the] hospital
On July 17, 1979 I am   called   by the owners from hospital

che si e' liberato   un posto e mi facevano   andare a fare
that itself is freed a place and me were making go to make
that a bed was available   and that they let me go to have

                            La
l'operazione   al cuore.   Un'operazione al cuore   era fatta
the operation at the heart. A operation   at the heart was made
heart surgery   A heart surgery   was made

            decidono
dal Dott.X. Il 24 decidere   di farmi   questa operazione, [a] me
by Dr.X.   The 24 to decide of making me this operation, [to] me
by Dr.X.   On the 24th decide to submit me to surgery,   me

e [a]   un altro   che stava nella camera operatoria.
and [to] an other   who was   in the room operating.
and   another guy who was   in the operating room.

                          trattengono
Io mi   fanno   l'operazione e me <u>trattengo</u> due giorni giu' di sotto.
I to me they make the operation and me retain two days down of below.
Me they make surgery and I keep me for two days downstairs.

(*) Meaning: the Administrative Office

Patient <u>F.D.</u> (H.O.I.)

Ecco   che io ero venuto [nel] tarda pomeriggio,
Here it is that I was come [in the] late (f.sg.) afternoon (m.sg.),
Here it is--I had come   late afternoon

e   <u>mi</u> ero un po' molto stanco. [Ero]   venuto [dal] lavoro   e
and myself was a bit very tired. [I was] come   [from the] work and
and I was me a bit very tired.   Come   work and

                     Ero
[ero]   molto stanco. <u>Era</u> anche un po' agitato. Era   [l'] 8 settembre,
[I was] very tired.   He was also a bit agitated. It was [the] 8 September,
   very tired.   He was also a bit nervous. It was September 8,

[una] giornata caldissima; ero tornato   a casa mia, io pensavo
[a]   day   very hot;   I was come back at house my, I was thinking
     very hot day;   I had come back to my house, I was planning

[di] fare un bagno caldo perche' cosi' potevo essere piu' calmo.
[of] to do a bath hot   because this way I could be calmer.
   take a hot bath   because in this way I could calm down.

Infatti [ho] aperto il bagno, [ho fatto uscire]   l'acqua calda..
In fact [I have]opened the bath,[I have made to come out]the water hot..
In fact turned the faucet,   hot water...

[la] [vasca]   [era] piena. Ho aperto   [la] finestra.
[the] [bathtub] [was] full. I have opened [the] window.
                       full. I opened the window.

Patient C.D.A. (A.D.L.)
                                                 ho dormito
Io [dormo] 5 ore. Alle 12 io ho dormito... io dormo (*). Alle 5 e mezzo
I [sleep] 5 hours. At the 12 I have slept... I sleep.   At the 5 and half
I5 hours.   At 12 I slept...   I sleep.   At 5:30

mi sono svegliato.   2 ore io... 5 ore io ho dormito. Alle 7 e mezzo
myself have awaken. 2 hours I... 5 hours I have slept. At the 7 and half
I woke up.   2 hours I... 5 hours I slept.   At 7:30

                                             sono alzato
la sveglia [ha suonato].   Alle 7 e mezzo mi alzo
the alarm clock [has rung]. At the 7 and half myself I get up
the alarm clock   At 7:30 I get up

                                             sono lavato
e sono andato in... nel bagno.   Poi mi   lavo   le mani e
and I am gone to... to the bathroom. Then myself I wash the hands and
and I went to...   to the bathroom. Then I wash   my hands and

                                             sono rasato
i piedi e il   fronte.   Poi io [mi]   rado.
the feet and the (m.sg.) forehead (f.sg.). Then I [myself] shave.
feet and forehead.   Then I shave.

                              da   sono vestito
Poi... dopo [sono andato] [in] la stanza di letto. Io [mi] vesto...
Then...later [I am gone] [in] the room of bed. I [myself] dress...
Then... Then   the bedroom.   I dress...

                              nella   ho preso
mi sono vestito.   Poi sono andato in la cucina e prende la colazione.
myself have dressed. Then I am gone in the kitchen and takes the
I dressed.   Then I went to the kitchen   and takes breakfast.
  breakfast.

```
                    sono uscito
Poi io usci'              a lavorare.
Then I went out (3rd sg.) to work.
Then I went out to work.
```

(*) Meaning: I go to sleep

Patient G.D.C. (H.O.I.)

```
Otto anni fa    [ero]  morto, secco.  Dopo, parecchi anni fa...
Eight years ago [I was] dead, dead.   Later, several years ago...
Eight years ago  dead, dead.   Later, several years ago...
```

```
                      parlo
pian piano   [ho fatto] ginnastica. Ora parlare  bene.
slowly slowly [I did]   exercise.   Now to speak well.
very slowly             exercise.   Now speak well.
```

```
Ero
Sono [a] F. ...T. si      chiama il medico,  T. [dell']     ospedale
I am [in] F. ...T.  himself calls  the physician, T. [from the] hospital
I am      F. ...T.  is called the physician,       T.        hospital
```

```
[di] F. Allora andavo a Roma,     [da un] medico   [del] R.
[in] F. Then I was going to Rome, [to a]  physician [of the] R.(hospital)
     F. At that time I used to go to Rome, physician  R.
```

```
Aspetta, il medico... ospedale... cervello... ginnastica... le mani...
Wait,    the doctor  hospital    brain      exercise     the hands...
Wait,    the doctor...hospital... brain...   exercise...  the hands...
```

```
Lavoro
Lavora [a] Milano.  [Il posto]  si    chiama la X.
He works [at] Milan. [The place] itself calls the x.
Works         Milan.            It is  called the X.
```

Patient E.D.U. (A.D.L.)

Mi   alzo verso 7 e mezza,   vado nel bagno,   mi [preparo]
Myself lift around 7 and half, I go in the bathroom, myself [prepare]
I get up at 7:30,   I go to the bathroom,

                 mangio
per la pulizia,   mange   [il] latte e poi dopo aiuto
for the cleaning, eat (nonword) [the] milk and then I help
to clean up,   eat   milk and then I help

                      spolvero   aiuto
la donna delle pulizie e cioe'   spolvera e aiuta a rifare i letti,
the woman of the cleaning and that is dusts and helps to remake the beds,
the maid   that is, dusts and helps to make the beds,

poi [vado] in cucina.   Legge un pochino, [cose]   leggere
then [I go] to kitchen.   Reads a little bit, [things] light (f.pl.)
then   to the kitchen. Reads a little bit,   light

      seguirle
che posso seguirlo   perche' le cose piu' difficili
that I can follow it because the things most difficult (f.pl.)
that I can follow it, because the most difficult things

        capirle
non posso capirlo,   non riesco [a] seguire il [filo].   Invece
non I can understand it, not manage [to] follow the [plot]. Instead
I can't understand it,   can't manage   follow the...   To the contrary

     le   leggere
con il   cose   piu' leggeri   riesco a leggere.
with the (m.sg.) things (f.pl.) most light (m.pl.) I manage to read.
with the lightest things   I manage to read.

Patient G.F. (A.D.L.)

Faccio   di
Fare il medico,   al   mattina   [vado] [in] ospedale.
To do the physician, at the (m.sg.) morning (f.sg.) [I go] [to] hospital.
Be a physician,   in the morning   hospital.

Poi [vado] [in] ufficio, [in] banca, [faccio] tutto,   ecco.
Then [I go] [to] office, [to] bank, [I do] everything, here.
Then   office,   bank,   everything, you see.

    comincio
Io cominciare alle 7 e mezzo, [lavoro] fino a mezzanotte. Quindi io avevo
I to start at the 7 and half, [I work] until midnight. Then I had
I start at 7:30,   until midnight. Then I had

tutta   andavo
tutto   un'attivita'   svolta. In piu' andare [in] ospedale,
all (m.sg.) an activity (f.sg.) done. In more to go [to] hospital,
all my activity done.   I addition go   hospital,

               Andavo
[sono] chirurgo, io [sono] ortopedico. Andare anche [in] ospedale
[I am] surgeon, I [am] orthopaedic. To go also [to]   hospital
       surgeon, I orthopaedics.   Also go   hospital

  operavo   andavo
[il] giorno. Alle 7 e mezza - 8 operare.   [Il] pomeriggio andare
[the] day. At the 7 and half - 8 to operate. [The] afternoon to go
     day. At 7:30 - 8:00 operate,   Afternoon go

piu' [in] ufficio che [in] ospedale.
more [to] office than [in] hospital.
more   office than   hospital.

Patient T.F. (H.O.I.)

                               sentivo Prendevo
[Sono] rivenuto dentro perche' dolore continuamente sentire. Prendere
     come again in   because pain   continuously to feel. To take
     Come back in here because pain continuously feel.   Take

                                                    miglioravo
(drug X) a casa, ma... altre pastiglie, ma non <u>migliorare</u>. Allora io
(drug X) at home, but... other pills,   but not to improve. Then I
(drug X) at home, but... other pills,   but not improve.   Then I

[sono] andato [dal] neurologo, anche perche' [il] cardiologo
        gone [to the] neurologist, also because [the] cardiologist
        gone neurologist,   also because   cardiologist

consigliava [di] [andare] [dal] neurologo. Allora [il] neurologo
recommended [to] [go] [to the] neurologist. Then [the] neurologist
recommended neurologist.   Then neurologist

        ha detto   avrebbe dato
[mi]   <u>dire</u> [che] [mi] <u>dare</u>   [una] pastiglia per dormire,
[to me] to say [that] [to me] to give   [a] pill for sleep,
        say   give   sleeping pill,

        dormivo   dormivo
ma io non <u>dormire</u> lo stesso; per due mesi notte e giorno non <u>dormire</u>
but I not to sleep the same; for two months night and day not to sleep
But I not sleep all the same; for two months night and day not sleep

ne'   con la camomilla   ne' con [le] pillole.
neither with the chamomile nor with [the] pills.
neither with the chamomile nor with pills.

Patient F.G. (H.O.I.)

Racconto il caso. Allora... Tanto lo sapete, quindi... Fumavo...
I tell the case. Then...   Anyway it you know, so... I was smoking...
I'll tell my case. Well... You know it, anyway, so... I was smoking a lot,

bevevo...   Allora entro in casa.   Il babbo [dice]:
I was drinking...   Then I enter in house. The dad [says]:
I was drinking a lot... Then I go home.   Dad

"Dove sei stato?"   "In giro - rispondo - con le ragazze"
"Where you are been?"   "In turn - I answer - with the girls"
"Where have you been?" "Around - I say - with some girls"

Il babbo non c'entrava   niente;   soltanto l'occhio sinistro
The dad not there was entering nothing; only   the eye left
Dad had nothing to do with it;   only my left eye

[si] [e']   aperto. [Mi] [hanno messo]   tre punti.
[itself] [is] opened. [To me] [they have put] three stitches.
          opened.   Three stitches.

                    contro il   sono andato
Probabilmente ho battuto nel   tavolo... e poi in coma.. ero.
Probably   I have hit in the table... and then in coma... I was.
Probably I hit the table...   and then in a coma... I was.

Gli amici [non] l'ho visti.   E' meglio che [non] [li] rintracci
The friends [not] them I have seen. Is better that [not] [them] find.
My friends I have   seen them. It's better if I find.

Patient G.G. (A.D.L.)

[Ero] [nei]   medi...   lui [era] [nei]   massimi.
[I was] [in the] middleweight... he [was] [in the] heavyweight.
              Middleweight... he   heavyweight.

Io [ero] forte, [ma] [avevo] difficolta' [a causa delle] donne,
I [was] strong, [but] [I had] difficulties [because of the] women,
I   strong,   difficulties   women,

[del]   bere,   [del]   fumo...   Io non c'ero... non riuscivo
[of the] drink, [of the] smoke... I not there was... not I was managing
         drinking,   smoke... My mind wasn't there... I could not

a fare... io [pensavo] [alle]   donne, [al]   bere, [al]   fumo...
to make... I [was caring] [about the] women, [to the] drink, [to the] smoke
make...   I   women,   drinking,   smoke

[ma] [il]   pugilato [e'] [un] lavoro serio. Amici,... X, Y, Z, e io...
[but] [the] boxing [is] [a]   job serious. Friends,... X, Y, Z, and I...
            boxing   serious job. Friends,... X, Y, Z, and I...

[eravamo] tutti pugili... pure io... [Avevo] [un] carattere litigioso
[were]   all boxers... also I... [I had] [a] temper bad
            all boxers... me too...   bad temper

Patient M.L. (H.O.I.)

Quel giorno [ad] un orario stabilito ci sono andato.
That day [at] a time established there I am gone.
That day I went there established time.

Lui m'ha portato in sala [da] operazione e... Ma io da allora
He me has taken in room [of] operation and... But I since then
He took me to the operating room and...   But since then I

ricordo solamente [il] suo viso. Allora da cio' che mi   e' stato detto
remember only [the] his face. Then from that that to me has been told
only remember his face.   Then from what has been told to me

sono subito...   Appena fatta l'anestesia...   L'operazione dicono
I am immediately... As soon done the anesthesia... The operation they say
I am immediately... As soon as the anesthesia was done... Surgery they say

che non [e'] riuscita.   In quel momento il cuore si era fermato
that not [has been] successful. In that moment the heart itself was stopped
that was not successful.   In that moment my heart stopped

[mi] pare due volte,   due o tre,   non ricordo bene.
[to me] it seems two times, two or three,   not I remember well.
   think two times,   two or three times, I do not remember well.

Patient A.M. (A.D.L.)

Subito [metto] [le]   scarpe. No! Prima... come si dice, ecco...
Right away [I put on] [the] shoes. No! Before... how it says, here...
Right away shoes.   No! Before... how do you say, here...

Dopo poi [vado] [al]   bagno   e come ho detto [faccio] [la] barba
After then [I go] [to the] bathroom and as I have said [I make] [the] beard
Then   bathroom and as I said   beard

                    pulisco pulisco
poi [i]   denti <u>pulire</u>... <u>pulire</u>   [i]   denti... poi [lavo] [i] capelli.
then [the] teeth to clean to clean [the] teeth... then [I wash] [the] hair.
then teeth clean...   clean teeth...   then   hair.

                    pulisco
Poi io... quindi <u>pulire</u>[mi],   va bene,... e poi...   e [metto]
Then I... then to clean [myself], goes well,... and then... and [I put on]
Then I...then clean,   all right,... and then... and

[i]   vestiti... Poi mi preoccupo [di] papa' che non fa niente.
[the] clothes... Then myself worry [of] dad   who not does nothing.
      clothes... Then I take care   dad   who does not do anything.

Devo aiutarlo io perche' non ha... E per papa'   vengo [a] mangiare
Must help him I because not he has... And because of dad I come [to] eat
I must help him myself because he hasn't... And because of dad I come eat

[a] [casa]...   Poi [vado] a scuola.(*)
[at] [home]... Then [I go] to school.
                Then   to school.

(*) Meaning: to therapy.

<u>Patient M.M.</u> (H.O.I.)

                                        gli
Dunque... [sono stato] ricoverato a S. per <u>i</u> esami.   Dopo 15 giorni...
Well...   [I have been] admitted to S. for the exams.   After 15 days...
Well...   admitted to S. for a check-up. 15 days later...

                            gli esami
Allora... un giorno... 15 giorni... <u>l'esame</u> a S.... dopo poi... prima di...
Then...   a day...   15 days... the exam at S.. after then..prior of...
Then...   one day... 15 days... the exam at S.. then later..before...

[a]l' orario della cena...   allora... sono svenuto, e allora...
[at] the time of the dinner... then... I am fainted, and then...
      dinnertime...   then... I fainted, and then...

[ho fatto]   [il]   ricovero a G.   [Sono stato]   un giorno a S. e poi
[I have made] [the] admission to G. [I have been] one day at S. and then
                           admission to G.   One day at S. and then

                                                 ero   ho
a G.   E [per] 4 o 5 giorni non e' cosciente.   Dopo poi ha preso
to G. And [for] 4 or 5 days not is conscious. After then has taken
to G. And 4 or 5 days is not conscious.   Then later has gained

                             mancava   Perdevo
coscienza.   Pero'... [mi] manca la forza.   Perdo   l'equilibrio.
consciousness. But... [to me] misses the strength. I lose the balance.
consciousness. But... strength is missing.   I lose balance.

[Per] 40 giorni [sono stato]   ricoverato a S. per broncopolmonite.
[For] 40 days [I have been]   admitted at S. for bronchopneumonia.
          40 days   admitted at S. for a bronchopneumonia.

Patient P.B. (C.T.)

La bambina é... ha fatto precipitare [i] biscotti. Poi l'acqua [cade]
The girl is...   has made to fall [the] cookies. Then the water [falls]
The girls is...   has caused cookies to fall.   Then the water [falls]

per terra.   Lavare, poi...   [con lo]   straccio lavare, asciugare poi...
for ground. To wash, then... [with the] mop to wash,   to dry then...
on the floor. Wash, then...   mop wash,   dry then...

ha
ho sporcato tutto.
I have dirtied everything.
have messed up everything.

(A.D.L.)

                                                 pulisco
Dunque [a]lle   6:30 [durante] la settimana pulire. [Ho]   5 camere
Well   [at] the 6:30 [during] the week to clean.   [I have] 5 rooms
Well   6:30   the week clean.   5 rooms

Pulisco

e accessori. Pulire tutto. [Faccio] la pizza, [i] funghi
and accessories. To clean everything. [I make] the pizza, [the] mushrooms
and accessories. Clean everything. The pizza, mushrooms

e [i] funghi, un chilo, un chilo e mezzo, tanti... la spesa
and [the] mushrooms, one kilo, one kilo and half, many... the shopping
and mushrooms, one, one and a half kilo, many... the shopping

tutto
[per] tutta il mese la compro.
[for] all (f.sg.) the month (m.sg.) it I buy.
all month I buy it.

Patient C.S. (A.D.L.)

Lavo prima tutto quanto. Alla mattina metto [la] gonna.
I wash first everything. At the morning I put on [the] skirt.
First a wash everything. In the morning I put on skirt.

Poi dopo [faccio] il bagno. [Mi] [asciugo] [con] l'asciugamano,
Then after [I make] the bath. [Myself] [dry] [with] the towel,
Then later the bath. The towel,

Poi dopo lavo, e poi dopo cosi'.Quindi [faccio] gli esercizi,
Then later I wash, and then like this. Then [I do] the exercises,
Then later I do the laundry, and then like this. Then the exercises,

[gli] esercizi sempre. E poi dopo la mia figlia si va a scuola.
[the] exercises always. And then the my daughter herself goes to school.
exercises always. And then the my daughter goes herself to school.

mi metto
Poi mangiamo e poi dopo si mette a dormire. E poi dopo
Then we eat and then later herself puts to sleep. And then later
Then we eat and then later goes to sleep. And then later

come si desta il sole (*), allora [faccio] la passeggiata.
as itself wakes the sun, then [I make] the walk.
as soon as the sun awakes, then the walk.
(*) Meaning: as soon as the sun sets.

Patient F.S. (A.D.L.)

   ritorno   a casa mia   la
Poi <u>ritorna</u> [a] <u>la</u> mia casa.   Poi io ascolto <u>il</u> televisione
Then returns [to] the my house. Then I hear the (m.sg.) television
Then returns my house.   Then I hear the television

      faccio   vivo
o poi   <u>fare</u> il pranzo perche', caro dottore, io <u>vive</u> solo!
or then to do the lunch because, dear doctor, I lives alone!
or then make lunch   because, dear doctor, I lives alone!

           ricevo faccio
Poi telefono,   <u>riceve</u>,   <u>fare</u>,   perche' <u>il</u>   giornate
Then I telephone, receives, to make, because the (m.sg.) days (f.pl.)
Then I telephone, receives, make,   bacause the days

      lunghe
[sono] <u>lungo</u>.   Poi ancora spesso <u>andare</u> [allo] studio.
[are] long (m.sg.). Then again often to go [to the] office.
     long.   Then again often go   office.

        i Parioli
[In] Via C.   [a] <u>il Pariolo</u> c'e'
[In] Street C. [at] il Pariolo there is
   Street C.   il Pariolo there is

il   mio   studio
<u>la</u>   <u>mia</u>   <u>studia</u>   ancora aperto.
the (f.sg.) my (f.sg.) office (f.sg. -incorrect N gender) still open (m.sg)
          my office   still open.

Patient L.S. (A.D.L.)

Prendo l'   friggo
<u>Prende</u> <u>una</u> olio, poi una cipolla. Poi [metto] [il] burro, poi [lo] <u>frigge</u>
He takes an oil, then an onion.   Then [I put] [the] butter,then [it] fries
Takes an oil, then an onion.   Then   butter, then   fries

dunque... poi va in acqua.   Dopo, ecco... pomodori e prezzemolo e
well...   then goes in water.   Then, here... tomatoes and parsley and
well...   then it goes in the water. Then, here... tomatoes and parsley and

                faccio bollire
ragú e sale.   Mescolo e bolle   piano piano. Allora metto
ragout and salt. I stir and it boils slowly.   Then I put
ragout and salt. I stir and it boils slowly.   Then I put

la pentola con [l'] acqua... no, [con] l'acqua e sale.   Butto dentro
the pan with [the] water... no, [with] the water and salt. I throw in
the pan with water...   no,   water and salt.   I throw in

la pasta.   Si mescola. [Si] mette ancora in pentola, poi [si] [aggiunge]
the pasta. It stirs.   [It] puts again in pan,   then [it] [adds]
the pasta. You stir.   Put again in the pan,   then

[il] ragú.   Poi [si] mescola, poi [si] [aggiunge] il formaggio.
[the] ragout. Then [it] stirs,   then [it] [adds]   the cheese.
      ragout. Then stir,   then   the cheese.

Patient M.U. (A.D.L.)

Mi
L'alzo   poi [vado] [in]   bagno   e poi metto   un po' di...
It get up   then [I go] [to the] bathroom and then I put a bit of...
I get it up then   bathroom and then I put a bit of...

il coso li'...   Lavo la faccia e poi vado in casa   e poi prendo
the thing there... I wash the face and then I go in house   and then I take
that thing there...I wash my face and then go in the house and then I take

un po' di caffè. E poi aspetto che la M. porta il campanello e vado via.
a bit of coffee. And then I wait that the M. brings the ring and go away.
some coffee.   And then I wait until M. brings the ring   and go away.

          vado   studio
Poi adesso quando andare alla... la M. perche' studiare [la] parola
Then now when to go to the... the M. because to study [the] word
Then now when go to the...   the M. because   study   word

       nel
e poi vado <u>in il</u> [Noun] sotto...   e poi vado...   <u>andare</u> al salotto
and then I go in the [Noun] below... and then I go... to go to the room
and then I go in the [Noun] below... and then I go... go to the room

       studia
E poi   viene E. e <u>studiare</u> anche lui   perche' parlare... perche' spesso
And then comes E. and to study also him because to talk... because often
And then E. comes and he study as well because to talk... because often

non parlo mica.
not I talk really.
I really don't talk.

NEUROPSYCHOLOGY AND COGNITION

The purpose of the Neuropsychology and Cognition series is to bring out volumes that promote understanding in topics relating brain and behavior. It is intended for use by both clinicians and research scientists in the fields of neuropsychology, cognitive psychology, psycholinguistics, speech and hearing, as well as education. Examples of topics to be covered in the series would relate to memory, language acquisition and breakdown, reading, attention, developing and aging brain. By addressing the theoretical, empirical, and applied aspects of brain-behavior relationships, this series will try to present the information in the fields of neuropsychology and cognition in a coherent manner.

Series Editor:

R. Malatesha Joshi, *Oklahoma State University, U.S.A.*

Publications:

1. P.G. Aaron: *Dyslexia and Hyperlexia.* 1989   ISBN 1-55608-079-4

2. R. M. Joshi (ed.): *Written Language Disorders.* 1991   ISBN 0-7923-0902-2

3. A. Caramazza: *Issues in Reading, Writing and Speaking.* A Neuropsychological Perspective. 1991   ISBN 0-7923-0996-0

KLUWER ACADEMIC PUBLISHERS – DORDRECHT / BOSTON / LONDON